The Infectious Diseases Manual

David Wilks
MA, MD, MRCP, DTM & H
Consultant Physician
Regional Infectious Diseases Unit
City Hospital
Edinburgh

Mark Farrington
MA, MB, BChir, MRCPath
Consultant Microbiologist
Clinical Microbiology and
Public Health Laboratory
Addenbrooke's Hospital
Cambridge

David Rubenstein
MA, MD, FRCP
University of Cambridge
School of Clinical Medicine
Addenbrooke's Hospital
Cambridge

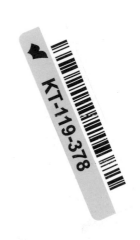

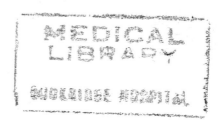

Blackwell
Science

© 1995 by
Blackwell Science Ltd
Editorial Offices:
Osney Mead, Oxford OX2 0EL
25 John Street, London WC1N 2BL
23 Ainslie Place, Edinburgh EH3 6AJ
238 Main Street, Cambridge
    Massachusetts 02142, USA
54 University Street, Carlton
    Victoria 3053, Australia

Other Editorial Offices:
Arnette Blackwell SA
    1, rue de Lille, 75007 Paris
    France

Blackwell Wissenschafts-Verlag GmbH
    Kurfürstendamm 57
    10707 Berlin, Germany

    Feldgasse 13, A-1238 Wien
    Austria

First published 1995

Set by Excel Typesetters Company, Hong Kong
Printed and bound in Great Britain
by Hartnolls Ltd, Bodmin, Cornwall

DISTRIBUTORS

Marston Book Services Ltd
PO Box 87
Oxford OX2 0DT
(*Orders*: Tel: 01865 791155
        Fax: 01865 791927
        Telex: 837515)

North America
    Blackwell Science, Inc.
    238 Main Street
    Cambridge, MA 02142
    (*Orders*: Tel: 800 215-1000
            617 876-7000
        Fax: 617 492-5263)

Australia
    Blackwell Science Pty Ltd
    54 University Street
    Carlton, Victoria 3053
    (*Orders*: Tel: 03 9347-0300
        Fax: 03 9349-3016)

A catalogue record for this title
is available from the British Library

ISBN 0-86542-844-1 (BSL)
ISBN 0-86542-670-8
(International Edition)

Library of Congress
Cataloging-in-Publication Data

Wilks, David.
    The infectious diseases manual/David Wilks,
Mark Farrington, David Rubenstein.
        p.   cm.
    Includes index.
    ISBN 0-86542-844-1
    1. Communicable diseases—Handbooks,
manuals, etc.   2. Infection—Handbooks,
manuals, etc.   3. Medical microbiology—
Handbooks, manuals, etc.
    I. Farrington, Mark.   II. Rubenstein, David.
III. Title.
        [DNLM: 1. Infection—handbooks.   WC 39
W688i 1995]
    RC111.W68   1995
    616.9—dc20
    DNLM/DLC
    for Library of Congress   95-6330
                                                CIP

Contents

Introduction

The Infectious Diseases Manual brings together detailed and practical information on all aspects of infectious diseases and microbiology. Common conditions are described in detail. The clinical presentation of rarely seen and usually tropical conditions is described in sufficient detail to allow recognition, whereas their treatment, which always requires specialist referral, is described in outline only.

Throughout the *Manual* we have grouped and classified information in ways that will be of most use to clinicians at the patient's bedside—thus pneumonia is a clinical topic in Section 1 with references to the numerous relevant micro-organisms within Section 2. In contrast, the clinical section on brucellosis is found in Section 2 by its specific bacterial cause, with cross-references from fever and other appropriate clinical syndromes in Section 1.

To make the best use of space we have used symbols and abbreviations, defined on the following pages. Throughout the text, the symbol (➤000) indicates that further information is available on the indicated page.

Information of less direct use for patient management (details of micro-organisms, pathogenesis and laboratory techniques) is to be found in Section 2, usually in short-note form.

Tables of antibiotics' doses and side effects are located in Section 3. Whilst every care has been taken to ensure that these tables contain no errors, we cannot accept responsibility for any that have occurred. The dose of any drug which is rarely used or unfamiliar should be checked by reference to local hospital formulary, the manufacturer's data sheet or the *British National Formulary*.

1

Abbreviations

βHS	β-haemolytic streptococcus	ERCP	endoscopic retrograde
AAD	antibiotic-associated diarrhoea		cholecystopancreatogram
ABG	arterial blood gas	ETEC	enterotoxigenic *E. coli*
ADC	AIDS dementia complex	FBC	full blood count
AE	acute endocarditis	FTA	fluorescent treponemal antigen test
AFB	acid-fast bacillus/bacilli	G6PD	glucose-6-phosphate dehydrogenase
AHF	Argentine haemorrhagic fever	GI	gastrointestinal
AIDS	acquired immunodeficiency	GN	glomerulonephritis
	syndrome	Gp	group(s)
ARDS	adult respiratory distress syndrome	h	hour
ASOT	antistreptolysin O titre	HAV	hepatitis A virus
AV	aortic valve	HBV	hepatitis B virus
BAL	bronchoalveolar lavage	HCV	hepatitis C virus
BHF	Bolivian haemorrhagic fever	HDCV	human diploid cell vaccine (rabies)
CAPD	chronic ambulatory peritoneal	HDV	hepatitis D virus
	dialysis	HEPA	high-efficiency particulate arrester
CCDC	consultant in communicable disease	HEV	hepatitis E virus
	control	HHV-6	human herpesvirus type 6
CDAD	*Clostridium difficile*-associated	Hib	*Haemophilus influenzae* type b
	diarrhoea	HIG	normal human immunoglobulin
CDSC	Communicable Disease	HIV	human immunodeficiency virus
	Surveillance Centre (Colindale)	HLGR	high-level gentamicin-resistant
CF	cystic fibrosis	hly	hourly
CL	cutaneous leishmaniasis	HPLC	high performance liquid
CMI	cell-mediated immunity		chromatography
CMV	cytomegalovirus	HPV	human papillomavirus
CNS	central nervous system	HSV	herpes simplex virus
CNSt	coagulase-negative staphylococci	IA	invasive aspergillosis
COAD	chronic obstructive airways disease	ICU	intensive care unit
CRS	congenital rubella syndrome	id	intradermal
CSF	cerebrospinal fluid	ID	infectious diseases
CT	computed tomography (scan)	IE	infective endocarditis
CXR	chest X-ray	IFAT	indirect fluorescent antibody test
DAEC	diffusely adherent *E. coli*	im/IM	intramuscular
DIC	disseminated intravascular	ip	intraperitoneal
	coagulation	IUD	intrauterine device
EAggEC	enteroaggregative *E. coli*	iv/IV	intravenous
EBV	Epstein–Barr virus	IVDU	intravenous drug use(r)
ECHO	echocardiogram	KS	Kaposi's sarcoma
EHEC	enterohaemorrhagic *E. coli*	LF	Lassa fever
EIEC	enteroinvasive *E. coli*	LGV	lymphogranuloma venereum
ELISA	enzyme-linked immunosorbent	LIP	lymphoid interstitial pneumonitis
	assay	LP	lumbar puncture
ENT	ear, nose and throat	LT	heat-labile toxin of
EPEC	enteropathogenic *E. coli*		*Enterobacteriacae*

MAI	*Mycobacterium avium-intracellulare*	RUQ	right upper quadrant
MBC	minimum bactericidal concentration	SBC	serum bactericidal concentration
		SBE	subacute bacterial endocarditis
MDa	megadalton	sc	subcutaneous
MIC	minimum inhibitory concentration	SDT	single-dose therapy
min	minute	SLE	systemic lupus erythematosus
MMR	measles/mumps/rubella vaccine	SPT	septic pelvic vein thrombosis
MOSF	multiorgan system failure	SRSV	small round structured virus
MRI	magnetic resonance imaging	SSSS	staphylococcal scalded-skin syndrome
MRSA	methicillin-resistant *Staphylococcus aureus*	ST	heat-stable toxin of *Enterobacteriacae*
MSU	midstream urine		
MV	mitral valve	STD	sexually transmitted disease
MW	molecular weight	TB	tuberculosis
NSAID	non-steroidal anti-inflammatory drug	TOA	tubo-ovarian abscess
		TPHA	*Treponema pallidum* haemagglutination assay
OM	otitis media		
OPV	oral polio vaccine	TSS(T)	toxic shock syndrome (toxin)
PCP	*Pneumocystis carinii* pneumonia	TV	tricuspid valve
PHLS	Public Health Laboratory Service	URTI	upper respiratory tract infection
PID	pelvic inflammatory disease	USS	ultrasound scan
PMC	pseudomembranous colitis	UTI	urinary tract infection
po	orally	VDRL	Venereal Disease Reference Laboratory
PSGN	poststreptococcal glomerulonephritis		
		VHF	viral haemorrhagic fever
PUO	pyrexia of unknown origin	VLM	visceral larva migrans
PVE	prosthetic valve endocarditis	VZV	varicella-zoster virus
RA	rheumatoid arthritis	WBC	white blood cell (count)
RF	rheumatic fever	WHO	World Health Organization
RS	Reiter's syndrome	YF	yellow fever
RSV	respiratory syncytial virus	ZN	Ziehl–Neelson
RTI	respiratory tract infection		

Symbols

Notifiable Diseases ⊠

In the United Kingdom the following diseases must be notified to the local authority, via the local consultant in communicable disease control (CCDC).

Acute encephalitis (➤78)
Acute poliomyelitis (➤250)
Anthrax (➤177)
Cholera (➤195)
Diphtheria (➤181)
Dysentery (amoebic
or bacillary) (➤44)
Food poisoning (➤44)
Leprosy (➤230)
Leptospirosis (➤226)
Malaria (➤268)
Measles (➤100)
Meningitis (➤74)
Meningococcaemia (➤74)
Mumps (➤102)

Ophthalmia neonatorum (➤83)
Paratyphoid fever (➤191)
Plague (➤211)
Rabies (➤257)
Relapsing fever (➤225)
Rubella (➤101)
Scarlet fever (➤108)
Smallpox (➤245)
Tetanus (➤217)
Tuberculosis (➤29)
Typhoid fever (➤191)
Typhus (➤236)
Viral haemorrhagic fever (➤256)
Viral hepatitis (➤48)
Whooping cough (➤108)
Yellow fever (➤253)

Chickenpox (➤ 103) is a notifiable disease in Scotland. Certain other diseases may be made **locally** notifiable.

Isolation

Isolation is a key technique for preventing spread of infectious diseases in hospitals. It can be physically and emotionally disturbing and disruptive of clinical care and therefore should be used only where there is proven or likely benefit. Strong evidence of efficacy is available for some infections, including MRSA and multiply resistant coliforms. Isolation policies are made at individual hospitals, and local protocols should always be consulted. If these are not available, consult your microbiologists ☎. Detailed instructions for nursing procedures are beyond the scope of this manual.

Source isolation is designed to prevent infected patients from transmitting their disease to others. It may generally be considered in four categories (Table 2).

Throughout the text, recommended levels of isolation are indicated by symbols (e.g. ④).

Protective isolation is used to prevent immunocompromised patients from acquiring infection. It is of less certain value, particularly because most infections in neutropenic patients are endogenous (➤133). Most units concentrate on protecting against specific organisms, e.g. nursing in HEPA-filtered air (vs. aspergillosis), antibiotic prophylaxis and microbiologically clean food (to avoid colonisation with new strains of Gram-negative bacteria).

Table 2 Levels of source isolation

Level of isolation	Examples	Route	Main suggested precautions
① Standard	*Neisseria meningitidis*, group A β-haemolytic streptococci	Airborne or direct contact	Separate room. Negative-pressure ventilation if available. Gowns, gloves ± masks for all entering room
② Body fluids	*Salmonella* spp., *Shigella* spp.	Contact with urine, faeces and secretions	Separate room. Gowns and gloves for patient contact
③ Infection risk from blood	Hepatitis B, HIV	Contact with blood or bloodstained body fluids*	Separate room only required if patients are bleeding, likely to bleed, undergoing major invasive procedure, incontinent or confused. Plastic aprons, gloves (± visors) for procedures where contact with body fluids is possible
④ Strict	Lassa fever	Airborne or direct contact	Strict isolation in specialist unit – usually regional infectious diseases centre. **Do not send any specimens without discussion with lab**

*Including CSF, pleural fluid, vaginal secretions, peritoneal fluid, synovial fluid, semen, pericardial fluid, amniotic fluid and breast milk.

Table 3 Recommendations for isolation. For category codes ⯈6

Disease	Category	See
Anthrax ⊠	④	177
Bordetella pertussis[1] ⊠	①	108
Borrelia recurrentis[2] ⊠	①	225
Bronchiolitis (RSV)[24]	①	249
Campylobacter jejuni[3]	②	196
Candida spp.[4]	②	291
Chickenpox ⊠[6]	①	103
Chlamydia trachomatis[5] (ophthalmia neonatorum ⊠, conjunctivitis, genital infection)	②	233
Cholera[7] ⊠	②	195
Clostridium difficile[8]	②	47
Coxsackie virus[9]	②	251
Creutzfeld–Jakob disease	②	260
Cryptosporidium parvum	②	263
Dermatitis[10] (severely infected)	①	88
Diarrhoea–unknown cause[12]	②	44
Diphtheria[11] ⊠	(①)	181
Dysentery ⊠ Amoebic[13] or bacillary[14]	②	44
Ebola virus ⊠	④	257
Eczema[10] (severely infected)	①	88
Encephalitis – unknown cause ⊠	①	78
Erysipelas[10]	①	89
Erythema infectiosum	①	107
Escherichia coli diarrhoea, travellers' diarrhoea, haemolytic uraemic syndrome (O157, VTEC, EIEC, EPEC, EAggEC, ETEC, etc.)	②	44
Exanthem subitum	①	107
Food poisoning ⊠		44
Undiagnosed cause[12]	②	
Campylobacter jejuni[3]	②	
Salmonella[15]	②	
Francisella tularensis[15]	①	212
Gastroenteritis, viral	②	258
Giardiasis	②	266
Gonococcal conjunctivitis[1]	②	82
Haemolytic streptococcus[10] Lancefield group A, B[3], C or G (*Streptococcus pyogenes*)	①	170
Hepatitis – unknown cause ⊠	②	
Hepatitis A	②	49
Hepatitis B, fulminant liver failure of undetermined cause	③	49

Disease	Category	See
Hepatitis C	②	52
Herpes simplex[17]	①	93
Herpes zoster[6]	①	105
HIV	③	114
Impetigo[10]	①	87
Lassa fever ⊠	④	256
Leprosy ⊠		230
Smear negative	–	
Smear positive	①	
Leptospirosis[1] ⊠	②	226
Lice, fleas[1]	②	
Listeriosis[18]	②	179
Marburg virus disease ⊠	④	257
Measles[19] ⊠	①	100
Melioidosis[15]	①	200
Meningitis ⊠		74
Neisseria meningitidis[1] (including meningococcal septicaemia/other invasive meningococcal infections)	①	
Neonatal	②	110
Viral[9]	①	77
Meningoencephalitis, acute (acute poliomyelitis) ⊠	①	250
MRSA[20]	①	167
Multiply resistant Gram-negative bacteria[20]	②	309
Mumps[9] ⊠	①	102
Ophthalmia neonatorum[1] ⊠	②	83
Parvovirus B19	①	107
Penicillin-resistant *Streptococcus pneumoniae*[11]	①	174
Pertussis[1] ⊠	①	108
Plague ⊠	④	211
Poliomyelitis, acute ⊠	①	250
Pseudomonas pseudomallei[15]	①	200
Psittacosis	①	22
PUO[21]	①	153
Rabies ⊠	④	257
Ratbite fever[1]	②	212
Relapsing fever[2] ⊠	①	225
Respiratory syncytial virus[24]	①	249
Rotavirus	②	258
Rubella[16] ⊠	①	101
Salmonellosis[15] (excluding typhoid and paratyphoid)	②	44

continued on p. 8

Table 3 Contd

Disease	Category	See	Disease	Category	See
Scabies[1]	①	73	Typhoid, paratyphoid and carriers[7] ⊠	②	190
Scarlet fever[10] ⊠	①	108	Typhus[2] ⊠	①	236
Smallpox[22] ⊠	④	245	Vaccinia, generalised	④	245
Staphylococcus aureus			Vancomycin-resistant	①	309
Pneumonia	①	25	Gram-positive organisms[20]		
Food poisoning ⊠	–	44	(usually Enterococcus		
Streptococcus pyogenes – see		170	faecalis or faecium)		
Haemolytic streptococcus			Varicella ⊠[6]	①	103
Syphilis (1° or 2° only)[1]	②	67	Vibrio parahaemolyticus[15]	②	195
Tapeworms	②	280	Viral haemorrhagic fever ⊠	④	256
Tuberculosis[23] (open pulmonary,	①	29	Whooping cough[1] ⊠	①	108
wound, urinary) ⊠			Yersinia enterocolitica and	②	194
Tularaemia[15]	①	212	pseudotuberculosis[15]		

[1] For first 24 h of treatment. [2] Until patient and contacts deloused. [3] Neonates only. [4] If part of proven outbreak. [5] For first 48 h of treatment. [6] Until vesicles are crusted and dry. Staff in contact should be immune. Notifiable in Scotland. [7] Until asymptomatic with three negative stool cultures. [8] Until asymptomatic for 3 days. [9] For 10 days after onset. [10] Until cultures known to be negative for β-haemolytic streptococci. [11] Until culture negative. [12] Until transmissible pathogens excluded. [13] Until asymptomatic and treated for cyst carriage. [14] Until asymptomatic and one negative stool culture. [15] Until asymptomatic. [16] Until 7 days after onset of rash. [17] Only for infants with disseminated infection. [18] Infants and mothers only. [19] Until 4 days after onset of rash. [20] Until agreed by microbiologist. [21] If outside Europe and N. America within past 4 weeks. [22] Even if only suspected. [23] For first 14 days of therapy. [24] Cohorting on children's ward whilst symptomatic.

Microbiological Specimens

Details of **sample collection** and transport vary from laboratory to laboratory, but a general summary of principles follows. Laboratories differ on the basis of local prevalence as to whether they routinely perform certain tests on particular specimens (e.g. *Clostridium difficile* toxin on all faeces). The importance of listing **full clinical details** has been emphasised throughout this book. **Always** give details of recent hospital in-patient stays and travel, and also occupation if the patient has diarrhoea or skin infection and works in catering, school or hospital. Similarly, **details of past, current and intended antibiotic therapy** are valuable for interpretation of many culture results. **Virus culture** is usually only worth attempting early in the course of infection. Specimens for **culture of bacteria and fungi** should always be taken **before antibiotic therapy is commenced**; after this sputum and swabs of mucosae and open wounds become colonised particularly rapidly with resistant bacteria.

- **Screening of contacts, or of cases for clearance**, is only occasionally useful for any pathogen out of hospital, and should always be done only according to locally written policies or after discussion with a microbiologist, ID physician or CCDC.
- Specimens are always best transported immediately to the laboratory. If delay is necessary, in general all samples should be refrigerated at 4°C, except those for gonococcal culture, which are best kept at room temperature, and inoculated blood culture bottles which should be incubated at 37°C.

Swabs, tissue and pus

Send pus, if available, in a sterile universal container because additional rapid tests can be performed (e.g. HPLC for short-chain fatty acids from anaerobes); a swab is an inferior substitute, upon which delicate organisms die. Use firm pressure when taking swabs and always use the appropriate swab transport medium (bacterial, viral, chlamydial). Use special **pernasal swabs** for *Bordetella pertussis* and **charcoal swabs** for *Neisseria gonorrhoeae* culture. Gonococcal culture plates are best inoculated at the bedside. Surface swabs of deeply infected lesions (e.g. sinus tracks from osteomyelitis) usually grow surface contaminants (e.g. coliforms and pseudomonads) and rarely grow the causative organism. Only isolation of *Staphylococcus aureus* from this type of specimen correlates with true deep infection. Culture of bone marrow, liver biopsies, etc. is occasionally useful, but should be discussed in advance with a microbiologist.

Medical devices

The tips of iv catheters suspected of being infected should be cut off with alcohol-wiped scissors and sent in a sterile universal container for semiquantitative culture. Growth of >15–20 colonies of coagulase-negative staphylococci or diphtheroids suggests infection, and any growth of other bacteria or fungi is likely to be significant. Small infected prostheses (e.g. heart valves) can be sent entire, but it is best to scrape adherent material from larger prostheses and send that.

Urine

Prepuce and labia should be held away from the urine stream, but periurethral cleaning does not additionally reduce contamination of MSUs from adults as long as the initial stream is discarded. Most laboratories supply universal containers with borate preservative, or dip-slides for urine collection in domiciliary practice. The former preserves both host and bacterial cells for 48 h. Dip-slides should be only dipped into urine, and the transport container should not be filled with it. Catheter urine specimens should be taken by aseptic puncture of the sampling area close to the patient. Culturing urinary catheter tips is a waste of time. Paediatric bag collection systems are often contaminated, but this is reduced by cleaning the perineum with antiseptic; a negative culture is useful, but positive results must be interpreted with care. Suprapubic aspiration is the gold standard for detecting bladder urine infection. Early-morning urine (EMU) specimens for AFB microscopy and culture should be ~150 ml volumes and taken on different days.

Sputum

Efforts, such as vigorous physiotherapy, to obtain expectorated sputum before antibiotics have been given improve the isolation rate of pneumococci and other significant pathogens. Three samples on successive days are needed to exclude open pulmonary tuberculosis. Bronchoalveolar lavage is the most sensitive diagnostic procedure, but induced sputum is simpler with adequate sensitivity for *Pneumocystis carinii* diagnosis. In ventilated patients, non-directed lavage allows recognition of significant isolates by quantitative culture ($>10^5$/ml).

Faeces

A walnut-sized sample is needed; this is most easily collected by passing stool on to folded toilet paper in the lavatory bowl, and scooping the sample into a universal container with a spatula attached to the inside of the lid. The best chance of isolating causative agents of acute diarrhoea is on the first sample, and only if it is taken early in the course of illness. Many pathogens are only transiently excreted (e.g. *Escherichia coli* O157), so multiple samples are only required for exclusion of some parasites

(e.g. *Giardia*) and to detect carriage of typhoid bacilli in food handlers (➤46). 'Hot' stool samples for visualisation of trophozoites of *Entamoeba histolytica* are only useful if the patient has dysentery, i.e. bloody diarrhoea.

Blood cultures

Blood cultures should be taken from any patient who is systemically ill in whom an infective diagnosis is being considered. Before venepuncture the skin must be carefully disinfected with an alcoholic antiseptic, which is allowed to dry. Most laboratories now use automated blood culture systems, which come with instruction sheets and should be inoculated with the specified volumes of blood (both over- and under-inoculation impair performance). Check the expiry date on the bottles and do not use if cloudy. Modern systems have greatly improved efficiency, and two or three cultures are sufficient for all indications except when the patient has received antibiotics recently. In this case when IE is suspected, it is worth taking two cultures on day 1 and daily cultures for the next 3–4 days. It is not necessary to change needles before injecting the culture bottles. Special bottles may be required for the isolation of *Neisseria meningitidis* (➤205).

CSF

Best taken in three consecutively labelled bottles and transported immediately to the laboratory. Take simultaneous blood glucose. For a reasonable chance of detecting AFB, 10 ml or more CSF is required.

Serum

Listing the **times of doses and samples** is important for interpretation of antibiotic assays. Specifying the **date of onset of illness** is vital for choosing and interpreting serological tests; acute and convalescent (10–14 days later) sera are often needed to prove recent infection. Most laboratories will store many such sera, issue a request for a convalescent sample and only perform the assays (in parallel) if a later serum is received. IgM assay diagnosis on single acute sera is possible for some infections (e.g. *Mycoplasma*, rubella, hepatitis viruses, *Toxoplasma*), and very high single titres are diagnostic for others (e.g. *Legionella*, respiratory *Chlamydia*, *Coxiella*). **Exposure history** and **date of leaving the endemic area** are essential for performance of tests for many geographically restricted infections (e.g. brucellosis, schistosomiasis).

Section 1:
Clinical Infectious Diseases

1: Upper Respiratory Tract Infections

Sinusitis

Most often affects the maxillary sinuses. May be acute or chronic and recurrent. Complications are due to the proximity of the orbits and intracranial structures.

Risk factors: Frequently secondary to: acute viral upper respiratory tract infection (URTI), complicating ~0.5% of childhood URTIs. Dental sepsis or procedures, nasal polyps or deviated septum, prolonged nasal intubation. Rarely, immunodeficiency (AIDS, IgG or IgA deficiency), cystic fibrosis, immotile cilia syndrome.

Clinical features: Facial pain, fever and purulent nasal discharge. Headache, nasal obstruction, halitosis, toothache and anosmia may occur. Cough is frequent in children.

Organisms: Acute: *Streptococcus pneumoniae Haemophilus influenzae, Mycoplasma pneumoniae,* viruses, *Moraxella catarrhalis,* rarely *Staphylococcus aureus.* **Chronic:** *Streptococcus pneumoniae, Haemophilus influenzae, Streptococcus 'milleri',* mixed oral anaerobes, *Staphylococcus aureus.*

Microbiological investigations: Nasal swabs are **not** helpful. Sinus aspiration to obtain material for Gram staining and culture, for persistent or recurrent infections.

Other investigations: Severe or persistent infection merits sinus X-rays. Fluid level or opacity suggests acute infection. Complete opacity or mucosal thickening alone may be seen in chronic infection. CT, MRI are sensitive indicators of sinusitis.

Differential diagnosis: Consider immunodeficiency, rare non-infectious causes (Wegener's, carcinoma, lymphoma), unusual infections (TB, leprosy, syphilis).

Antibiotic management: Amoxycillin **or** co-amoxiclav **or** cefotaxime.

Supportive management: Nasal decongestants: oxymetazoline hydrochloride nasal spray, 0.05%, one or two sprays each nostril 8-hly, **or** pseudoephedrine hydrochloride, 60 mg 8-hly,

po. ENT referral for persistent or recurrent infection.

Complications: Rare but serious. Orbital cellulitis (➤85), osteomyelitis of facial bones (➤97), intracranial abscess (➤79), meningitis (➤74), cavernous and superior sagittal sinus thrombosis, orbital fissure syndrome (sphenoid sinus).

Comments: Chronic recurrent sinusitis reflects impaired drainage from the sinuses and merits ENT referral. Infection is usually due to mixed aerobic and anaerobic oral flora and responds poorly to antibiotic therapy alone. Immunocompromised patients and diabetics may develop fungal sinusitis (*Aspergillus* spp., *Mucor* spp. and relatives ➤290). ENT referral is required.

Otitis media (OM)

Risk factors: Frequently follows URTI. Common in children because of short, straight Eustachian tubes and blockage secondary to lymphoid hyperplasia.

Clinical features: Fever and earache. Otorrhoea if perforation has occurred. Presentation may be non-specific in infants. Tenderness over the mastoid process and redness and bulging of the tympanic membrane, which may have perforated.

Organisms: *Streptococcus pneumoniae, Haemophilus influenzae, Mycoplasma pneumoniae, Moraxella catarrhalis.* Approximately 30% are viral, frequently due to respiratory syncytial virus. *Staphylococcus aureus* and group A β-haemolytic streptococci are seen rarely. Chronic infection may proceed to cholesteatoma with involvement of *Proteus* spp. and pseudomonads.

Microbiological investigations: In uncomplicated cases, none. See below for guidance on management of persistent and recurrent infections.

Antibiotic management: Amoxycillin **or** trimethoprim **or** co-amoxiclav.

Complications: Mastoiditis, meningitis, intracranial abscess.

Comments: Although up to 20% of *Haemophilus influenzae* are resistant to amoxycillin, only 10–25% of cases of OM will involve this organism so the overall chance of treatment failure due to amoxycillin-resistant *Haemophilus influenzae* is low. Indications for **not** choosing amoxycillin would be recent failure to respond to amoxycillin, local prevalence of amoxycillin-resistant *Haemophilus influenzae*, culture results suggesting infection with a resistant organism or penicillin allergy. Recurrent OM may be treated with short-term prophylaxis (e.g. amoxycillin 20 mg/kg 24-hly).

> **Practice point:** ENT referral for consideration of tympanocentesis or myringotomy is indicated for severely ill patients (and those with severe pain or persistent infection despite antibiotics), neonates and the immunodeficient, or if a suppurative complication is suspected. Also refer patients with persistent (often asymptomatic) middle ear effusion (chronic secretory OM) for greater than 3 months and those with persistent infection and perforation (chronic suppurative OM).

Otitis externa

A hypersensitivity reaction of the skin lining the external auditory canal. Symptoms include itching, pain and a feeling of fullness. On otoscopy, oedema and redness of the walls of the meatus. Often responds to careful cleansing and topical steroids. If infection is present it is usually mixed due to diphtheroids, pseudomonads and coliforms. Neomycin and hydrocortisone drops may be used. If there is evidence of local skin infection, such as a boil, flucloxacillin is given. Perforation must be excluded before drops are prescribed. *Aspergillus* and other fungal infections are best treated with clotrimazole drops.

Malignant otitis externa is a rare infection with *Pseudomonas aeruginosa* which affects elderly diabetics and the immunocompromised. It has a significant mortality, due to infection of adjacent bone and soft tissue, and requires aggressive systemic treatment with antipseudomonal antibiotics and surgical debridement. Urgent ENT referral is essential.

Dental and oral infections

Dental caries is related to acid production from fermentation of dietary carbohydrates by bacteria including *Streptococcus mutans* and lactobacilli. Its significance for the physician lies in its effects on nutrition and as a risk factor for gingival disease, dental abscesses and Vincent's angina.

Vincent's angina

Risk factors: Poor oral hygiene, poor nutrition, smoking and severe intercurrent illness.

Clinical features: Oral pain, gingival bleeding, halitosis, fever and anorexia. On examination there is necrosis and pseudomembrane formation on tonsils and gums. There may be local lymphadenopathy and excess salivation.

Organisms: Mixed infection due to *Leptotrichia* spp., *Bacteroides* spp. and *Fusobacterium* spp.

Differential diagnosis: Candidiasis (➤291), herpes simplex stomatitis (➤102), diphtheria (➤181).

Microbiological investigations: Gram stain of scrapings from the affected area. Throat swab for *Candida albicans* and *Corynebacterium diphtheriae* if suspected.

Antibiotic management: Penicillin V/amoxycillin + metronidazole **or** co-amoxiclav.

Supportive management: Attention to oral and dental hygiene.

Complications: In the severely malnourished or immunocompromised patient progression to severe gangrenous stomatitis occurs rarely.

> **Practice point:** Patients with agranulocytosis may present with severe oral and pharyngeal ulceration due to *Candida* spp., herpes simplex or *Capnocytophaga* spp. infection, which may act as a portal of entry for oral streptococcal bacteraemia.

Dental abscess

Risk factors: Poor dental hygiene, pregnancy.

Clinical features: Fever, toothache, facial pain and swelling.

Organisms: Mixed oral aerobes and anaerobes.

Microbiological investigations: None routinely.

Antibiotic management: Penicillin V/amoxycillin + metronidazole **or** co-amoxiclav.

Pharyngitis

Infection of the posterior oral cavity, often involving the lymphoid tissue of Waldeyer's ring. Most cases are viral; management is aimed at avoiding the immunological sequelae of streptococcal infection, and recognising acute bacterial epiglottitis and, rarely, diphtheria.

Clinical features: Fever, malaise, sore throat and myalgia. On examination, erythema and oedema of the tonsils and pharyngeal mucosa. It is usually impossible to determine the cause clinically. Cough and coryza suggest influenza or rhinoviruses whereas conjunctivitis suggests adenovirus. Vesicles and ulceration affecting both the pharynx and mouth are seen in HSV stomatitis; in Coxsackievirus A herpangina (➢108) small vesicles and ulcers are usually confined to the posterior pharynx. Purulent tonsillar exudate and a rash suggest streptococcal infection or EBV; the latter is often accompanied by generalised lymphadenopathy and/or hepatosplenomegaly. Purulent tonsillar exudate is rare in influenza or rhinovirus infection.

Organisms: Rhinovirus, coronavirus, adenovirus, influenza A and B, parainfluenza, herpes simplex virus, Coxsackievirus A, EBV and CMV infection. **Gp A β-haemolytic streptococci (βHS)**, less often group C or G. Rarely, *Arcanobacterium haemolyticum*, *Neisseria gonorrhoeae*. Very rarely, *Corynebacterium diphtheriae*.

Microbiological investigations: Throat swab to exclude βHS. Latex agglutination tests for the rapid diagnosis of Gp A βHS antigens in throat swabs are widely used in the USA and are specific and quite sensitive but expensive. A rise in ASOT may give retrospective confirmation of streptococcal infection. If diphtheria is suspected liaison with the microbiology department is essential ☎. Viral culture may be positive, particularly in HSV infection. Viral serology may be useful in retrospect.

Differential diagnosis: Diphtheria is extremely rare in the developed world, but should be suspected in an unimmunised patient who is unwell, particularly if there is a grey tonsillar exudate spreading from the tonsils to involve the uvula, palate or posterior pharyngeal wall (➢181).

Antibiotic management: Penicillin V **or** erythromycin.

> **Practice point:** Patients with 1° EBV infection develop a widespread maculopapular rash after treatment with ampicillin or amoxycillin. These antibiotics should be avoided in sore throat unless the diagnosis of bacterial infection has been firmly established.

Complications: Bacterial chest infection, quinsy, otitis media, sinusitis. Rapid deterioration with cough, dyspnoea and hypoxia in a patient with URTI due to influenza A or B may be due to viral or secondary bacterial pneumonia.

Comments: **Scarlet fever** ✉, now rare in the UK, is caused by streptococcal erythrodermic toxin, which may be produced in streptococcal infection at any site. Clinical features include 'strawberry tongue' and a rash which spreads from the face (sparing the circumoral area) to the trunk and limbs, and is accentuated in the skin folds (Pastia's lines). This usually lasts 6–9 days, following which it may desquamate, particularly over the palms and soles. During desquamation there is often an eosinophilia (➢108).

Lemierre's disease

'Anaerobic tonsillitis': Severe pharyngitis associated with fever, septicaemia, metastatic pulmonary infection and jugular vein thrombosis is rarely seen in young adults and is caused by *Fusobacterium necrophorum* (➢222).

Laryngitis

In addition to the symptoms of pharyngitis, some patients with URTI may develop hoarseness and odynophagia. Laryngitis is usually viral in aetiology, although it may accompany infection by streptococci. Persistent hoarseness is usually due to non-infectious causes but may indicate chronic granulomatous laryngitis. Causes include *Candida albicans* and herpes simplex virus; diagnosed on biopsy.

Croup (acute laryngotracheobronchitis)

Croup typically affects children from a few months old to the age of 3 years, and occurs in epidemics in autumn and early spring. During the course of a viral URTI, most often due to parainfluenza virus, inspiratory stridor and a distinctive 'seal's bark' cough develop. Cyanosis and intercostal recession indicate more severe airway obstruction. Hypoxia is common. Antibiotics and mist inhalation have not been shown to be of value but steroids (prednisolone 2 mg/kg 24-hly for three days) reduce severity and duration of illness without side-effects. Sicker children should also be given nebulised adrenaline (1:1000, 0.5 ml/kg to a maximum of 5 ml 2-hly). Careful observation is needed, with a view to timely intubation should airway obstruction progress. The important differential diagnosis is acute epiglottitis.

Bacterial tracheitis

Retrosternal discomfort commonly accompanies viral URTI. Rarely, bacterial tracheitis may follow with fever, dyspnoea and stridor with purulent sputum. Gram stain and culture of sputum and blood culture are required if severe. Infection is most often due to *Staphylococcus aureus*, Gp A βHS and *Haemophilus influenzae* type b. Lateral soft-tissue X-ray of neck may show subglottic narrowing with a normal epiglottis ('pencil sign'). Bacterial tracheitis may follow intubation and trauma.

Antibiotic management: Co-amoxiclav or cefotaxime or flucloxacillin–to be guided by the results of sputum culture.

Quinsy

Quinsy (peritonsillar abscess) usually follows bacterial pharyngitis. It is usually polymicrobial in origin, with oral anaerobes and Gp A βHS predominating. Patients present with abrupt increase in pain and dysphagia. On examination there is asymmetrical tonsillar enlargement with swelling in the neck and often a palpable fluctuant mass. Management consists of ENT referral for consideration of surgical drainage and parenteral benzylpenicillin or co-amoxiclav or cefotaxime.

Acute epiglottitis

Inflammation, oedema and obstruction of the supraglottic structures including the epiglottis due to *Haemophilus influenzae* type b (rarely other capsular types) typically affecting children aged 3–7 years.

Clinical features: Abrupt onset, over hours, of severe sore throat and fever. Children are unwell, with stridor, drooling and dysphagia. They may adopt a typical posture, sitting up and leaning forward. The swollen, cherry-red epiglottis may be visible but **attempts to use a tongue depressor should be avoided as this may precipitate fatal acute total obstruction**.

Organisms: *Haemophilus influenzae* type b.

Antibiotic management: Due to the possibility of ampicillin/amoxycillin resistance, cefotaxime iv or amoxycillin + chloramphenicol is given. Rifampicin prophylaxis should be given to the patient and all household and nursery/day-care contacts including adults if there are other susceptible children in the family (≻77).

Supportive management: Management of the airway is paramount. **Elective intubation is associated with reduced mortality, as emergency intubation may be very difficult.** Do not attempt to visualise the epiglottis. Arrange for urgent intubation in theatre by an experienced person. Give oxygen and be prepared for urgent intubation or tracheostomy if complete obstruction supervenes. Do not attempt iv access or blood tests until airway is secure.

Other investigations: Lateral soft-tissue neck X-ray may show the engorged epiglottis (the 'thumb sign').

Differential diagnosis: It is essential to distinguish between viral croup and epiglottitis. Salient features are the abrupt onset, toxic

appearance, dysphagia and drooling associated with epiglottitis. Diphtheria and inhaled
foreign body may also need to be considered.

Complications: Systemic spread, bacteraemia,
meningitis, arthritis and cellulitis.

Comments: This condition has been reported
rarely in adults. All forms of invasive
Haemophilus influenzae type b are less common with the introduction of the Hib vaccine.

Thyroiditis

Sudden onset of pain, tenderness and swelling in
the thyroid due to infection by *Staphylococcus
aureus*, *Streptococcus pneumoniae* or mixed oral
anaerobes. ENT referral for consideration of
needle aspiration (send for culture). Acute
suppurative thyroiditis is rare. Often associated
with a persistent thyroglossal duct, or a third or
fourth branchial arch anomaly with a congenital
fistula from the pyriform fossa to the thyroid.
Confirmation by barium swallow. Inflammation
is more often subacute, related to recent viral
infection (e.g. mumps, measles, influenza and
EBV).

2: Lower Respiratory Tract Infections

Acute bronchiolitis/viral pneumonia in children ①

Viral URTI may progress to acute bronchiolitis and pneumonia in children under 5 years. Pneumonia is usually viral in this age-group. Acute bronchiolitis is seen most often under the age of 24 months. There is inflammation of bronchioles 75–300 μm in diameter with loss of cilia and oedema leading to obstruction of the lumen by cellular debris and secretions. It occurs in epidemics, usually in winter, and is frequently accompanied by viral pneumonia.

Clinical features: After symptoms of URTI, cough, dyspnoea and wheeze develop. Very young children may present with refusal to feed and apnoeic attacks. On examination, there is fever, tachycardia, tachypnoea and sometimes cyanosis. Clinical hyperinflation and intercostal recession suggest bronchiolitis. On auscultation there are widespread crepitations and wheezes.

Organisms: Respiratory syncytial virus (RSV) accounts for the majority of cases. Parainfluenza, adenoviruses and influenza are less common. Some cases follow rhinovirus and coronavirus infection. Cytomegalovirus has been reported as a cause of viral pneumonia in very young children.

Microbiological investigations: Nasopharyngeal secretions for viral culture and rapid diagnostic tests for RSV. Serology may be positive in retrospect.

Other investigations: The chest X-ray shows hyperinflation, characteristic of acute bronchiolitis, with or without infiltrates, which may be due to concomitant pneumonia or atelectasis. Pulse oximetry.

Differential diagnosis: Asthma, inhaled foreign body, bacterial pneumonia, pertussis.

Antibiotic management: Most recover without specific antiviral therapy. In severe cases, inhaled nebulised ribavarin may be used. This is active against RSV, but has little action against other viruses listed. Steroids do not improve the prognosis. Systemic antibiotics (e.g. cefotaxime) are often given in case of bacterial superinfection.

Supportive management: Humidified oxygen to maintain O_2 saturation ≥93%. Nasogastric or iv fluids often required. Nebulised bronchodilators may help.

Complications: Less than 1% require ventilation. Infection may be particularly severe in children with pre-existing cardiopulmonary disease.

Viral pneumonia in adults

Risk factors: Viral pneumonia is rare in adults although secondary bacterial pneumonia commonly follows viral URTI.

Clinical features: After symptoms of URTI, cough and alterations in pulmonary function tests are common, but frank pneumonia occurs only rarely. On examination, there is tachycardia, tachypnoea and sometimes cyanosis. Auscultation reveals crepitations and wheezes. Hypoxia may be severe and difficult to reverse. Infection can be particularly severe if there is pre-existing cardiopulmonary disease.

Organisms: Influenza A virus accounts for almost all cases. Pneumonia is occasionally seen as part of other specific viral syndromes, including infectious mononucleosis and primary varicella zoster virus infection (chickenpox).

Microbiological investigations: Nasopharyngeal secretions for viral culture and rapid diagnostic tests for RSV. Serology may be positive in retrospect. Suspected chickenpox may be confirmed by electron microscopy of vesicle fluid. Sputum and blood cultures are essential to exclude a secondary bacterial pneumonia, which is much more likely.

Other investigations: Chest X-ray shows diffuse patchy shadowing.

Differential diagnosis: Bacterial pneumonia.

Antibiotic management: As it is usually impossible to exclude secondary bacterial pneumonia, most patients will receive antibiotics (e.g. cefotaxime + erythromycin). Chickenpox pneumonia should be treated with high-dose intravenous acyclovir, as well as prophylactic antistaphylococcal antibiotics.

Supportive management: Oxygen and bronchodilators are needed if severe.

Complications: Bacterial pneumonia often follows viral URTI, and can complicate viral pneumonia. Commonest organisms are *Streptococcus pneumoniae*, *Haemophilus influenzae* and *Staphylococcus aureus*.

Comments: Vaccination against influenza is recommended for all elderly patients and those with cardiac or pulmonary disease (➤337).

Acute exacerbation of chronic bronchitis

Chronic bronchitis is defined as a productive cough for greater than 3 months of more than 2 consecutive years. It is usually accompanied by emphysema, which is defined pathologically as dilatation of the air spaces distal to the terminal bronchioles with destruction of alveolar septa. These two entities are usually referred to together as chronic obstructive airways disease (COAD). Acute infective exacerbation of COAD is a very common cause of hospital admission in the UK.

Risk factors: Smoking, environmental pollution, occupational exposure to dust and noxious gases, α_1-antitrypsin deficiency. Infective exacerbation often follows viral URTI. Postoperative exacerbations are common —due to the effects of the anaesthetic and diaphragmatic splinting by abdominal surgery.

Clinical features: Patients have pre-existing features of COAD with persistent productive cough, dyspnoea on exercise and physical signs of hyperexpansion. During infective exacerbations, sputum increases in volume and becomes purulent and dyspnoea becomes more severe. Pleurisy and haemoptysis may occur. On examination the following are often present: fever, tachycardia, cyanosis, tachypnoea, signs of hyperexpansion (reduced cricothyroid distance, barrel chest), signs of airways obstruction (pursed lips

breathing, poor chest movement, reduced air entry with added crepitations and wheezes) and changes in mental state ranging from agitation to toxic confusional state. Signs of secondary pneumonia or of heart failure (congestive cardiac failure or cor pulmonale) may also be seen. Signs of hypercarbia (confusion, bounding pulse and peripheral vasodilatation, flap) may be present.

Organisms: Often mixed. *Haemophilus influenzae* (non-capsulate) *Streptococcus pneumoniae*, *Moraxella catarrhalis* and *Mycoplasma pneumoniae*. Less severe cases may be viral.

Microbiological investigations: Gram stain and culture of sputum if severe or first-line treatment fails. Blood culture if systemic sepsis suspected.

Other investigations: Sick patients will require full blood count (FBC), urea, electrolytes and blood glucose. Chest X-ray typically shows evidence of COAD without obvious consolidation. Arterial blood gas (ABG) analysis should be performed in all patients as a baseline and repeated if the clinical situation deteriorates. Many patients with COAD have respiratory failure, due to alveolar hypoventilation and ventilation/perfusion mismatch. Po_2 is reduced and Pco_2 is increased. In this situation they are used to a high Pco_2 and depend on hypoxia for their ventilatory drive. Uncontrolled oxygen therapy may abolish this 'hypoxic drive', resulting in hypoventilation and CO_2 retention.

Differential diagnosis: Bacterial and viral pneumonia.

Antibiotic management: The new macrolides (e.g. clarithromycin) are active against the 'atypical' agents as well as *Haemophilus influenzae* and *Streptococcus pneumoniae*. Alternatives for less severe cases include amoxycillin, trimethoprim, tetracycline, co-amoxiclav and oral cephalosporins such as cefuroxime axetil, cefaclor and cefixime. Ciprofloxacin is not a suitable first-line agent due to its inferior performance against *Streptococcus pneumoniae*. Severe cases admitted to hospital should be treated as for pneumonia (i.e. cefotaxime + erythromycin ➤26).

Supportive management: Nebulised **broncho-dilators** should be given: salbutamol 2.5–5 mg neb. 4-hly, ± ipatropium bromide 400 μg neb. 4-hly. Intravenous **aminophylline** 0.5 mg/kg/h. **Steroids**, prednisolone 40 mg od, po, are usually given but their efficacy in this situation is disputed. **Physiotherapy**, including suction if necessary. **Controlled oxygen therapy**: give 24% oxygen by mask. Measure ABG after 1 h. If $P\text{co}_2$ has not risen, increase to 28%. Repeat the process and increase to 35% if necessary. Try to increase $P\text{o}_2$ to around 8 kPa. Avoid sedation. Patients who fail to respond may require intubation and ventilation. If they have severe pre-existing respiratory failure, it may prove difficult to wean them from the ventilator. Respiratory stimulants (e.g. doxapram 1.5–3 mg/min iv) are used in some centres for patients who are likely to progress to ventilation.

Complications: Progression to pneumonia. Pulmonary hypertension and cor pulmonale. Polycythaemia. Pneumothorax and pulmonary collapse secondary to retained secretions should be excluded.

Practice points: It is vital to ascertain the patient's exercise tolerance and lung function when well. Many patients with COAD live close to end-stage respiratory failure, and their premorbid condition is an important factor when deciding about intubation and ventilation.

Patients with COAD should receive influenza and pneumococcal vaccine, and be encouraged to start antibiotic therapy at the first signs of an infective exacerbation.

Pneumonia

Lower respiratory tract infections account for a large proportion of GP attendances and hospital admissions. It is impossible to distinguish between the different causative organisms on clinical grounds. Therefore the pathogenesis and clinical features of each type of pneumonia are discussed first, followed by guidelines for management of pneumonia in general.

Bacterial pneumonia

The majority of bacterial pneumonias result from 'microaspiration' of virulent bacteria such as *Streptococcus pneumoniae* colonising the upper respiratory tract (in contrast to aspiration pneumonia, which involves less virulent organisms aspirated in much larger quantities).

Risk factors: Bacterial pneumonia is more common in the elderly, in alcoholics and during any severe intercurrent illness. Other factors include recent URTI, recent anaesthetic, particularly if intubated, COAD and/or smoking, heart failure, immunocompromised patients (including HIV+ patients, transplant recipients and asplenic patients). *Streptococcus pneumoniae* classically causes lobar pneumonia in young adults with no previous ill health, but, in general, infection by this organism is more often associated with bronchopneumonia in patients with one of the risk factors listed above.

Organisms: Different patients are at particular risk from different organisms (Table 4).

The term '**atypical pneumonia**' was initially coined to describe pneumonia which failed to respond to penicillin or sulpha drugs and in which bacteriology failed to provide a diagnosis. Infection with *Mycoplasma pneumoniae* accounts for at least 20% of community-acquired pneumonias in the UK, particularly in previously healthy individuals, occurring with increased frequency during epidemics, which typically occur every 3–4 years. It affects all age-groups although it is commoner in young adults. Infection occurs by person-to-person droplet spread. There is an incubation period of approximately 3 weeks. *Legionella pneumophila* (≻24) accounts for between 1 and 20% and *Chlamydia* spp. account for a much smaller percentage. Unlike the agents of bacterial pneumonia, these organisms are not respiratory tract colonisers. *Chlamydia pneumoniae* (formerly 'TWAR agent') has recently been identified as a cause of pneumonia, particularly in young adults. It causes a similar clinical picture to *Mycoplasma pneumoniae* and is spread from person to person. Approximately 40% of young adults have serological evi-

Table 4 Organisms causing pneumonia in different risk groups

Risk factors	Organisms
None	*Streptococcus pneumoniae, Mycoplasma pneumoniae, Chlamydia psittaci, Chlamydia pneumoniae*, rarely *Legionella pneumophila*
None: infection occurring in outbreaks	*Legionella pneumophila, Chlamydia psittaci, Chlamydia pneumoniae, Mycoplasma pneumoniae*
Recent URTI	*Streptococcus pneumoniae, Staphylococcus aureus, Haemophilus influenzae*
Aspiration (➤25)	*Streptococcus pneumoniae, Staphylococcus aureus, Haemophilus influenzae, Streptococcus 'milleri'*, non-sporing anaerobes
Cystic fibrosis	*Streptococcus pneumoniae, Staphylococcus aureus, Pseudomonas aeruginosa, Pseudomonas (Burkholderia) cepacia*
HIV+ patients (➤119)	*Streptococcus pneumoniae, Mycoplasma pneumoniae, Haemophilus influenzae, Pneumocystis carinii*
Alcoholics, malnourished	*Streptococcus pneumoniae, Klebsiella pneumoniae* (also at risk of aspiration pneumonia)
COAD (➤21)	*Streptococcus pneumoniae, Haemophilus influenzae* (less often *Moraxella catarrhalis, Staphylococcus aureus*)
Neutropenia (➤133)	Coliforms, *Aspergillus* spp.
Ventilated patients	Coliforms, pseudomonads

dence of past infection. *Chlamydia psittaci* is a zoonosis, usually acquired from ill birds. Respiratory psittacosis can be a mild flu-like illness or a severe, sometimes fatal pneumonia. Σ ~200; grossly underdiagnosed.

Practice point: Recent influenza, particularly in patients with pre-existing lung disease such as COAD, predisposes to *Staphylococcus aureus, Streptococcus pneumoniae* and *Haemophilus influenzae* pneumonia.

Clinical features: Relatively rapid onset of fever and rigors, accompanied by a dry cough and pleuritic chest pain. Tachycardia and tachypnoea. As the disease progresses sputum volume and purulence increase with or without haemoptysis. On examination there may be signs of consolidation with bronchial breathing, dull percussion note and crepitations. Pleural effusion is present in up to 50% of cases and may become secondarily infected (empyema ➤28). Elderly patients may be afebrile and present with a toxic confusional state. In severe cases, signs of severe systemic

sepsis supervene, with confusion progressing to multiorgan system failure. In the preantibiotic era, recovery from classical lobar pneumonia occurred rapidly after the illness had reached its 'crisis'.

Patients with 'atypical' pneumonia classically have prominent constitutional symptoms suggestive of URTI, including sore throat, headache and rhinorrhoea. Auscultation may be normal, even in patients who are unwell or have definite chest X-ray changes. However, prospective studies have shown that it is not possible to distinguish pneumo-coccal from 'atypical' pneumonias by clinical features or investigations at presentation.

Microbiological investigations: Positive Gram stain and culture of **sputum** is helpful, but is dependent on patient's ability to produce an adequate specimen. This is less likely in the very young and the very old. Gram stain is poorly predictive, but culture is useful to assess antibiotic sensitivity. Positive **blood cultures** are diagnostic. **Thoracocentesis** if pleural effusion is large or persistent. In severe infection which fails to respond to antibiotic therapy, bronchoscopy with **broncho-alveolar lavage** and bronchial brushings provides material for microscopy, culture and histology.

The diagnosis of *Mycoplasma pneumoniae* or *Chlamydia* spp. infection is usually made retrospectively on the basis of **serology**, which becomes positive ~10 days after the onset of illness. *Mycoplasma pneumoniae* infection is often accompanied by the formation of **cold agglutinins**, which are present in serum from early in the illness; in the context of acute respiratory illness, their presence strongly favours infection by this organism.

Other investigations: Patients usually have a neutrophil leucocytosis, but with overwhelming infection, patients can be neutropenic initially. Leucocytosis is seen in 25% of patients with 'atypical' pneumonia. Mild renal failure is common in the elderly; many have hyponatraemia, which occurs in pneumonia from any cause. In severe illness, arterial blood gas analysis shows hypoxia, with hypercapnia in the presence of COAD.

Chest X-ray may show classical lobar infiltration, but usually shows bronchopneumonia, with patchy shadowing and air bronchograms indicating consolidation. Complications include lung abscess and empyema. In 'atypical' pneumonia, CXR is normal or shows diffuse changes with reticulonodular shadowing extending from the hilum to the lung base, which are bilateral in 25% of cases.

CXR changes may take several months to resolve.

Practice point: Cavitation on the chest X-ray suggests lung abscess, a cavitating neoplasm, *Staphylococcus aureus, Klebsiella pneumoniae* or *Mycobacterium tuberculosis.*

Complications: Empyema, metastatic infection (meningitis, arthritis, endocarditis), severe sepsis, ARDS and multiorgan system failure (MOSF). *Mycoplasma pneumoniae* infection is very rarely associated with acute neurological complications including meningoencephalitis, acute cerebellar ataxia, mononeuritis multiplex affecting the cranial nerves and brachial plexus or Guillain–Barré syndrome, cold agglutinin-mediated haemolytic anaemia, pericarditis, Stevens–Johnson syndrome and erythema nodosum.

Legionellosis (Legionnaire's disease)

Initially described after a dramatic outbreak of pulmonary disease in Philadelphia in 1976 at a meeting of American war veterans. Infection due to *Legionella pneumophila* has been implicated in 1–20% of community-acquired pneumonias. **Pontiac fever** is a self-limiting non-pulmonary febrile illness caused by *Legionella pneumophila* or *Legionella feeleii.*

Legionella pneumophila (➤207) colonises water-piping systems, including wet areas within air-conditioning. Infection is acquired by inhalation and there is an incubation period of 2–10 days. Human-to-human transmission does not occur.

Risk factors: Host factors are important predictors of infection, including male sex, age, smoking, COAD, immunosuppressive drugs and recent anaesthetics (particularly if intubated).

Clinical features: Presents as severe community-acquired pneumonia with fever, rigors, headache, myalgia and a non-productive cough. Chest pain, dyspnoea, purulent sputum and haemoptysis may follow. Up to 50% have abdominal pain, nausea and diarrhoea. Toxic confusional state. Focal neurological deficits occur rarely. Renal and hepatic dysfunction are common in legionellosis. This may reflect the severity of infection rather than a specific effect. May progress to fulminant respiratory failure, accompanied by other features of MOSF.

Microbiological investigations: Gram stain and culture of sputum to exclude other pathogens. Diagnosis is usually made retrospectively on serology which becomes positive approximately 10 days after the onset of illness but 25% fail to seroconvert. Detection of *Legionella pneumophila* serogroup 1 antigens in urine and

respiratory secretions is available (+).
Culture (takes 2–10 days) is possible from
sputum, tracheal aspirates and blood:
laboratories will inoculate appropriate
media if requested ☎.

Complications: Rare extrapulmonary complications include renal and cutaneous
abscesses, peritonitis, endocarditis and
haemodialysis fistula infection.

Aspiration pneumonia

Aspiration pneumonia describes the pulmonary consequences of 'macroaspiration'
of larger quantities of oral and gastric contents and/or water from the environment.
This results in chemical damage and/or
infection with oral flora, particularly
anaerobes.

Risk factors: Reduced level of consciousness
and depressed gag reflex, dysphagia due to
local oesophageal or neurological disease,
intubation and nasogastric feeding,
oesophageal dysmotility and reflux, persistent vomiting. Alcoholics and those severely obtunded by intercurrent illness are
at particular risk.

Clinical features: Aspiration of gastric contents causes acute chemical injury to
the lungs. Patients may present immediately after an aspiration event, particularly if it occurs in hospital, for example perioperatively. More often, a patient
with one or more risk factors presents
several days after the event with symptoms and signs suggestive of pulmonary
infection. Severe cases proceed to lung
abscess, empyema and bronchopleural
fistula. Inhalation of small foreign bodies
(typically peanuts) can cause localised
bronchial obstruction with distal abscess
formation.

Organisms: Mixed oral flora including
anaerobic streptococci, *Fusobacterium
nucleatum* and *Bacteroides* spp. Almost
any organism can be involved if it was previously colonising the upper airways.

Microbiological investigations: Gram stain
and culture of sputum and blood to exclude other organisms. Thoracocentesis if
pleural effusion is large or persistent.
Bronchoscopy may be required to provide
material for microscopy and culture and to
exclude an inhaled foreign body.

Table 5 Less common causes of pneumonia

Organism	Risk factors	Clinical features	Comments
Staphylococcus aureus	Post-influenza. Septic emboli in IVDU (often with endocarditis). Intubated or tracheostomy patients	Fever, cough, chest pain, haemoptysis. Bilateral disease and cavitation common. High mortality	*Staphylococcus aureus* commonly colonises the upper airways and is regularly grown from sputum; it **rarely** causes pneumonia.
Klebsiella pneumoniae ('Friedlander's bacillus')	Typically affects elderly men with diabetes, alcoholism or pre-existing cardiac or pulmonary disease	Often rapid onset, with bloodstained and gelatinous sputum. Typically upper lobes	CXR may show bulging of fissures due to expansion in volume of affected lobe. Cavitation and abscess formation common
Pseudomonas aeruginosa	Neutropenic patients and those on long-term ventilation are most at risk	Bilateral lower-zone pneumonia, sometimes with abscess formation	Histological examination shows characteristic periarterial invasion

continued on p. 26

Table 5 contd

Organism	Risk factors	Clinical features	Comments
Other Gram-negative aerobic bacilli	Usually hospital-acquired, in patients on long-term ventilation, elderly debilitated patients and those with underlying lung disease	Often severe. May cavitate	If sputum microscopy and culture does not show Gram-negative aerobic bacilli, infection with these organisms is unlikely

Other extremely rare causes of pneumonia include anthrax (≻177), plague (≻211), tularaemia (≻212), Q fever (≻234) and melioidosis (≻200).

Management of pneumonia

The causative agent is usually unknown when therapy is commenced. Management depends on a careful assessment of severity. The following factors (particularly the first three) are associated with increased mortality: respiratory rate > 30/min, diastolic BP < 60 mmHg, urea > 7 mmol/l, age > 60, confusion, atrial fibrillation, underlying disease, serum albumin < 35 g/l, Po_2 < 8 kPa, WBC < 4 × 10^9/l or > 20 × 10^9/l, positive blood cultures.

Investigations have been discussed above, and include chest X-ray, full blood count, urea, electrolytes and liver function tests, urinalysis, sputum and blood cultures, arterial blood gas analysis and serology for viral and atypical agents.

Antibiotic management:

Severe pneumonia (⩾ two of the features listed above): Initial **parenteral** therapy: cefo-taxime 2 g 8-hly + erythromycin 1 g 6-hly.

When well enough, change to **oral** therapy (Table 6).

Mild pneumonia: Give oral treatment initially if possible—aim to be on oral drugs within 48 h or when temperature is < 38°C.

Initial **parenteral** therapy: ampicillin 1 g 6-hly + erythromycin 1 g **12-hly** (substitute flucloxacillin for amoxycillin if influenza likely).

Initial **oral** therapy: amoxycillin 250 mg 8-hly (+ clarithromycin or erythromycin if no response to amoxycillin after 72 h).

Initial **oral** therapy if influenza suspected: flucloxacillin 500 mg 6-hly + clarithromycin 250 mg 12-hly.

Thereafter, see Table 7.

Sulphonamides, tetracyclines and quinolones should be avoided because of pneumococcal resistance and inferior efficacy.

Table 6 Oral continuation therapy for severe pneumonia

Microbiological result	Therapy (standard doses ≻318)
Streptococcus pneumoniae or ampicillin-susceptible *Haemophilus influenzae*	Amoxycillin
Mycoplasma or chlamydia	Clarithromycin **or** erythromycin
No microbial confirmation	Amoxycillin + clarithromycin (substitute flucloxacillin for amoxycillin if influenza likely)

Table 7 Oral continuation therapy for mild pneumonia

Microbiological result	Therapy
Streptococcus pneumoniae	Benzylpenicillin iv or amoxycillin orally
Ampicillin-susceptible *H. influenzae*	Ampicillin iv or amoxycillin orally
Mycoplasma or chlamydia	Clarithromycin **or** erythromycin
Influenza suspected or proven	Flucloxacillin + clarithromycin
No microbial confirmation	Amoxycillin + clarithromycin or erythromycin if no response to amoxycillin after 72 h

For **specific unusual** pathogens, see Table 8.

Table 8 Therapy for specific uncommon causes of pneumonia

Situation	Recommended therapy
Staphylococcus aureus	Flucloxacillin 2 g qds iv ± rifampicin, gentamicin or fucidin
Legionella pneumophila	Erythromycin 1 g qds iv ± rifampicin 600 mg 12-hly po
Coxiella burnetii (➤234)	Doxycycline or chloramphenicol
Aspiration pneumonia	Cefotaxime and metronidazole

Supportive management: Oxygen therapy should be given to keep $Po_2 > 8\,kPa$ or O_2 saturation $> 90\%$. Careful attention should be paid to fluid balance.

Pneumonia in children

Acute respiratory tract infections are more common in childhood and may be severe, particularly in children with pre-existing illness such as congenital cardiac disease, bronchopulmonary dysplasia, severe asthma or cystic fibrosis.

The clinical features and likely causative organisms of pneumonia differ at different ages. In small babies, pneumonia is often accompanied by air-trapping leading to wheeze and hyperinflation (see acute bronchiolitis ➤20).

Pneumonia is more likely to be viral in aetiology in children. Other organisms are also seen more often in children (Table 9). *Chlamydia trachomatis* causes pneumonia in children from 3 weeks to 4 months (➤113).

Table 9 Causes of pneumonia in children

Age-group	Common organisms
Birth to 3 weeks	Gp B β-haemolytic streptococci, coliforms, *Listeria monocytogenes*, *Streptococcus pneumoniae*. Viral infection unusual
3 weeks to 4 months	*Chlamydia trachomatis*, respiratory syncytial virus, parainfluenza, *Staphylococcus aureus*, *Streptococcus pneumoniae*, *Haemophilus influenzae*
4 months to 5 years	Respiratory syncytial virus, parainfuenza, adenovirus, influenza A and B, *Haemophilus influenzae*, *Streptococcus pneumoniae*, *Staphylococcus aureus*, *Mycoplasma pneumoniae* (unusual)
5 years to 15 years	*Mycoplasma pneumoniae*, *Streptococcus pneumoniae*, *Haemophilus influenzae*

Lung abscess

Necrosis of lung parenchyma due to bacterial infection, leading to a cavitated pus-containing lesion.

Risk factors: Following aspiration pneumonia or trauma. Secondary to local bronchial obstruction by clots, pus, foreign body or tumour. Following specific bacterial pneumonias which tend to cavitate: *Staphylococcus aureus, Klebsiella pneumoniae, Pseudomonas aeruginosa*. Septic pulmonary emboli, often due to *Staphylococcus aureus* occur in IVDUs, particularly in the presence of tricuspid valve endocarditis. *Nocardia* spp. and *Aspergillus* spp. in immunocompromised patients.

Clinical features: Risk factors for aspiration pneumonia (➤25). Onset varies from acute, within days after a recognised aspiration event or pneumonia, to insidious, over weeks. Fever, fatigue, cough, sputum (often copious and offensive). Weight loss, clubbing and anaemia.

Organisms: After aspiration: upper respiratory tract anaerobic organisms (*Peptostreptococcus* spp., *Bacteroides* spp. (not *fragilis* group), *Fusobacterium* spp.), *Streptococcus* 'milleri', and Gram-negative aerobic bacilli. After pneumonia: *Staphylococcus aureus, Klebsiella pneumoniae, Pseudomonas aeruginosa*. Rare causes include *Actinomyces israelii, Nocardia asteroides* and fungi.

Microbiological investigations: Gram stain and culture of sputum. This may be unhelpful in predominantly anaerobic infections. Blood cultures. If there is an associated pleural effusion, thoracocentesis is indicated to exclude empyema. Bronchoscopy is usually indicated to obtain material for culture, to assist drainage and to exclude the presence of bronchial obstruction. Percutaneous aspiration (CT-guided).

Other investigations: Neutrophil leucocytosis is usual, but may wane in chronic cases. Chest X-ray shows a cavitating pulmonary lesion with a fluid level. Multiple peripheral lesions suggest septic pulmonary emboli. CT scan is a sensitive method of diagnosis and a guide to fine-needle aspiration for culture and cytology.

Antibiotic management: Benzylpenicillin + metronidazole are used initially, but therapy should then be guided by the results of microbiology and specialist chest referral is recommended. Duration of therapy is controversial—at least 1 month.

Supportive management: Bronchoscopy and physiotherapy may be required to assist drainage. Surgical resection is required rarely for lesions that fail to respond to antibiotics.

Complications: Metastatic infection. Empyema. Bronchopleural fistula.

Empyema

Pus within the pleural cavity.

Risk factors: Secondary to bacterial pneumonia, particularly after infection with *Staphylococcus aureus*, anaerobes or Gram-negative aerobic bacilli. Empyema is now unusual after pneumococcal pneumonia unless treatment is delayed. Pulmonary infections with *Actinomyces israelii* and *Nocardia asteroides* tend to involve the pleura. Secondary to ruptured oesophagus, subphrenic or hepatic abscess. Postthoracic surgery or penetrating chest injury. Pleural tuberculosis may present as empyema.

Clinical features: Persistent fever in one of the situations listed above. Weight loss, and dyspnoea if the empyema is large. Purulent sputum if there is a bronchopleural fistula. On examination, clubbing and signs of pleural effusion.

Organisms: Dependent on the clinical situation: upper respiratory tract anaerobic organisms (*Peptostreptococcus* spp., *Bacteroides* spp. (not *fragilis* group), *Fusobacterium* spp.), *Staphylococcus aureus, Klebsiella pneumoniae, Pseudomonas aeruginosa, Streptococcus pneumoniae* and *Streptococcus* 'milleri'. Rarely, *Actinomyces israelii, Nocardia asteroides, Mycobacterium tuberculosis*.

Microbiological investigations: Diagnostic aspiration of fluid through a wide-bore needle. Delivery of pus in a sealed syringe allows the microbiology department to culture anaerobes.

Other investigations: Neutrophil leucocytosis. Chest X-ray and CT scan will delineate the extent of the infection.

Management: Drainage via intercostal tube is nearly always essential, and resolution is more rapid if loculated collections are broken down. The role of systemic and instilled antibiotics is unclear but most recommend an initial course of antibiotics. Amoxycillin + metronidazole is rational initial therapy and can be guided by the results of culture. Prolonged therapy is rarely required.

> **Practice point: Sterile** parapneumonic effusion is a common cause of persistent fever during treatment of pneumonia, and often requires aspiration.

Tuberculosis (TB) ⊠

TB infection may be defined as a state in which *Mycobacterium tuberculosis* (or *bovis* etc. ➤229) has established itself in the body, without symptoms or evidence of disease, in contrast to **TB disease**, where there are symptoms and signs of damage to one or more organs. TB remains a major cause of mortality in the developing world, particularly in countries with a high prevalence of HIV infection. In developing countries (and in the UK in the past) most children are infected by TB, but only ~10% progress to clinical disease. Currently in the UK TB infection is rare in childhood; most infected persons are middle-aged or elderly, or are immigrants from endemic areas including Africa and the Indian subcontinent. Reactivation of pulmonary TB is therefore usually seen in patients from these risk groups; factors predisposing to reactivation include alcoholism, diabetes mellitus, malnutrition, immunosuppression (drugs, HIV, cytotoxic therapy) and malignancy. Σ ~6000; ~300 deaths.

Pathogenesis: Infection is initially acquired by the respiratory aerosol route. Organisms replicate in the lung and travel to the hilar lymph nodes, from where they are disseminated throughout the body. Further replication is usually halted at this stage by the development of cell-mediated immunity (CMI), but complete eradication of organisms does not

take place. Later in life infection can reactivate, particularly if CMI is impaired by one of the risk factors listed above.

Pulmonary tuberculosis
Clinical features

Primary infection is usually asymptomatic in the healthy well-nourished individual, manifested only by a conversion from tuberculin-negative to positive (see below). Some patients, especially children, may complain of fever, cough and dyspnoea. CXR is usually normal or may show areas of infiltration (usually in the middle or lower zones) with unilateral hilar or paratracheal lymphadenopathy ('Ghon complex'). Of patients with abnormal CXR, 15% have bilateral hilar lymphadenopathy. Rare allergic manifestations associated with primary infection include erythema nodosum (➤93), phlyctenular conjunctivitis and a sterile polyarthritis (Poncet's disease). Primary infection is usually curtailed by host CMI. Occasionally, particularly in children under 5 years, massive dissemination occurs, resulting in miliary TB (see below). Approximately 10% of young adults with symptomatic primary tuberculosis progress within a few months to cavitary TB. This **progressive primary TB** is similar to reactivated disease (see below)–the presence of lymphadenopathy or a recent conversion from tuberculin-negative to positive may suggest progressive primary rather than reactivated disease. Patients are often very unwell, with fever, cough and weight loss.

Miliary TB (so called because of the millet-seed-sized lesions that form in all areas of high blood flow, particularly the viscera, bone marrow and eyes) occurs following dissemination of bacilli, typically in children with acute infection. Miliary TB may also occur during reactivation (**late generalised TB**), particularly in elderly or immunocompromised patients, in which case its onset is more insidious, e.g. as a PUO (➤153), although patients may experience sudden severe deterioration. Symptoms include fever, night sweats and weight loss. Anaemia, leucocytosis or leucopenia, thrombocytopenia and DIC may occur. Miliary lesions may be visible on the CXR as

2–4 mm nodules, but these are absent particularly during the first 10 days of disease. TB meningitis (see below), usually presenting with headache, may occur as a complication.
Reactivated TB presents months to years after primary infection. Symptoms include cough, haemoptysis (~25%), fever (15–40%), night sweats (60%), fatigue (60%), anorexia and weight loss. Approximately 20% of patients with radiological evidence of active TB are asymptomatic. CXR usually shows consolidation with cavitation and fibrosis, most commonly in the upper zones. Lymphadenopathy is rare. Fibrosis, calcification and loss of volume is seen in chronic disease. Disease may progress very rapidly over months, or insidiously over years.

Pulmonary complications

TB pleurisy may occur shortly after 1° infection or during reactivated disease. Fever, pleuritic chest pain and dry cough are common. AFB are rarely seen in pleural fluid. Diagnosis is made by culture or, more often, by histology of pleural biopsy. Spontaneous resolution frequently occurs, but there is a high risk of reactivated disease in the following 5 years and treatment is indicated.
Empyema (➤28) results from rupture of tuberculous cavity into the pleural cavity. **Bronchiectasis** results from compression of bronchi (usually middle lobe) by enlarged lymph nodes. **Haemoptysis** is usually mild and recurrent, but severe life-threatening episodes occur rarely from erosion of a pulmonary artery by a TB cavity. **Aspergilloma** (➤290) develops rarely in a healed TB cavity, causing haemoptysis. Antifungal treatment is usually unsuccessful and resection of the affected lobe is often required.

Extrapulmonary tuberculosis

TB lymphadenitis ('scrofula') is commonest in Asian and African immigrants. Lymph nodes of the head and neck are almost always affected (~5% have mediastinal lymphadenitis). Disease is bilateral in 25%, and only ~20% have constitutional symptoms. Usually presents as a discrete rubbery non-tender lymph node ('cold abscess'), which discharges, giving rise to a chronic sinus.

Genitourinary TB results from reactivation of bacilli disseminated during 1° infection. Renal parenchymal disease, with progressive destruction of the kidney, is usually clinically silent. Involvement of the ureter and bladder follow, with obstructive uropathy and ulceration, fibrosis and shrinkage of the bladder. Symptoms include dysuria, frequency, haematuria and flank pain. Sterile pyuria is typical, and TB should be considered in all patients with this. Diagnosis is by microscopy and culture of early-morning urine (positive in ~90% if three samples are sent). In later stages IVU shows renal calcification, short rigid ureter, thick-walled non-distensible bladder and urethral stricture. Salpingitis, endometritis and epididymo-orchitis also occur. Adrenal involvement usually occurs in association with miliary disease and rarely causes hypoadrenalism.

Gastrointestinal TB results from swallowed bacilli, most commonly causing ileitis with anorexia, weight loss, altered bowel habit and abdominal pain. Perforation, obstruction and fistula formation may follow. Peritoneal TB, which usually spreads from an infected mesenteric lymph node, presents insidiously with fever, weight loss, anorexia, abdominal swelling and irregular bowel habit and is not usually associated with pulmonary disease.

Bone and joint involvement: most commonly the vertebral column (50%), hip (15%), knee (15%) and other large joints are affected. Vertebral disease ('Pott's disease') typically affects the anterior part of the lower thoracic or lumbar vertebral bodies with back pain, fever and weight loss progressing to kyphosis or paraplegia. Extension to form paravertebral or psoas abscess may occur. Mycobacteria are typically present in very low numbers in bony lesions and cultures of bone aspirations and biopsy are often negative or slow to become positive.

CNS involvement typically causes a basal meningitis with entrapment of cranial nerves and vasculitis affecting cerebral arteries. Onset is usually insidious over several weeks, but can be acute, especially in children. Headache, fever and altered mental state are the commonest presenting symptoms. Less frequently, cranial nerve lesions (esp. VI, III and IV) and evidence of raised intracranial pressure occur, followed by progression to coma and fits. Cerebral vasculitis, typically affecting the anterior and middle cerebral arteries, results in infarction and hemiplegia. AFB are seen in smears of CSF in < 20% of cases; yield is increased if a large volume ($\geqslant 10$ ml) of CSF is sent for examination. Other CSF changes include low glucose, markedly raised protein and usually lymphocytic pleocytosis (➤75). Rarer neurological complications of TB include acute transverse myelitis and radiculitis.

Pericarditis may occur with pulmonary TB or as the sole manifestation of infection. It may present with pericardial pain and a friction rub or with massive effusion and tamponade. Steroids speed resolution and are given in addition to chemotherapy. Constrictive pericarditis may follow acute pericarditis within weeks or may occur many years later. It typically presents insidiously with dyspnoea, oedema, hepatosplenomegaly, raised venous pressure on inspiration and pericardial calcification on CXR. Surgical pericardectomy is usually required.

TB and HIV: HIV infection predisposes to reactivation of TB, which occurs at any time during the course of HIV disease, and often precedes other opportunistic infections. TB at any site including the lungs is an AIDS-defining illness (➤116). Extrapulmonary TB and involvement of the lower lung fields are commoner in HIV patients. Treatment is with standard anti-TB drugs. Infection with atypical mycobacteria also occurs in HIV infection (➤128). Outbreaks of multiple-drug-resistant TB have been reported in large US cities, but this has not yet been seen in UK (➤229).

Organisms: *Mycobacterium tuberculosis* currently accounts for almost all UK TB. *Mycobacterium bovis* is now very rare and usually acquired from human-to-human spread.

Microbiological investigations: Diagnosis depends on microscopy and culture of mycobacteria, and on histological findings.

Special stains (Ziehl–Neelson, auramine phenol) are used. In suspected pulmonary TB three sputum specimens should be examined. Other relevant specimens include early-morning urine ($\geqslant 150$ ml) and gastric washings. Fibre-optic bronchoscopy, with bronchoalveolar lavage and transbronchial biopsy, has a high yield of positive results. In suspected extrapulmonary TB relevant tissue samples should be examined but microscopy is frequently negative, and diagnosis is often made on histology of tissue samples (esp. pleural biopsy, lymph node, liver, bone marrow) showing caseating granulomata or AFB. Culture confirmation allowing speciation and sensitivity testing may take up to 8 weeks. Serological tests and direct detection of mycobacterial products and DNA remain experimental.

Tuberculin testing is the demonstration of cell-mediated immunity to purified mycobacterial proteins ('tuberculin') by intradermal injection. It may be performed by a number of means. The Heaf test uses a special multipronged injector. Reactions are graded 0–4; $\geqslant$ grade 2 is regarded as positive. For routine ward use the Mantoux test is more convenient: 0.1 ml of tuberculin (1:10 000 containing 1 tuberculin unit (TU)) is injected intradermally in the upper third of the flexor aspect of the forearm. The injection site is carefully marked and read at 48–96 h. *Palpable* induration > 5 mm in diameter constitutes a positive response. If negative, the test should be repeated with 0.1 ml of 1:1000 tuberculin (10 TU). Tuberculin testing varies in usefulness depending on the population studied. Previous BCG immunisation will cause a positive result. The test may be negative in up to 25% of patients with active TB, particularly in miliary disease. In the UK it is most useful in children who have not received BCG and in the surveillance of contacts of cases, in whom a conversion from negative to positive indicates recent infection and a need for prophylactic therapy (see below).

Other investigations: Normochromic normocytic anaemia, hyponatraemia due to inappropriate ADH secretion, mild hypercalcaemia and a raised ESR are common.

Management of TB
Principles of anti-TB chemotherapy: Multidrug therapy is required to prevent the emergence of resistant organisms especially in high inoculum disease and to kill organisms metabolising at different rates in different cellular environments. Thus, isoniazid is good at killing mycobacteria that are actively dividing, but it is less effective against semidormant organisms. Pyrazinamide is particularly active against mycobacteria which are semidormant in acid intracellular environments, and rifampicin is considered effective against intermittently metabolising organisms because of its very rapid onset of action.

Antituberculous drugs
First-line drugs for use against TB in the UK (Table 10)
Rifampicin: broad range of activity including many mycobacteria, staphylococci, streptococci, neisserias, *Haemophilus* spp., *Brucella* spp., *Legionella* spp., *Chlamydia* spp., *Coxiella burnetii*. One-step mutation to resistance of target RNA polymerase, hence use in combination for all indications except meningococcal and haemophilus prophylaxis. Well absorbed orally (iv available); CSF ✓, urine ✓. Available in combination with other antituberculous drugs to aid compliance. Transiently raised hepatic transaminases common, but significant hepatotoxicity infrequent except in those with pre-existing liver disease. Usually mild rashes and GI disturbance (occasional *Clostridium difficile*-associated diarrhoea); orange-coloured urine, saliva and tears (stains soft contact lenses); induction of liver microsomal enzymes interferes with activity of oral contraceptives and other steroids, phenytoin, sulphonylureas, anticoagulants, cyclosporin. Rare thrombocytopenia. Intermittent treatment associated with side-effects in up to 30%: influenza-like syndrome, shortness of breath, thrombocytopenia, hypotension, renal failure. **Rifabutin** is similar to rifampicin, and is used for prophylaxis of MAI infection in patients with AIDS and low CD4 counts, and for treatment of other mycobacterial infections.
Isoniazid: used for treatment and prophylaxis

of *Mycobacterium tuberculosis*; other mycobacteria usually resistant. Oral and parenteral preparations available; CSF ✓, urine ✓. Causes peripheral neuropathy (particularly likely in alcoholics, diabetics, malnourished and patients with chronic renal failure and is preventable by giving pyridoxine 10 mg 24-hly). Rare hepatotoxicity, optic neuritis, psychosis, nausea, vomiting, rashes, fever. Potentiates phenytoin, ethosuximide and carbamazepine.
Ethambutol: active against tubercle bacilli and other mycobacteria. Oral only; CSF ✓ with meningitis, urine ✓. Dose-dependent visual disturbance (loss of acuity, visual fields or colour-blindness)−rare at 15 mg/kg. Check vision with Snellen chart before treatment and warn patients to stop drug and report any change in vision. Avoid in patients with renal failure and in children or patients with language difficulties who may not report visual symptoms.
Pyrazinamide: active against *Mycobacterium tuberculosis*, especially against intracellular organisms at acid pH, and early in the course of treatment. Inactive against *bovis* and MAI. Well absorbed orally; CSF ✓, urine ✓. Common mild arthralgia. Occasional hepatotoxicity, rashes, nausea.

Other antituberculous agents sometimes used because of resistance or drug allergy include capreomycin, clofazimine, cycloserine, ethionamide, kanamycin, para-aminosalicylic acid (PAS), thioacetazone and streptomycin. For financial reasons, several of these agents are still in widespread use in developing countries.

Primary drug resistance (resistance at presentation) commoner in developing world, but rare in UK (2.3% in 1988 to ⩾ one drug in indigenous cases, 4.5% in immigrants from Indian subcontinent). Relapses (up to 3%) most commonly involve organisms with same sensitivity as the primary isolate, probably due to failure of compliance.

Intermittent supervised therapy (see Table 11 for regimens) is recommended for patients who may be non-compliant.

Table 10 BTS recommendations for treatment of TB (*Thorax* (1990) 45:403–8)

	Initial phase	Months	Continuation phase	Months
Adults				
Pulmonary TB	I,R,P, (E)*	2	I, R	4
Meningitis	I, R, P	2	I, R	10
TB lymphadenitis	I, R, P	2	I, R	4
Bone and joint	I, R, P	2	I, R	7
Pericarditis	I, R, P, E	2	I, R	4
Other extrapulmonary TB	I, R, P, E	2	I, R	4
Children				
Pulmonary TB	I, R, P	2	I, R	4
or	I, R	9		
Non-pulmonary	As above			

I = isoniazid, R = rifampicin, P = pyrazinamide, E = ethambutol.
* Ethambutol is added if there is reason to suspect drug-resistant organisms. **Liver function tests** (LFTs) should be checked before starting therapy. Transient asymptomatic increases in serum transaminases are very common after starting treatment. Discontinuation is **not** indicated unless there are symptoms of hepatitis (anorexia, vomiting, hepatomegaly) or jaundice. It is not necessary to monitor LFTs except in patients known to have pre-existing liver disease. **Steroids** are used in life-threatening or widespread TB in an attempt to reduce acute inflammation and allow time for drugs to work. They are usually indicated for pericarditis, extensive pulmonary disease, moderate or severe meningitis, ureteric TB and pleural effusion.

Table 11 Doses of antituberculous drugs

	Daily therapy	Intermittent supervised therapy	
Drug	Dose	Dose	Frequency
Isoniazid	300 mg od Child: 10 mg/kg	15 mg/kg	3 times weekly
Rifampicin	Weight <50 kg: 450 mg od, ≥50 kg: 600 mg od Child: 10 mg/kg	600–900 mg Child: 15 mg/kg	3 times weekly
Pyrazinamide	Weight <50 kg: 1.5 g od ≥50 kg: 2 g od Child: 35 mg/kg	Weight <50 kg: 2 g, ≥50 kg: 2.5 g Child: 50 mg/kg	3 times weekly
Ethambutol	15 mg/kg	30 mg/kg	3 times weekly
Streptomycin	Weight <50 kg: 750 mg od ≥50 kg: 1 g od Child: 15 mg/kg	Weight <50 kg: 750 mg, ≥50 kg: 1 g Child: 15 mg/kg	3 times weekly

Table 12 Treatment of TB in special circumstances

Circumstances	Regimen
Chemoprophylaxis (>34)	Isoniazid alone for 6 months **or** isoniazid/rifampicin for 3 months (standard doses)
Diabetes mellitus	Standard therapy (note interaction with sulphonylureas)
Liver disease	Standard therapy, but monitor liver function
Pregnancy	Avoid streptomycin
Lactation	Standard therapy
Chronic renal failure	Rifampicin, isoniazid and pyrazinamide may be given in standard doses. Streptomycin and ethambutol should be avoided; if unavoidable, give reduced dose and monitor serum levels. For doses for patients on dialysis (>331)
HIV infection and AIDS	Standard therapy for extended duration, usually 9 months for pulmonary disease. After treatment lifelong isoniazid prophylaxis is recommended by some experts
Isoniazid resistance	If resistance is known prior to starting therapy give streptomycin, pyrazinamide, rifampicin and ethambutol for 2 months, and continue rifampicin and ethambutol for further 7 months. If isoniazid resistance arises during therapy, a total of 12 months' treatment with rifampicin and ethambutol should be given with pyrazinamide as well for the first 2 months

Control and prevention of TB

Approximately 10% of household contacts of sputum smear-positive ('open') TB cases develop active disease. This figure is ~2% for smear-negative and extrapulmonary cases. Smear-positive cases are considered non-infectious after 2 weeks' therapy which includes isoniazid and rifampicin.

Control of TB in hospital: Smear-positive patients should be nursed in a single room for the first 2 weeks of treatment. No further precautions (such as gowns or masks) are necessary, but it is sensible to wear masks during respiratory physiotherapy. Adults with smear-negative and extrapulmonary disease can be nursed on the open ward. Children should be nursed in a single room until the source case has been identified as it is likely that this person will be among those visiting the child. If a patient in a general ward is found to have TB, then other patients should be followed up as close contacts (see below).

Prevention of TB in health professionals: Staff in contact with patients, laboratory workers and those handling clinical material are regarded as at risk. Similar guidelines apply to hospital, private hospital, prison and old people's home employees. Staff working with infants and young children must be screened to detect infectious TB. Pre-employment screening includes history of BCG, Heaf test and CXR and should follow the guidelines of the British Thoracic Society (BTS).[1] Stringent protective measures have been recommended in the USA to prevent acquisition by staff of drug-resistant TB.

Examination of contacts is the responsibility of the local authority (health board in Scotland) and is usually undertaken by a designated chest physician. Notification is essential. Close contacts are defined as those sharing a household with the index case — occasionally a contact at work will also be regarded as close. Close contacts of all cases of TB should be examined. Casual contacts are at low risk, but should be examined if they are unusually sus-

[1] *Br Med J* (1990) 300:995–9.

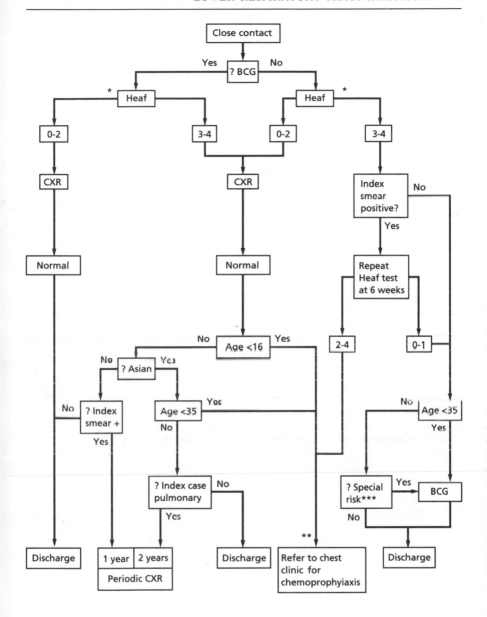

Fig. 1 Management of close contacts of tuberculosis cases. Redrawn with permission from *Br Med J* (1990) 300:995–9.

ceptible (e.g. children or immunosuppressed adults) or if the index case is thought to be highly infectious. Examination of contacts is aimed at detecting cases of pulmonary TB, offering BCG to those who are tuberculin-negative and chemoprophylaxis (>34) to those without evidence of active disease but who may have been infected. Detailed BTS guidelines should be followed. Whilst this work is usually undertaken by designated specialists, guidelines are summarised for information in Fig. 1. Children under 5 years who are contacts of smear-positive cases should receive chemoprophylaxis irrespective of tuberculin status and be given BCG afterwards, if they have not already been vaccinated.

Immigrants from the Indian subcontinent, Africa and other high-risk areas such as Vietnam should be evaluated for TB infection and disease. If tuberculin-negative they should be offered BCG. If tuberculin-positive they should be referred for CXR and clinical assessment. Chemoprophylaxis is recommended for children and adults under 35 years with Heaf test grades 3 or 4 (2–4 if there is no history of BCG). BCG should be offered at birth to all children of immigrants from high-risk areas.

BCG immunisation uses a live attenuated strain of *Mycobacterium bovis* (Bacillus Calmette–Guérin). It is contraindicated in patients with immunosuppression (incl. steroids, cytotoxics and HIV), malignancy, hypogammaglobulinaemia, pregnancy, intercurrent febrile illness, tuberculin positivity or generalised septic skin infection. The efficacy of BCG varies with different populations, probably due to patterns of previous exposure to *Mycobacterium tuberculosis* and atypical mycobacteria, and it is best given before the age of maximum incidence of generalised TB infection in a population. In British children it is estimated to give ~70% protection. It is currently recommended in the UK for members of the following groups if they are tuberculin-negative and have no history of successful BCG vaccination: children aged 10–13 years, students, health care professionals, veterinary staff dealing with animals known to harbour tuberculosis, contacts of patients with active disease, immigrants from endemic areas (esp. Indian subcontinent, Vietnam, sub-Saharan Africa), travellers to Asia, Africa or Central and South America who intend to stay for > 1 month. Children born to immigrants from India, Africa, Vietnam and other high-risk areas should be offered BCG at birth. BCG also offers partial protection against *Mycobacterium leprae*.

3: Cardiac Infections

Infective endocarditis (IE)

Definition: Bacterial, fungal, rickettsial or chlamydial infection of heart valves or mural endocardium. The term IE encompasses the whole spectrum of illness. The terms acute endocarditis (AE) and subacute endocarditis (SBE), which describe disease at both ends of the spectrum of IE, remain clinically useful but have limited microbiological predictive value. Infection of the vascular endothelium of patent ductus arteriosus, A-V fistulae and coarctation produce a similar clinical pattern.

Risk factors: AE describes an acute presentation (hours to days), due to virulent organisms such as *Staphylococcus aureus*, which can adhere to normal endothelium. Infection by less virulent organisms such as 'viridans' streptococci normally presents less acutely (weeks) and usually infects previously damaged endocardium. Platelet thrombi adhere to damaged endocardium and provide a nidus for bacterial adhesion and invasion.

Predisposing cardiac lesions: Endocardial damage arises in areas of turbulence, where a high-pressure jet of blood enters a low-pressure chamber, e.g. on the atrial side of the mitral valve (MV) and the wall of the left atrium in mitral regurgitation. Classically, IE affects valves damaged by rheumatic heart disease, but this is becoming less common (~30% of recent published series). Congenital and degenerative heart disease and mitral valve prolapse predispose to IE. In 20–40% of cases there is no identifiable lesion.

Source of bacteraemia: 'Viridans' streptococci are oral commensals and patients often have a history of periodontal disease or recent dental work. In hospital patients, intravenous catheters, in particular central lines, are sources of infection. Urinary and GI tracts are common sources in the elderly, particularly of enterococci.

Age: Incidence increases with age; IE often presents insidiously in the elderly.

Clinical features: AE presents acutely over days, with swinging fever, rigors and arthralgia. Commonly *Staphylococcus aureus* AE presents as fever, collapse and meningism in the elderly with no localising clues. SBE presents insidiously over weeks with weakness, anorexia, fatigue, sweats, weight loss and arthralgia. Fever is usually remitting and low-grade in SBE. IE is unlikely if fever is absent. **Heart murmur** is present in ~85% of cases; the aortic valve (AV) and MV are most often affected. Tricuspid valve (TV) endocarditis is rare except in IVDUs. **Changing murmurs** are rare—any change is usually due to worsening AV or MV regurgitation in the context of worsening heart failure. A murmur is often absent early in AE, in mural endocarditis, in congenital bicuspid AV IE, in the elderly and in isolated TV IE. Approximately 30% of *Staphylococcus aureus* AE have no murmur noted at presentation.

Classical peripheral signs include splenomegaly (~30%), petechiae (~30%) (particularly conjunctival), Osler's nodes (10–25%), Janeway lesions, clubbing (~10%) and splinter haemorrhages. One or more of these signs are present in ~50% of cases.

Embolism to the limbs, kidneys, mesentery and CNS (leading to stroke, brain abscess, mononeuritis, meningitis, mycotic aneurysm) occurs in 30–50% of cases.

Organisms: For native valve endocarditis: 'viridans' streptococci (~40%), enterococci (~10%), other streptococci (~20%). Group A βHS are rare. *Staphylococcus aureus* (AE) and *Staphylococcus epidermidis* (often nosocomial) account for ~20%. Miscellaneous others include *Haemophilus* spp., *Streptococcus pneumoniae* and *Neisseria gonorrhoeae*. Gram-negative aerobic bacilli including *Pseudomonas aeruginosa* are rare except in PVE or nosocomial IE. Rarely, *Coxiella burnetti*, *Brucella* spp. or fungi (uncommon except in the context of IVDU, severe intercurrent illness or PVE).

Microbiological investigations: Blood cultures are positive in ~90% of cases. Bacteraemia is usually continuous, so in AE three sets may be taken from separate venepunctures in 1 hour prior to starting therapy. In SBE, three or four sets should be sent over a 48-hour period. With 'viridans' streptococci three blood cultures of adequate volume (15–20 ml) give ~98% pick-up rate. Failures usually follow antibiotic treatment. If IE is suspected in a patient who has already received antibiotics, further cultures should be taken daily over a 4–5-day period after therapy has been stopped. If blood cultures are negative after 48 hours' incubation, consider the causes of culture-negative IE (*Coxiella burnetii, Brucella* spp., fungi, nutritionally variant streptococci, other fastidious organisms). Serology for *Coxiella burnetii, Chlamydia* spp., *Brucella* spp. and fungi may be required. Close liaison with the microbiology laboratory is essential. The laboratory may arrange detailed antibiotic sensitivity tests (MIC, MBC and possibly serum bactericidal levels ➤308) to guide therapy.

Other investigations: Raised ESR and C-reactive protein. Normochromic, normocytic anaemia. Normal or raised neutrophil count. Thrombocytopenia. Positive rheumatoid factor. Microscopic haematuria. **Echocardiography** may show vegetations, but a normal ECHO does *not* exclude IE. The value of ECHO lies in determining the site and extent of cardiac damage and the need for surgical intervention. Transoesophageal ECHO is more sensitive than transthoracic.

Complications: Immune complex-mediated effects include **arthritis** and **glomerulonephritis** (GN). GN is usually focal, with haematuria and proteinuria but normal renal function. Rarely, diffuse GN with impairment of renal function develops. **Cardiac** complications include heart failure due to valve damage, conduction defects (due to extension of infection from the valve ring into the conducting system), arrhythmias and MI due to coronary embolism. **Peripheral emboli** and metastatic abscesses may occur at presentation or during treatment.

Indications for surgery in IE: Valve replacement is indicated for progressive severe heart failure, especially with AV rupture or regurgitation, or evidence of other structural damage such as ruptured chordae; persistent bacteraemia despite appropriate antibiotic therapy (which usually implies valve ring abscess or a difficult to treat organism such as an enterococcus); relapse after second course of antibiotics; extension of infection into the conducting system with refractory heart block or bundle branch block, or into the pericardium with septic pericarditis. After surgery at least 2 weeks' antibiotic therapy is given, extended to 4 weeks if Gram stain or culture of the resected valve shows bacteria, or if blood cultures are positive at the time of operation.

Response to treatment: Prolonged administration of bactericidal antibiotics is required for cure and to prevent relapse. Anaemia and splenomegaly take months to resolve. Recurrent fever be due to microbiological treatment failure, line infection, drug fever or metastatic abscess. Consider also deep-vein thrombosis, urinary tract infection and other complications of hospital admission.

Practice point: Refer all patients with IE for expert dental assessment during their inpatient treatment. Their current episode may not be of dental origin, but future relapses may be.

Antibiotic management: Close liaison with the microbiology department is essential in all cases since antibiotic sensitivity *in vitro* determines treatment (Table 13).

Differential diagnosis: Most other febrile illnesses but also, rarely, atrial myxoma and acute rheumatic fever.

Bacteraemia without evidence of IE: Patients with *Staphylococcus aureus* bacteraemia and no obvious source should be assessed for IE and treated for at least 2 weeks. Repeat blood cultures daily for 3–5 days. If there is prolonged bacteraemia or still no obvious source of infection, IE should be strongly suspected

Table 13 Antibiotic treatment of native valve IE

Organism	Comments	Treatment	For penicillin-allergic patients
'Viridans' streptococci, *Streptococcus bovis*	Usually highly sensitive to benzylpenicillin (MBC < 1 mg/l). If *S. bovis*, investigations for colonic polyp or carcinoma are indicated	Benzylpenicillin 7.2 g/day + synergy dose gentamicin △ for 2 weeks, then benzylpenicillin or oral amoxycillin (1 g 8-hly) for 2 weeks thereafter	Vancomycin △ 1 g 12-hly + synergy dose gentamicin △ for 4 weeks
	If MBC > 1 mg/l	Benzylpenicillin 12 g/day + synergy dose gentamicin △ for 4–6 weeks	
Enterococci	MBC for benzylpenicillin usually > 1 mg/l	Benzylpenicillin 12 g/day + synergy dose gentamicin △ for 4–6 weeks	Vancomycin △ 1 g 12-hly + synergy dose gentamicin △ for 4–6 weeks
Staphylococci (non-MRSA)	Clinical trials show no convincing benefit from prolonged gentamicin, which may be omitted after 5 days if there is a relative contraindication such as renal impairment	Flucloxacillin 12 g/day + treatment dose gentamicin △ for 2 weeks, then flucloxacillin alone for 2–4 weeks thereafter. Fucidin 500 mg po 8-hly or rifampicin 600 mg po daily may be added in place of gentamicin	Vancomycin △ 1 g 12-hly for 4–6 weeks
Methicillin resistant staphylococci (MRSA) ☎	Consider combination with oral fucidin or rifampicin	Vancomycin △ 1 g 12-hly for 4–6 weeks	Vancomycin △ 1 g 12-hly for 4–6 weeks
Streptococcus pneumoniae, Neisseria meningitidis		Benzylpenicillin 20 MU/day for 4–6 weeks	Cefotaxime 2 g 8-hly for 4–6 weeks
Haemophilus spp. and other fastidious Gram-negative rods	Guided by results of culture and sensitivity	Ampicillin 2 g 6-hly + treatment dose gentamicin △ or cefotaxime 2 g 8-hly for 4–6 weeks	
Pseudomonas spp. ☎	Largely a disease of IVDUs and PVE. Right-sided IE worth trying antibiotics alone. Left-sided IE merits immediate valve replacement followed by 6 weeks of antibiotics	Azlocillin 15 g/day + treatment dose gentamicin △ for 6 weeks	Ceftazidime 2 g 8-hly + treatment dose gentamicin △ for 4–6 weeks

△ Gentamicin and vancomycin levels must be measured at least twice weekly (≻314). For recommended starting doses of gentamicin for synergy and treatment ≻314, 322.

and treatment should be extended to 4 weeks. **Sustained** bacteraemia with 'viridans' streptococci or *Staphylococcus epidermidis* is treated as IE.

IE in intravenous drug users

Intravenous drug users with IE usually have no history of cardiac disease and the clinical picture is atypical in several respects:

Clinical features: Tricuspid valve IE accounts for more than 50% of cases. Presentation is often with septic pulmonary emboli, causing cough, dyspnoea and pleurisy. Tricuspid murmurs are usually absent. If AV or MV is affected presentation is more typical.

Organisms: *Staphylococcus aureus* (60%), streptococci and enterococci (20%). Less often, *Pseudomonas* spp., aerobic Gram-negative rods, *Candida* spp.; 5% of IE in this group is polymicrobial.

Other investigations: Chest X-ray may show multiple peripheral lesions with a tendency to cavitate.

Prosthetic valve endocarditis (PVE)

This affects mechanical valves more commonly than bioprosthetic grafts, and affects the AV more than the MV. With mechanical valves, infection consists of ring abscess in tissue behind the valve, with extension into adjacent structures. The valve may leak (commonly presenting as aortic regurgitation) or become obstructed (commoner with MV). Conduction defects also occur. Infection of bioprosthetic valves is usually confined to the valve leaflets; ring abscesses are less common.

Clinical features: Fever and cardiac findings (e.g. an aortic regurgitant murmur), embolic phenomena and heart failure. In *Candida* spp. IE blood cultures may take 72–96 h to become positive. *Aspergillus* IE is almost always blood culture-negative and usually presents as peripheral embolus, the diagnosis being confirmed on histology of the resected embolic material.

Organisms: Infection occurring less than 3–4 months after operation is normally acquired perioperatively and is usually caused by *Staphylococcus aureus*, *Staphylococcus epidermidis*, aerobic Gram-negative rods, coryneforms or fungi. Concomitant sternal wound sepsis is common. Later infections are due to a similar spectrum of organisms as native valve IE and are acquired in the same ways.

Antibiotic management: Guided by microbiological results. Empirical treatment is vancomycin + treatment dose gentamicin △.

> **Practice point:** A normal ECHO does **not** exclude IE.

> **Practice point:** Don't wait to treat suspected bacteraemia. Take three sets of blood cultures and start treatment immediately (➤160).

Table 14 Prophylaxis against IE

Procedure	Recommended regimen	If penicillin-allergic*
Dental extractions, scaling or periodontal surgery under **local or no anaesthesia** (fillings and other procedures not causing gum trauma do **not** require prophylaxis)	Amoxycillin 3 g po, under supervision, 1 h prior to procedure. Children 5–10 yrs: $\frac{1}{2}$ adult dose; <5 yrs: $\frac{1}{4}$ adult dose	Clindamycin 600 mg po, under supervision, 1 h prior to procedure. Children 5–10 yrs: 300 mg; <5 yrs, 150 mg **or** erythromycin stearate, 1.5 g po, under supervision, 1 h prior to procedure plus 0.5 g 6 h later. Children 5–10 yrs: $\frac{1}{2}$ adult dose; <5 yrs: $\frac{1}{4}$ adult dose

continued on p. 41

Table 14 contd

Procedure	Recommended regimen	If penicillin-allergic*
Dental extractions, scaling or periodontal surgery under **general anaesthesia**	Amoxycillin 1 g im (in 2.5 ml 1% lignocaine hydrochloride) or iv (in water for injection) just before induction plus 0.5 g po under supervision, 6 h later. Children <10 yrs: $\frac{1}{2}$ adult dose **or** amoxycillin 3 g po under supervision, 4 h before anaesthesia followed by 3 g po as soon as possible after operation. Children 5–10 yrs: $\frac{1}{2}$ adult dose; <5 yrs: $\frac{1}{4}$ adult dose **or** amoxycillin 3 g po and probenecid 1 g po under supervision, 4 h before anaesthesia	See below under Special-risk patients
Special-risk patients who should be referred to hospital: (i) patients with prosthetic valves who are to have a general anaesthetic; (ii) patients who are to have a general anaesthetic and who are allergic to penicillin or have had penicillin more than once in the preceding month; (iii) patients with a previous history of endocarditis	Amoxycillin 1 g im (in 2.5 ml 1% lignocaine hydrochloride) or iv (in water for injection) plus gentamicin 120 mg im just before induction, then amoxycillin 0.5 g po 6 h later. Children < 10 yrs: amoxycillin, $\frac{1}{2}$ adult dose plus gentamicin 2 mg/kg	Teicoplanin 400 mg iv plus gentamicin 120 mg iv just before induction or 15 min before surgical procedure. Children < 14 yrs: teicoplanin, 6 mg/kg iv plus gentamicin 2 mg/kg iv **or** clindamycin 300 mg iv over 10 min just before induction or 15 min before surgical procedure plus 150 mg po or iv 6 h later. Children 5–10 yrs: $\frac{1}{2}$ adult dose; <5 yrs: $\frac{1}{4}$ adult dose **or** vancomycin 1 g by slow iv infusion over 60 min followed by gentamicin 120 mg iv. Children < 10 yrs: vancomycin, 20 mg/kg iv plus gentamicin 2 mg/kg iv
Surgery or instrumentation of upper respiratory tract	As for dental procedures, but postoperative antibiotics may need to be given parenterally due to difficulty in swallowing	
**Genitourinary surgery or instrumentation and obstetric, gynaecological and gastrointestinal procedures in patients with prosthetic valves	Amoxycillin 1 g im (in 2.5 ml 1% lignocaine hydrochloride) or iv (in water for injection) plus gentamicin 120 mg im just before induction, then amoxycillin 0.5 g po 6 h later. Children < 10 yrs: amoxycillin, $\frac{1}{2}$ adult dose plus gentamicin 2 mg/kg	Teicoplanin plus gentamicin as above under Special-risk patients **or** vancomycin plus gentamicin as above under Special-risk patients

* Or if prescribed penicillin more than once in the preceding month.
** If urine is known to be infected, prophylaxis should be extended to include cover against the pathogens involved ☞.
Recommendations of the British Society for Antimicrobial Chemotherapy Working Party, *Lancet* (1990) 335:89, *Lancet* (1992) 339:1292.

Prophylaxis against infective endocarditis

Prophylaxis is indicated for patients with a history of rheumatic heart disease, congenital heart disease (except uncomplicated atrial septal defect), other forms of valvular heart disease including a history of native value repair, mitral valve prolapse (if there is a systolic murmur), surgically constructed systemic–pulmonary shunt, and hypertrophic obstructive cardiomyopathy (Table 14). Patients with prosthetic valves and previous history of endocarditis are at particularly high risk.

Viral pericarditis

Clinical features: A flu-like illness is typical. Onset is usually acute with substernal pain relieved by sitting forward. There may be a pericardial rub, and in the presence of large amounts of pericardial fluid, signs of cardiac tamponade (hypotension, tachycardia, muffled heart sounds, raised venous pressure which rises further on inspiration).

Organisms: Most cases are due to enteroviruses, in particular, Coxsackie A and B and echo-viruses. Influenza, mumps, varicella-zoster and EBV are all reported as rare causes.

Microbiological investigations: Serology for viral causes. If effusion is large and tamponade present, pericardiocentesis is required. Fluid obtained must be examined for bacteria including mycobacteria.

Other investigations: ECG shows widespread concave-upwards ST wave elevation. Chest X-ray may show cardiomegaly. Echocardiography may show pericardial fluid.

Differential diagnosis: Non-infectious causes of pericarditis include uraemia, myocardial infarction, Dressler's syndrome, trauma, connective tissue diseases, acute rheumatic fever, malignant infiltration.

Supportive management: Aspirin or indomethacin. Most cases resolve spontaneously after 2–6 weeks.

Complications: There is recurrence in 15–20% of cases. There may be associated myocarditis.

Pyogenic pericarditis

Risk factors: Bacterial pericarditis nearly always arises in the context of severe intercurrent illness, e.g. after thoracic surgery, by contiguous spread from infection in the pleura, lungs, subphrenic space or endocardium, or by haematogenous spread from septic foci elsewhere.

Clinical features: Presentation is acute with fever, tachycardia and signs of cardiac decompensation. Features of viral pericarditis such as pain relieved by sitting forward, rub and typical ECG changes are usually absent.

Organisms: *Streptococcus pneumoniae, Staphylococcus aureus*. Gram-negative aerobic bacilli. Less often, *Neisseria meningitidis, Neisseria gonorrhoeae, Haemophilus influenzae*. Many other organisms have been reported as very rare causes.

Microbiological investigations: Blood culture. Pericardiocentesis may be required for diagnosis or for relief of tamponade.

Other investigations: If pericardial effusion is present, the chest X-ray shows cardiomegaly. Echocardiography will show pericardial fluid.

Differential diagnosis: Tuberculous or viral pericarditis. Acute rheumatic fever. Non-infectious causes of pericarditis.

Antibiotic management: Prolonged intravenous antibiotics guided by sensitivity testing, similar to regimens listed for IE.

Supportive management: Most patients are extremely unwell and require intensive investigation, supportive management and intensive care.

Tuberculous pericarditis ⊠

Risk factors: Pericarditis can be the sole manifestation of TB, although many patients have history of concurrent pulmonary tuberculosis.

Clinical features: Onset is usually insidious with slow accumulation of pericardial fluid, with fever, weight loss and fatigue. Rarely TB pericarditis presents as an acute fibrinous pericarditis.

Organisms: *Mycobacterium tuberculosis, Mycobacterium bovis*.

Microbiological investigations: Diagnosis is often difficult since acid-fast bacilli are not usually seen in the pericardial fluid. Pericardial biopsy is most likely to be diagnostic. Granulomatous pericarditis is due to tuberculosis until proven otherwise.

Management: (➤32).

Myocarditis

Myocarditis is inflammation of cardiac muscle. Most cases are viral, although myocarditis is also seen in Lyme disease.

Clinical features: Presentation ranges from a symptomless finding to fulminant heart failure. Patients are usually febrile and tachycardic, with dyspnoea and fatigue. On examination there may be cardiomegaly and murmurs of mitral and tricuspid regurgitation. There may be hypotension and signs of congestive cardiac failure. Arrythmias and heart block may occur. There may be associated features of pericarditis.

Organisms: Coxsackievirus A and B, echovirus. Many other viruses have been reported as rare causes. *Borrelia burgdorferi*. Myocarditis is also a feature of systemic infections including *Trypanosoma cruzi*, *Toxoplasma gondii*, *Neisseria meningitidis*, *Corynebacterium diphtheriae*.

Microbiological investigations: Serology including for Lyme disease (➤224).

Other investigations: ECG may show widespread ST and T wave changes. Most patients recover fully. Myocardial biopsy is required in those who do not.

Differential diagnosis: Pericarditis. ˒Idiopathic congestive cardiomyopathy. Acute rheumatic fever.

Supportive management: Rest and anti-inflammatory agents.

Comments: Sudden death occurring in the convalescent phase of influenza may be due to myocarditis, and it is sensible to advise against extreme physical exertion during this period.

4: Gastrointestinal Infections

Normal bowel flora

A knowledge of the constituents of the normal bowel flora is useful in the understanding of intra-abdominal sepsis (Table 15).

Infectious diarrhoea

'Infectious gastroenteritis' may be due to true infection or it may be the result of ingestion of toxin preformed in food. It is often possible to infer which organism is involved from the clinical features of the illness, the risk factors present, particularly exposure to specific foods, common exposure history in affected contacts and knowledge of other cases current in the community. Infectious diarrhoea is classified into secretory diarrhoea and invasive enteritis.

✉ Food poisoning (bacterial, viral or toxic) and dysentery are notifiable diseases.

Risk factors: Usually acquired by ingestion of the infectious agent in food; some are at higher risk (previous gastric surgery, hypochlorhydria, immunodeficiency). Recent antibiotic use predisposes to antibiotic-associated diarrhoea. Diagnosis is suggested by the clinical features (see Tables 16 and 17), other cases in the community and the travel and food history.

Microbiological investigations: Stool microscopy for blood and pus cells. Pus cells are absent in viral gastroenteritis. Examination for ova, cysts and parasites is indicated if there is a history of travel. Stool electron microscopy is used to confirm viral gastroenteritis. Stool culture for specific pathogens including *Salmonella* spp., VTEC, *Shigella* spp. and *Campylobacter jejuni.* ☎ Always inform the laboratory of travel history and if diarrhoea is bloody. Modified Ziehl–Neelson stain is used to demonstrate *Cryptosporidium parvum* (➤263, Σ ~5000), which is particularly common in children under 5 years and the immunocompromised.

Other investigations: Sigmoidoscopy will reveal changes of pseudomembranous colitis (due to *Clostridium difficile* ➤47) and ulceration due to *Entamoeba histolytica* and allow biopsy to exclude non-infectious causes of diarrhoea such as inflammatory bowel disease (IBD).

Differential diagnosis: IBD, diverticulosis, colonic carcinoma, ischaemic colitis, malabsorption.

Antibiotic management: Antibiotics are rarely indicated for infectious diarrhoea. They are useless against toxin preformed in food, and in some infections, such as uncomplicated

Table 15 Normal bowel flora

Region	Flora
Stomach	Usually sterile, unless achlorhydric, when flora resembles that of small intestine
Small intestine	Usually contains small numbers of lactobacilli, enterococci and diphtheroids. Diabetes or abnormal anatomy (e.g. following surgery to create a blind loop, or in diverticulosis) may allow bacterial overgrowth with malabsorption and diarrhoea
Large intestine	Bacteria account for 30% of the wet weight of faeces. **Strict anaerobes outnumber the aerobic Gram-negative rods ('coliforms') by at least 100:1**

Table 16 Predominantly secretory diarrhoea

Organism	Incubation period	Typical duration (days)	C	V	F	B	Comments
Bacillus cereus ⊠ (➤178) Σ ~130	1–6h	<1	+	++	–	–	Heat-stable toxin preformed in food, typically rice or meat. Incubation period extended and diarrhoea worse if toxin produced by bacterial multiplication in gut
Clostridium perfringens (➤216) ⊠ Σ ~1000	8–12h	1	+	±	+	–	Toxin produced in gut. Usually after ingestion of food, typically meat, kept warm to allow germination of spores and bacterial growth
Staphylococcus aureus (➤165) ⊠ Σ ~70	2–7h	<1	+	++	±	–	Toxin preformed in food. Typically dairy produce, meat products
E. coli (enterotoxigenic (ETEC) and other adherent strains, e.g. EAggEC, DAEC (➤187)	12–72h	2–4	+	–	–	–	No routine therapy is indicated although oral ciprofloxacin shortens the duration of the attack. Typically transmitted by meat, salads, milk, water ⊠
Vibrio cholerae (➤194) ⊠	1–5 days	Variable	–	+	–	–	Severe secretory diarrhoea. Diagnosis suggested by travel to endemic/epidemic area. Ciprofloxacin shortens duration of diarrhoea. Faeco-oral transmission
Viral diarrhoea (rota-, adeno-, calici-, Norwalk agent and SRSVs and astroviruses) (➤258)	1–3 days	3–9	+	+	+	–	Sporadic viral gastroenteritis of infants is usually caused by rotavirus, adenoviruses, caliciviruses and astroviruses. Epidemic diarrhoea affecting older children and adults more often due to Norwalk agent. Treatment is supportive. These agents are highly infectious and prevention of nosocomial spread may require isolation. Faeco-oral and respiratory spread

C = cramps, V = vomiting, F = fever, B = blood in stools, SRSV = small round structured virus.

salmonella gastroenteritis, they predispose to the carrier state.

Antibiotics **are** indicated in the following circumstances:

• **Salmonellosis** with bacteraemia or severe illness. Ciprofloxacin is the drug of choice in the UK at present, particularly as clinical trials suggest that it does not predispose towards the carrier state. Amoxycillin and trimethoprim may be used but resistance is common (➤191).

• **Shigellosis** due to *Shigella dysenteriae* is treated with ciprofloxacin or trimethoprim

(➤192), although milder cases, due to *Shigella sonnei*, usually resolve without antibiotics.

• *Campylobacter jejuni* infection may respond to erythromycin if given early in the course of a severe infection (➤196).

• **Antibiotic-associated diarrhoea** due to *Clostridium difficile* is treated with oral metronidazole or vancomycin (➤47).

Supportive management: Rehydration is the key to management of diarrhoea from whatever cause. Oral rehydration is adequate for the majority of cases, and is best given as a solution containing both salt and sugar, which

Table 17 'Invasive' enteritis

Organism	Incubation period	Typical duration (days)	C	V	F	B	Comments
Shigellae (➤192) ⊠ Escherichia coli (EIEC ➤187)	12–96 h	5–7	+	+	+	+	Very small infective dose. Faeco-oral spread. Complications include toxic megacolon, reactive arthritis. Antibiotics for severe infection (➤45)
Yersinia enterocolitica (➤194)	3–7 days	10–14	+	+	+	−	Requires special culture techniques. Unusual in UK. Extraintestinal manifestations are common. Usually from pork or dairy produce
Vibrio parahaemolyticus	24–72 h	2–10	+	+	+	+	Usually transmitted by shellfish (➤195)
Campylobacter jejuni (➤196)	1–10 days	2–20	+	+	+	+	From meat, esp. poultry, and dairy produce. Severe attacks may be shortened by erythromycin
Escherichia coli (VTEC, syn. EHEC ➤188)	1–5 days	1–4	+	+	+	+	Bloody diarrhoea due to verotoxin production. Associated with HUS, especially in children
Giardia lamblia (➤266)	7–21 days	Variable	+	+	±	−	May cause chronic steatorrhoea and malabsorption. Metronidazole is indicated
Entamoeba histolytica (➤267) ⊠	Variable 14–28 days	Variable	+	±	±	+	Diagnosis suggested by travel history; very rarely acquired in UK. Complications include liver abscess, amoeboma, cutaneous ulceration
Non-typhoidal Salmonella spp. (➤191)	8–48 h	4–7	+	+	+	±	May rarely cause systemic illness with bacteraemia and metastatic infection. Antibiotics are indicated for this, but not usually for uncomplicated gastroenteritis (➤45)

C = cramps, V = vomiting, F = fever, B = blood in stools, HUS = haemolytic uraemic syndrome.
In children, consider also Henoch–Schönlein purpura (➤110)

are actively taken up together in the small intestine. Commercial **rehydration fluids** are available (Dioralyte). Home-made recipes are widely used in developing countries: e.g., 4 tablespoons of sugar, ¾ teaspoon of salt, 1 teaspoon of sodium bicarbonate mixed in 250 ml of orange juice made up to 1 litre with water.

Antispasmodic agents such as loperamide may be used for mild diarrhoea without blood, but should not be used if there are features to suggest dysentery.

Control of gastrointestinal infections

Responsibility for investigation and control of GI infections in the community rests with the consultant in communicable disease control (CCDC). National PHLS guidelines are published but local rules, which may be less stringent, often exist.

• ⊠ Notification is required for all cases of food poisoning (bacterial, viral and toxic), dysentery (amoebic and bacillary), typhoid, paratyphoid and viral hepatitis.

• No one with diarrhoea or vomiting should be at work or school. All cases should submit a stool sample to allow identification of the causative organism.

• Certain groups are at high risk of passing on infection to others:

Group 1: Food handlers whose work involves touching unwrapped foods to be consumed raw or without further cooking.

Group 2: Health care, nursery and other staff

who have direct contact, or contact through serving food, with highly susceptible patients or persons.

Group 3: Children <5 years attending playgroups, nurseries or similar groups.

Group 4: Older children and adults who are unable to implement good standards of personal hygiene.

In the absence of specific local rules, the recommendations listed in Table 18 may be applied.

Antibiotic-associated diarrhoea (AAD) ①

Certain agents, notably clindamycin, ampicillin/ amoxycillin, co-amoxiclav and the parenteral or broad-spectrum cephalosporins are particularly likely to cause diarrhoea, although almost all antibiotics have been implicated. Most cases are due to infection by toxin-producing *Clostridium difficile*, growth of which is promoted by alteration in other bowel flora (>220). *Clostridium difficile* produces a colitis, which in its most severe form causes colonic ulceration with pseudomembrane formation ('pseudomembranous colitis'−PMC). AAD is an important and expensive cause of nosocomial morbidity and mortality.

Risk factors: Antibiotic use, particularly those listed above. (*Clostridium difficile*-associated diarrhoea (CDAD) has rarely been reported

Table 18 Recommendations for exclusion from work/school and follow-up of patients with GI infections

Organism	Cases may return to work/school	Contacts: action needed
Food poisoning (culture-negative) All high-risk groups	48h after symptoms cease	None
Campylobacter, Giardia, Cryptosporidium	When symptom-free	None
Salmonella (other than typhoid and paratyphoid) Group 1 Groups 2–4	48h after symptoms cease[1] When symptom-free	Stool sample from contacts who are in group 1. Others: none
Shigella sonnei Group 1 All others	48h after symptoms cease[1] When symptom-free	Advice on personal hygiene[2,3]
Other shigellae Groups 1–4 Others	After three negative stools 48h after symptoms cease	Advice on personal hygiene[2]. Stool samples from all in high-risk groups[4]
Typhoid/paratyphoid Group 1 and water supply workers Groups 2–4 Others	After 12 negative stools[4] After three negative stools When symptom-free[5]	Advise to seek attention if unwell within 4 weeks
Hepatitis A	1 week after onset of jaundice	Exclude household contacts who are group 1

[1] Three negative samples should be obtained if there is reason to doubt personal hygiene.
[2] Because of the ease with which it may be transmitted by personal contact, guidelines for control of *Shigella sonnei* place great emphasis on high standards of personal hygiene, particularly hand washing with soap and water after toilet use and before preparing or eating food.
[3] Screening of other contacts may be required in the case of an outbreak.
[4] Eight in the first 2 months, then four at monthly intervals, two after magnesium sulphate purges. Urine should also be cultured. Screening should continue for 6 months after return to work.
[5] Three negative stool and urine samples should be obtained, but patients need not be excluded from work/school.

in the absence of antibiotic use, e.g. in association with anticancer chemotherapy.) Age, GI surgery and previous medical procedures, including enemas and the use of stool softeners, also predispose. *Clostridium difficile* can be recovered easily from surfaces within the rooms of patients with AAD, especially if they are incontinent, and from the hands of their medical attendants. The carriage rate in hospital patients on admission is ~1% and the organism is usually acquired nosocomially. CDAD is rising in incidence (Σ 4000 in 1993).

Clinical features: Asymptomatic carriage is common. Diarrhoea varies from mild to very severe, with abdominal cramps, fever and leucocytosis. Sigmoidoscopy shows ulceration and pseudomembranes in severe cases, although disease can be restricted to ascending colon. Toxic megacolon and perforation occur rarely. Relapse after apparently successful treatment is common (~25%), and persistent diarrhoea leading to hypoalbuminaemia can occur.

Microbiological investigations: Assay for *Clostridium difficile* toxin in stool ($\succ$220). Culture is also possible, but is slower and not specific for the disease. Avoid sending multiple repeat faecal samples from patients with symptomatic relapse, or to assess 'clearance' because continued presence of toxin or organism is common (~25%) and not predictive of response or relapse.

Other investigations: CT scan may show characteristic thickening of colon, with contrast trapped in folds ('accordion sign').

Antibiotic management: Stop the precipitating antibiotic whenever possible. Metronidazole 400 mg 8-hly, **po**, **or** vancomycin 125 mg 6-hly, **po**. Vancomycin is much more expensive and might encourage colonisation by vancomycin-resistant enterococci, but is slightly more effective. Either agent should be given for 10 days, and if there is no response the other may be substituted. Relapse should be treated with a further course. Various strategies have been suggested for preventing relapse, but none has been subjected to clinical trial. These include tapering doses of vancomycin over several weeks, very low-dose vancomycin therapy for 3 weeks post-treatment, cholestyramine and

even enemas containing normal bowel organisms. About 50% of relapses are in fact due to reinfection, and infection control measures are important.

Prevention: Patients should be isolated whilst they have diarrhoea and for 3 days thereafter. The use of gloves for routine handling of all body fluids has been shown to reduce the transmission of *Clostridium difficile* and the incidence of AAD. Ward bedpan washers do not kill the spores of *Clostridium difficile*, and bedpans used by infected patients should not be returned to general circulation until they have been autoclaved. Control of antibiotic prescribing. Cleaning of rooms after discharge or transfer of patients is essential.

Antibiotic-associated diarrhoea without *Clostridium difficile*: Patients with antibiotic-associated diarrhoea and negative tests for *Clostridium difficile* toxin tend to be less ill, with few constitutional symptoms. Other putative causes of AAD include *Clostridium perfringens, Staphylococcus aureus* and *Candida* spp.

Traveller's diarrhoea

International travellers frequently develop diarrhoea. A wide range of organisms are responsible, including ETEC, shigellae, salmonellae, *Campylobacter* spp., *Giardia lamblia* and rarely *Entamoeba histolytica*. Travellers who will have difficulty obtaining medical attention should carry stand-by medication ($\succ$138).

Viral hepatitis

The clinical features of acute viral hepatitis A–E are similar for all hepatitis viruses, although they differ considerably in severity, tempo and likelihood of progression to chronic infection. Many other viruses cause hepatitis as part of systemic infection, including EBV, CMV and yellow fever virus. Hepatitis also occurs with bacterial infections, either as part of a specific syndrome, such as leptospirosis, or as a non-specific feature of severe sepsis. Acute hepatitis is also caused by drugs, e.g. paracetamol, alcohol, chlorpromazine, antituberculous drugs and halothane.

Clinical features: Anorexia, nausea and vomiting. Fever, chills, headache, fatigue and myalgia. Right-upper-quadrant pain and tenderness. Jaundice develops in a proportion of patients, initially with pale stools and dark urine. The speed of onset and clinical course varies depending on the virus involved. Patients usually feel better with the onset of jaundice.

Fulminant hepatitis describes the development of liver failure during viral hepatitis.

Cholestatic hepatitis is characterised by prolonged severe jaundice with pruritis persisting for several months after the acute attack.

Hepatitis A (HAV) ≈ ②
Virus: ssRNA picornavirus (➤249).
Synonyms: Infectious hepatitis. Epidemic hepatitis. Epidemic jaundice.
Transmission: Faeco-oral, either by contaminated water/food or person-to-person. Infection is widespread in the developing world, affecting mainly children. In the UK, infection is commoner with low socio-economic status. Outbreaks occur in institutions, particularly primary schools.
Incubation period: Two to 6 weeks.
Clinical features: Usually asymptomatic under 2 years of age. Jaundice occurs in 70% of adults, with onset over days.
Progression to chronic liver disease: Does not occur.
Complications: Fulminant hepatitis is rare (<0.2%). Cholestatic hepatitis (very rare). Relapsing hepatitis occurs but is very rare.
Serodiagnosis: Total Ig or IgG indicate previous exposure. Anti-HAV IgM indicates recent infection and is required for diagnosis of current hepatitis.
Immunisation: Active immunisation is available, with an inactivated virus vaccine (➤142). It is recommended for travellers to endemic areas whose trip will not be confined to tourist areas, occupational groups at particular risk (e.g. sewage workers) and contacts of cases. Active immunisation gives effective, long-lasting immunity. Due to the relatively high seroprevalence of HAV antibodies, pooled human immunoglobulin (HIG) contains sufficient protective antibodies to reduce the risk of infection. Passive immunisation with HIG gives only partial, short-lived immunity, but takes effect immediately after injection.
Treatment of contacts: Close personal contacts should receive HIG. They should also receive active immunisation with an accelerated schedule. Immunisation may also be required to terminate outbreaks in institutions.
Isolation policy: If patients require hospitalisation, ②. Virus is present in stools for 1–2 weeks before the onset of jaundice and for 1 week after.

Hepatitis B (HBV) ≈ ③
Virus: dsDNA hepadnavirus (➤247).
Synonyms: Serum hepatitis. Australia antigen hepatitis.
Transmission: Parenteral. Transmission occurs through percutaneous exposure (needle-stick, needle-sharing, blood transfusion), sexual contact and vertically by maternal–neonatal infection. Maternofetal transmission occurs but accounts for only 5% of vertical transmission.
Risk factors: Groups at risk of HBV infection in the developed world include IVDUs, homosexual men, prostitutes, health care workers. Haemodialysis patients are now regularly screened.
Incubation period: Two to 6 months.
Clinical features: Usually asymptomatic in infants. Jaundice occurs in 25% of adults. Onset usually insidious. Occasionally associated with 'serum sickness' like illness attributed to immune complex deposition with symmetrical distal polyarthritis, angio-oedema, urticaria and rarely glomerulonephritis.
Complications: Fulminant hepatitis is rare (~1%). Cholestatic hepatitis (very rare).
Progression to chronic liver disease: There is complete recovery in 95% of acute cases. Chronic infection with development of chronic active hepatitis develops in 1–3%. In these patients there is an estimated annual incidence of cirrhosis of ~2.5% (~15% at 5 years).
Serodiagnosis: There are many serological markers of HBV infection. See Table 19 for serodiagnosis in practice. The time course of development of clinically useful markers is illustrated in Fig. 2.

Table 19 Serological markers of HBV infection

Marker	Structure	Comments
Dane particle	The whole infectious virion. 42 nm lipid enveloped structure	Detectable by electron microscopy in many cases. Implies infectivity
HBV core	The 28 nm core of the Dane particle	Contains the viral DNA
HBV surface antigen (HBsAg) (syn. 'Australia antigen')	The surface antigen of the Dane particle. Also found on smaller particles and viral filaments in serum	Taken as the **main indicator of infectivity**. Patients may have HBsAg and be non-infectious but this is not discernible in practice
HBV core antigen (HBcAg)	Antigen associated with HBV core	No commercial test available for this antigen
HBV-associated DNA polymerase	Associated with the Dane particle	Implies continuing viral replication and infectivity
HBV e antigen (HBeAg)	Antigen derived from HBV core	Correlated strongly with **high infectivity** and progression to chronic liver disease
Anti-HBs	Antibody to HBsAg	Taken as a marker of protective immunity
Anti-HBC	Antibody to HBcAg	Marker of previous exposure
Anti-HBe	Antibody to HBeAg	Indicates relatively low infectivity in HBsAg-positive blood

Serodiagnosis in practice

• **Diagnosis of cause of jaundice:** HBsAg is present in serum from 1 to 7 weeks before the onset of jaundice and for up to 6 weeks thereafter in uncomplicated cases. Approximately 15% of cases will be HBsAg-negative by the time they present. They will have IgM anti-HBC antibodies. IgG anti-HBC indicates previous exposure but does not establish cause of recent disease.

• **Assessment of infectivity and risk of progression:** HBsAg indicates that the patient is potentially infectious and is at risk of progression to chronic hepatitis. Of patients developing chronic hepatitis 99% are HBsAg-positive. HBeAg implies very high infectivity and increased risk of progression. Anti-HBe suggests low infectivity.

• **Clinical staff doing 'exposure-prone' procedures:** Current Department of Health guidelines stipulate that all such staff must be immunised against HBV infection. Staff who are HBeAg-positive are considered to rep-

resent a hazard to patients and must not carry out such procedures. Staff with evidence of HBV infection but who are HBeAg-negative may continue to work as normal.

Management: Interferon is used for a subset of patients identified on the basis of histological appearances, liver function tests and serological results; referral for specialist hepatology opinion is recommended. Liver transplantation is usually followed by reinfection of the graft, but 5-year survival is better than in patients who are not transplanted. Transplantation in this context remains controversial.

Immunisation: Active immunisation is now achieved using vaccine produced by recombinant DNA technology. Protection is effective and long-lived. In the UK it is usual to check serological response and advise booster vaccination if low, but it is not clear at what level protection becomes inadequate. Immunisation is advised for all risk groups listed above (three doses at 0, 1 and 6 months; check

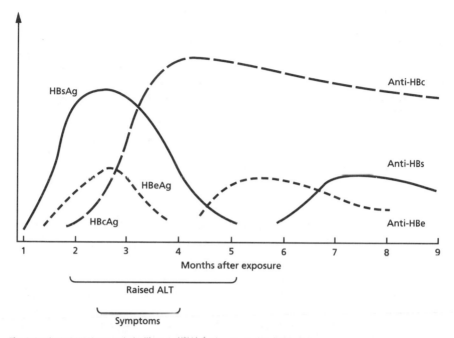

Fig. 2 Serological events associated with acute HBV infection. See text for abbreviations.

antibody response 2–4 months thereafter; booster required every 5 years).

Treatment of contacts: After needle-stick or other parenteral exposure to infectious individual, sexual contact or for neonates of infected mothers, an accelerated schedule of active immunisation with simultaneous administration of HBV-immune globulin is advised. In some countries with high rates of endemicity, immunisation of all neonates has been started in an effort to break the chain of vertical transmission, but the high cost of vaccine makes this impracticable in those countries worst affected.

Isolation policy: ③ Hospital isolation policies often dictate side-room isolation for HBsAg-positive patients, especially those likely to bleed. Careful attention to handling of body fluids and contaminated sharps is of greater importance. At home, transmission may occur by sharing of razors, toothbrushes, etc. and patients should be made aware of this. Vaccination is recommended for close household

contacts. Haemodialysis patients should be regularly screened.

Hepatitis D (HDV) ⊠

Virus: An RNA virus which is defective in the sense that it requires HBV for its replication.

Synonyms: Delta virus.

Transmission: As for HBV.

Incubation period: Days to weeks.

Clinical features: Acute hepatitis often in a patient previously known to be HBsAg-positive. Infection with HBV and HDV may be simultaneous, in which case there is increased severity and mortality, with fulminant hepatitis in up to 10%. Simultaneous infection results in a biphasic illness with two peaks of elevated ALT.

Progression to chronic liver disease: The risk of progression to CAH and cirrhosis is increased by HDV infection compared with HBV infection alone, particularly when HDV superinfection on top of previous HBV infection occurs.

Serodiagnosis: Anti-HDV IgG and IgM can be demonstrated in serum.
Immunisation: Not available.

Hepatitis C (HCV) ⊠

Virus: An ssRNA flavivirus.
Synonyms: Parenterally transmitted non-A non-B hepatitis (PT-NANB). Non-B transfusion-associated hepatitis.
Transmission: Parenteral, usually via blood, because until recently no serological test was available. HCV accounts for 90% of transfusion-associated hepatitis, although this will fall following the introduction of HCV antibody screening of donated blood. Infection is also common in IVDUs. Sexual transmission appears to be very infrequent.
Incubation period: Two to 26 weeks.
Clinical features: Acute hepatitis often following blood transfusion. Frequently asymptomatic. Less than 25% of adults are jaundiced.
Complications: Fulminant hepatitis occurs, probably more frequently than with HBV.
Progression to chronic liver disease: Chronic infection with progression to CAH and cirrhosis is much more common with HCV than with HBV. Estimates vary from 20 to 70% depending on the study group and methods employed to diagnose persistent infection. Of those with CAH, up to 20% will develop cirrhosis. Cofactors such as alcohol are important. Interferon has not been shown to produce any lasting benefit in HCV+ patients but clinical trials are in progress.
Serodiagnosis: First-generation antibody tests ('C-110 3' tests) were relatively non-specific with high rates of false positives, and typically became positive 3–6 months after illness. Second-generation tests are positive in ~90% of cases with shorter time to positivity (typically 4 weeks). PCR for HCV RNA is also available ➔; positive PCR is usually associated with histological abnormalities on liver biopsy.
Immunisation: Not available.
Treatment: Interferon remains experimental. Hepatology referral is recommended.

Hepatitis E (HEV) ⊠

Virus: A newly recognised RNA virus, with similarities to caliciviruses (➤258).

Synonyms: Enterically transmitted non-A non-B hepatitis (ET-NANB).
Transmission: Faeco-oral, as for HAV. Typically waterborne. Prevalent in the developing world, where it is the commonest cause of hepatitis in adults.
Incubation period: Twenty to 40 days.
Clinical features: Usually more severe than HAV, with a much higher incidence of fulminant hepatic failure. The mortality is particularly high during pregnancy, up to 40%.
Progression to chronic liver disease: Does not occur.
Serodiagnosis: Not routinely available in most laboratories, but tests exist for research studies.

Hepatitis F and G

The terms HFV and HGV have been coined to describe cases of parenterally transmitted hepatitis which are not due to HBV, HCV or HDV. These agents have not been isolated, and it is likely that there are many undiscovered viruses capable of producing the same clinical picture.

Granulomatous hepatitis

The discovery of granulomata at liver biopsy is not unusual. Often the diagnosis is obvious in the context of the patient's other signs. In many cases this is not so, and the diagnosis may be found among the conditions listed in Table 20. In most series ~10% remain undiagnosed.

Cholecystitis

The biliary tract is normally sterile; infection becomes established secondary to stones or anatomical abnormality, such as malignant or inflammatory strictures. Bacteria may reach the bile via the ampulla of Vater or from the portal or systemic circulations.
Risk factors: Cholecystitis is associated with calculi in ~95% of cases. Acalculous cholecystitis typically occurs in elderly debilitated patients with severe intercurrent illness. Cholecystitis is a complication which may

Table 20 Causes of granulomatous hepatitis

Category	Conditions
Infections	
Mycobacteria	***Mycobacterium tuberculosis*** (the commonest cause worldwide ➤229), *Mycobacterium leprae* (➤230), atypical mycobacteria (➤231)
Bacteria	*Brucella* spp. (➤209), *Francisella tularensis* (➤212), *Yersinia enterocolitica* (➤194), *Pseudomonas pseudomallei* (➤200)
Spirochaetes	*Treponema pallidum* (➤67)
Fungi	Blastomycosis (➤293), histoplasmosis (➤293), coccidioidomycosis (➤293), cryptococcosis (➤292)
Protozoa	*Leishmania major* (➤274), ***Toxoplasma gondii*** (➤264)
Helminths	***Schistosoma* spp.** (➤285), *Toxocara canis* (➤279), *Ascaris lumbricoides* (➤277)
Rickettsia	*Coxiella burnetii* (➤234), *Rickettsia conori* (➤235)
Viruses	EBV (➤243), CMV (➤243)
Non-infectious causes	
Chemicals	Beryllium, copper, drugs
Others	**Sarcoidosis**, Crohn's disease, ulcerative colitis, primary biliary cirrhosis, hypogammaglobulinaemia, systemic lupus erythematosus, **Hodgkin's lymphoma**

Commoner causes in **bold** type.

follow any operation, due to biliary stasis associated with recumbency and dehydration.

Clinical features: Fever, rigors, nausea and vomiting, right-upper-quadrant pain. On examination, tender right upper quadrant and possibly a tender, palpable, enlarged gall-bladder. There may be evidence of associated bacteraemia with hypotension and confusion. Emphysematous cholecystitis is a rare condition due to infection by *Clostridium perfringens*, sometimes in mixed culture with Gram-negative aerobes. There is gas formation within the gall-bladder and risk of gangrene and perforation.

Organisms: Bowel flora, usually in mixed culture: coliforms, enterococci and anaerobes, including *Bacteroides fragilis* and *Clostridium perfringens*.

Microbiological investigations: Blood culture. Culture of bile if available (e.g. during ERCP or surgical intervention).

Other investigations: Ultrasound scan (USS) and radionuclear HIDA scan are the investigations of choice for confirming the diagnosis.

USS demonstrates bile-duct obstruction, detects 95% of stones and allows assessment of the gall-bladder wall, which is usually thickened. The HIDA scan is a sensitive test for acute cholecystitis.

Antibiotic management: In mildly ill patients, give co-amoxiclav. In more severe cases, use benzylpenicillin + gentamicin + metronidazole **or** cefotaxime + metronidazole. No antibiotic regimen will reliably sterilise an obstructed biliary tree. Antibiotics which usually penetrate well into bile do not do so in this situation.

Supportive management: Initial management of acute cholecystitis is with antibiotics, analgesia, fluid therapy and nasogastric suction if the patient is vomiting. The timing of cholecystectomy after cholecystitis is a matter of controversy and requires experienced surgical judgement.

Complications: Septicaemia, ascending cholangitis, pancreatitis, liver abscess, perforation and peritonitis. Complications are more frequent in the elderly.

Ascending cholangitis

Ascending cholangitis is associated with partial or complete biliary obstruction due to stones or strictures (malignant or inflammatory). The classic features are fever with rigors, abdominal pain and jaundice ('Charcot's triad'). There may be associated evidence of bacteraemia and sepsis syndrome with shock and confusion. Liver abscess, frequently multiple, may develop. This severe infection requires combined surgical and medical treatment. Antibiotic therapy should be as above. Surgical decompression of the gallbladder is usually urgently required, and may often be achieved endoscopically.

Peritonitis

Localised or generalised inflammation of the peritoneal cavity, due to micro-organisms or irritant chemicals (e.g. bile, stomach contents).
Risk factors: Ruptured viscus (e.g. appendix, diverticulum, peptic ulcer, perforated bowel as a complication of enteric fever), ischaemic bowel (e.g. vascular insufficiency, strangulated hernia), trauma, postoperative infection or leakage, pelvic inflammatory disease (including perihepatitis in Fitz-Hugh–Curtis syndrome ➤66), ruptured abscess. Unusual causes include spontaneous bacterial peritonitis, peritoneal dialysis peritonitis and tuberculous peritonitis.
Clinical features: Fever, vomiting, abdominal pain with tenderness, guarding and evidence of paralytic ileus (absent bowel sounds). Hypotension and tachycardia are initially due to hypovolaemia due to loss of intravascular fluid into the peritoneal cavity. If bacteraemia and sepsis syndrome (➤158) develop, then they also contribute to hypotension and confusion.
Organisms: Mixed infection with bowel flora: coliforms, anaerobes, *Enterococcus* spp., *Streptococcus 'milleri'*.
Microbiological investigations: Culture of blood and peritoneal fluid.
Other investigations: Leucocytosis, abnormal liver function tests and raised amylase are common. Chest and abdomen X-ray show

subdiaphragmatic gas if there has been perforation of a viscus.
Differential diagnosis: The differential diagnosis of the 'acute abdomen' includes appendicitis, perforated peptic ulcer, cholecystitis, pancreatitis, renal and biliary colic, inflammatory bowel disease, gynaecological causes, including ruptured ectopic pregnancy and ovarian torsion, retroperitoneal haemorrhage and leaking aortic aneurysm. Non-surgical causes include basal pneumonia; others, such as familial Mediterranean fever and porphyria, are very rare.
Antibiotic management: Benzylpenicillin + gentamicin + metronidazole **or** cefotaxime + metronidazole **or** co-amoxiclav. Vancomycin + gentamicin + metronidazole in the penicillin- and cephalosporin-allergic patient.
Supportive management: Antibiotics are used to speed recovery and prevent bacteraemia – definitive treatment requires surgery for the underlying cause. Instillation of topical antibiotics at operation has not been shown to be of benefit.

Peritoneal dialysis (CAPD) peritonitis

Patients on chronic ambulatory peritoneal dialysis (CAPD) have a permanent indwelling catheter in the peritoneal cavity. Fluid is instilled and withdrawn three or four times daily, and there is therefore a risk of peritoneal infection. Scrupulous attention to aseptic technique is essential when handling CAPD catheters, and reduces the incidence of peritonitis to well below one episode per patient-year.
Clinical features: Abdominal pain and cloudiness of the peritoneal fluid.
Organisms: A vast range, of which the commonest are *Staphylococcus epidermidis, Staphylococcus aureus*, coliforms, *Streptococcus* spp.
Microbiological investigations: Microscopy showing >100 cells/µl suggests infection. Gram stain is positive in 50% of cases, more commonly with Gram-positive infection.
Antibiotic management: All renal units will have a local protocol for the management of CAPD peritonitis. If this is not available, the following regimen, which gives two intraperitoneal

(ip) doses of vancomycin 7 days apart, is suggested:

Send whole bag of peritoneal fluid to laboratory for culture.

Into the first bag of dialysis fluid give vancomycin 2 g (adjusted for body weight as below) + heparin 1000 iu ip. Fluid should be instilled over at least 30 min and remain in peritoneal cavity for ≥6 h. Also give ciprofloxacin 1 g po stat.

Start ciprofloxacin 500 mg po 12-hly thereafter.

Continue heparin whilst bags remain cloudy.

Dose of ip vancomycin: 20–40 kg, 1 g; 40–70 kg, 1.5 g; ≥70 kg, 2 g. Subsequent dose of vancomycin is given on day 7. Levels should be measured between days 1 and 7. These are likely to be higher than usually encountered, but doses should only be reduced if levels exceed 60 mg/l.

If Gram-positive organism is isolated, discontinue ciprofloxacin and continue vancomycin for 14 days (i.e. two doses). If Gram-negative organism is isolated, stop vancomycin and continue ciprofloxacin for 14 days (or modify according to results of culture). If there is no growth after 4 days and there have been no previous episodes of Gram-negative peritonitis, stop ciprofloxacin and continue vancomycin for 14 days.

Spontaneous bacterial peritonitis

Risk factors: Cirrhosis, nephrotic syndrome, girls under 10 years with no previous history of ill health.

Clinical features: As for peritonitis above, although presentation in the cirrhotic patient may be clinically silent.

Organisms: Cirrhosis: coliforms, *Streptococcus pneumoniae*, other *Streptococcus* spp. Nephrotic patients and young girls: *Streptococcus pneumoniae*, β-haemolytic streptococci.

Microbiological investigations: Culture of blood and peritoneal fluid. Peritoneal aspiration should always be carried out in cirrhotic and nephrotic patients who are non-specifically unwell. WBC >250 cells/μl suggests infection.

Antibiotic management: Initially cefotaxime **or** benzylpenicillin + gentamicin, then guided by the results of culture.

Intra-abdominal abscess

Risk factors: Appendicitis, diverticulitis, pancreatitis, genitourinary tract disease, biliary disease. Less commonly, tumour, trauma, perforated peptic ulcer.

Clinical features: Fever, abdominal pain and sometimes localising signs such as a palpable mass depending on the underlying pathology.

Organisms: Coliforms, anaerobes, *Streptococcus* '*milleri*', *Enterococcus* spp. Actinomycosis may develop in long-standing abscesses (➤222).

Investigations: Blood culture. Aspiration of pus if possible. Ultrasound, CT and radiolabelled white cell scans are used to establish the size and site of the abscess.

Antibiotic management. In the absence of material for microbiology, benzylpenicillin + gentamicin + metronidazole **or** cefotaxime + metronidazole **or** co-amoxiclav. Vancomycin + gentamicin + metronidazole in the penicillin- and cephalosporin-allergic patient.

Supportive management: Drainage is almost always required; in some cases this can be achieved by percutaneous drainage under radiological guidance. For a well-localised appendix abscess, when there is no evidence of generalised peritonitis, patients are frequently treated with antibiotics and observed. Two-thirds will settle and can then have elective appendicectomy. If the clinical state deteriorates, urgent surgery is required.

Management of abscesses at particular sites such as in the pancreas, spleen or liver is discussed separately below.

Diverticulitis

Diverticula are small herniations of the colonic mucosa. Diverticulosis is commoner with increasing age. Perforation of a diverticulum leads to diverticulitis, which results from pericolic inflammation and microabscess formation. Generalised peritonitis or abscess are serious complications.

Clinical features: Abdominal pain and tenderness, frequently in left lower quadrant ('left-sided appendicitis'), fever, nausea and vomiting. There may be a palpable mass. Rectal bleeding, which can be severe.

Organisms: As for intra-abdominal abscess.

Microbiological investigations: Blood cultures if systemically unwell.

Other investigations: Usually none acutely. After acute symptoms have settled, sigmoidoscopy and barium enema to confirm diagnosis and exclude colonic carcinoma.

Differential diagnosis: Carcinoma of the colon, inflammatory bowel disease, mesenteric ischaemia and pelvic inflammatory disease.

Antibiotic management: Intravenous antibiotics as for intra-abdominal abscess.

Supportive management: Nasogastric aspiration. Intravenous fluids.

Pyogenic liver abscess

A collection of pus within the liver parenchyma, usually secondary to infection elsewhere in the abdomen.

Risk factors: Cholangitis, haematogenous spread from the gut via the portal vein ('portal pyaemia') secondary to appendicitis, direct extension from contiguous infection, post-traumatic, secondary infection of liver tumour. The cause is unknown in 20% of cases. Compared with amoebic abscess, patients are older and lack a recent travel history, and pyogenic abscesses are often multiple/multilocular.

Clinical features: Fever, nausea and vomiting, weight loss. Right-upper-quadrant tenderness, hepatomegaly, jaundice, raised right hemidiaphragm and pleural effusion.

Organisms: Frequently mixed: coliforms, anaerobes, streptococci (in particular *Streptococcus 'milleri'*), *Enterococcus* spp., rarely *Staphylococcus aureus* or *Pseudomonas* spp.

> **Practice point:** Suspect amoebic liver abscess (➤267) in a patient with high fever and rigors and a travel history. Early liver USS is required.

Microbiological investigations: Culture of abscess contents is essential. Blood culture.

Other investigations: Leucocytosis, raised alkaline phosphatase, milder elevations of transaminases and bilirubin. Reduced albumin. Ultrasound or CT will be required to establish the size and site and guide aspiration.

Differential diagnosis: Cholangitis, amoebic liver abscess, subphrenic abscess, tumour.

Antibiotic management: Guided by the results of microbiology: initial therapy as for intra-abdominal abscess above. Prolonged oral therapy is required to prevent relapse: at least 1 month, increasing to 4 months in the case of multiple abscesses.

Supportive management: Drainage is the most important component of therapy preferably by percutaneous drain insertion under CT control.

Pancreatic abscess

Acute pancreatitis is a sterile process, and antibiotics do not accelerate recovery, except in the presence of intercurrent biliary disease. Pancreatic abscess refers to a collection of infected pus in the pancreas or due to an infected pseudocyst. Abscess complicates ~5% of cases of acute pancreatitis, and is commoner when pancreatitis is secondary to biliary disease. Prophylactic antibiotics do not reduce this incidence.

Clinical features: Fever, abdominal pain and tenderness, ileus persisting for greater than 10 days in a patient presenting with acute pancreatitis.

Organisms: Coliforms, enterococci, occasionally *Staphylococcus aureus*. Anaerobic infection is unusual, but superinfection with yeasts (particularly *Candida albicans*) is common.

Microbiological investigations: Blood culture and culture of aspirated pus if possible.

Other investigations: Leucocytosis and raised serum amylase are common but do not distinguish from acute non-infective pancreatitis. Air bubbles in the pancreas on plain X-ray are pathognomonic. CT scan is the modality of choice, and also allows guided aspiration and drainage. USS and white cell scan will also demonstrate the collection.

Antibiotic management: Antibiotics are given

to prevent bacteraemia and aid healing. Benzylpenicillin + gentamicin **or** cefotaxime. Metronidazole is added if clinical response is poor or if investigation of aspirated material suggests anaerobic infection.

Supportive management: Drainage, either at laparotomy or percutaneously under radiological control, is required.

Complications: Probably as a result of activated pancreatic enzymes, pancreatic abscesses have a tendency to spread, unlike other intra-abdominal collections. Extension occurs along the retroperitoneum in any direction and rarely pancreatic abscesses extend and discharge at distant sites, e.g. the scrotum or the neck.

Splenic abscess

Risk factors: Splenic abscesses arise in three situations:

• Metastatic seeding during bacteraemia. This accounts for the majority of cases and is particularly common in IVDUs and may accompany IE (➤40).

• Secondary to infection associated with infarction from blunt trauma or haemoglobinopathy.

• By direct extension from contiguous infection in the abdomen.

Clinical features: Fever, left-upper-quadrant pain. Left-sided chest signs, e.g. pleural effusion. Splenomegaly is present in 50%. Splenic rub is rare. Multilocular splenic abscesses are much more likely to be clinically silent and carry a higher mortality.

Organisms: Depending on the clinical situation: *Staphylococcus aureus* (~25%, particularly likely in IVDUs), coliforms (~25%), enterococci (~10%), *Salmonella* spp. (particularly in patients with AIDS, who may also develop splenic abscess due to MAI ➤128).

Fungi (*Candida* spp., *Aspergillus* spp.) are increasing in frequency and are often hospital-acquired. Anaerobes (~20%). Mixed infections are common.

Microbiological investigations: Culture of blood and pus. Resected spleen should be submitted for culture.

Other investigations: Ultrasound, radionuclear white cell scan and CT scan are equally good for diagnosing unilocular abscess. CT is superior for multilocular abscesses.

Antibiotic management: As for intra-abdominal abscess, then guided by microbiology results. Blood culture is positive in ~50% of cases.

Supportive management: Splenectomy is indicated in all cases (➤132).

Retroperitoneal abscess

Risk factors: Direct extension of pyelonephritis, spinal osteomyelitis, other intra-abdominal sepsis, traumatic haemorrhage, bacteraemia.

Clinical features: Fever, abdominal pain, flank and lumbar pain. A palpable mass may be present. If extension into the psoas sheath has occurred there may be pain on hip flexion.

Organisms: *Staphylococcus aureus* often with a history of cutaneous infection. Coliforms, particularly if secondary to pyelonephritis. Less often mixed infections including anaerobes. See also vertebral osteomyelitis (➤98). Rarely *Mycobacterium tuberculosis*.

Microbiological investigations: Culture of blood and pus.

Other investigations: Plain X-ray, CT and radionuclear white cell scan.

Antibiotic management: Benzylpenicillin + gentamicin + metronidazole **or** cefotaxime + metronidazole, depending on risk factors and guided by microbiology.

Supportive management: Surgical drainage.

5: Kidney and Urinary Tract Infections

Urinary tract infection (UTI)

UTI covers a spectrum of illness from asymptomatic bacteriuria to acute pyelonephritis (APN) with Gram-negative bacteraemia. **Cystitis** or lower UTI describes a superficial mucosal infection confined to the lower urinary tract (UT). **APN** is due to infection and inflammation of the renal parenchyma. **Chronic pyelonephritis** (CPN) is a histological pattern of diffuse interstitial inflammation due to many causes, some of them infective. It follows acute pyelonephritis in childhood, particularly in association with vesicoureteric reflux (VUR).

UTI is classified into uncomplicated (acute cystitis in females) and complicated (UTI with APN in females, all UTIs in males). Special cases include children, UTI during pregnancy and catheter-associated infections.

Community-acquired UTI usually results from ascending infection following colonisation of the vagina, periurethral area and anterior urethra by uropathogenic bacteria.

Risk factors: Risk factors vary with age
- Neonates–1 year: functional or anatomical abnormalities of the UT (e.g. congenital stenosis, urethral valves).
- Aged 1–15 years: infection more common in girls, particularly associated with VUR. Infection during first 5 years is associated with VUR or congenital abnormalities and gives rise to renal scarring and subsequent risk of CPN.
- Aged 16–35 years: risk of infection increases in females, associated with sexual intercourse. Diaphragm and spermicide use convey higher risk.
- After 35 years the sex incidence starts to equalise—risk factors include gynaecological surgery and bladder prolapse in women, prostatic hypertrophy and chronic prostatitis in men, and UT stones, tumours and catheter use in both sexes.
- Prolonged recumbency, catheter use, dehydration and antibiotic use, which promotes introital colonisation and cross-infection by uropathogenic strains, increase the risk of UTI for hospital inpatients.

UTI is normally prevented by mucosal defences (e.g. secreted proteins which prevent bacterial adhesion), the composition of the urine (low pH, high urea, high osmolarity) and mechanical factors (e.g. regular complete emptying of the bladder).

Clinical features: Adults: Dysuria, urgency, frequency, low-grade fever, suprapubic discomfort and cloudy, bloodstained urine. Flank pain and tenderness with rigors and vomiting suggest APN, but lack of these clinical features does not reliably exclude it. **Young children** present more non-specifically with fever, abdominal pain, vomiting and poor feeding. **Infection in neonates** presents as failure to thrive, vomiting, fever and jaundice and is frequently associated with bacteraemia. **UTI in the very elderly** is common and often presents non-specifically with nocturia, incontinence or confusion.

Organisms: *Escherichia coli* (80%)—a limited range of *E. coli* serogroups which have surface molecules that allow them to adhere to UT epithelium ('adhesins') are 'uropathogenic', accounting for most UTIs (➤189). Other coliforms such as *Klebsiella* spp., *Proteus* spp., *Enterobacter* spp. are isolated less often but are more likely to be antibiotic-resistant. *Staphylococcus saprophyticus* is a relatively common cause of uncomplicated UTI in young women. Hospital infections (particularly catheter-associated or in patients on antibiotics) are associated with a wider range of organisms including *Pseudomonas aeruginosa*, *Staphylococcus epidermidis*, yeasts and *Enterococcus* spp. *Staphylococcus aureus* bacteriuria suggests haematogenous seeding of the kidney from infection elsewhere. Adenovirus infection is a rare cause of epidemic haemorrhagic cystitis in children.

Microbiological investigations: It is good practice to send a midstream urine (MSU) for microscopy and culture in all patients before starting therapy. Some question the cost-effectiveness of this in uncomplicated UTI, but the incidence of ampicillin resistance in community-acquired *Escherichia coli* is now >30%. Dipsticks are useful screens if results are positive, but all miss ~25% true positives.

Interpreting the results of MSU: Epithelial cells suggest contamination of the specimen by skin organisms. Pus cells are usually present in UTI. Their absence favours contamination. Pyuria without bacterial growth occurs following previous antibiotics or with tumour, stones, urethritis or tuberculosis. A bacterial count of $>10^5$ organisms/ml is considered to indicate UTI, but many patients with clinical evidence of infection have lower counts. Some authorities consider counts over 10^2 organisms/ml significant if they represent a pure growth of a known urinary pathogen, but few laboratories perform urine cultures to detect this low level. Suprapubic puncture is rarely used, but is useful if an aseptically taken specimen is essential, and any growth is significant. Blood cultures should be taken if systemic infection is a possibility.

Other investigations: Urological assessment (ultrasound scan, in the first instance, followed by IVP) for **stones, tumours** and **anatomical abnormalities** should be carried out in recurrent uncomplicated UTI, all complicated UTIs and in all children and infants. Rectal examination is required in men.

Differential diagnosis: Urethritis is suggested by pyuria without bacteriuria. Historical clues include a change of sexual partner, gradual onset of relatively mild dysuria, urethral or vaginal discharge and associated cervicitis (➤66). Candidal or bacterial vaginitis often causes burning 'external' dysuria. Genitourinary tuberculosis should be considered, especially in the elderly and in immigrants.

Antibiotic management: All symptomatic UTIs should be treated. For **uncomplicated UTI** a large range of oral antibiotics is available: trimethoprim, co-amoxiclav, oral cephalosporin (e.g. cephalexin), norfloxacin or ciprofloxacin. Amoxicillin is less suitable due

to >30% resistance rates. Single-dose oral therapy (SDT) with co-amoxiclav (500/125 mg), norfloxacin (400 mg), co-trimoxazole (1920 mg) or trimethoprim (400 mg) is slightly less effective than treatment for 7 days but has a lower incidence of side-effects. Three-day treatment regimens are as effective as 7-day schedules with no more side-effects than SDT, and these are recommended for uncomplicated UTI, when there is no suggestion of upper tract involvement, or complications such as pregnancy. Short-course therapy is not suitable for children. For **complicated UTI** 7–14 days' treatment is recommended (APN: 14 days). In **severe illness**, intravenous therapy is required initially. Amoxicillin + gentamicin **or** co-amoxiclav **or** cefotaxime **or** ciprofloxacin is suitable whilst awaiting the results of urine and blood cultures.

Supportive management: Patients should drink as much fluid as possible. Intravenous rehydration is necessary if vomiting and dehydration are prominent symptoms.

Complications: Renal abscess, bacteraemia with sepsis syndrome.

Asymptomatic bacteriuria

Pregnant women should be screened for bacteriuria at booking and treated if two MSUs are positive, since UTI is common during pregnancy, often develops into APN (~30%) and may result in prematurity and fetal loss. Amoxicillin, cephalexin and nitrofurantoin are safe. **Avoid** tetracyclines (dental discoloration), fluoroquinolones (possible foetal arthropathy) and trimethoprim (risk of teratogenicity) during pregnancy, and sulphonamides (risk of neonatal jaundice) during the last trimester. There is little evidence that treating adults, including the elderly, with asymptomatic bacteriuria is beneficial except in patients with neutropenia or immunosuppression. Children should be treated with antibiotics and investigated for UT abnormality.

Catheter-associated UTI

The risk of bacteriuria with an indwelling catheter is proportional to duration since insertion, and is reduced by careful asepsis during insertion and maintenance of a closed system of drainage. Infection is often asymptomatic, but is the commonest cause of hospital-acquired Gram-negative bacteraemia. Scrupulous aseptic technique at insertion is essential. Many recommend a single dose of intravenous gentamicin at catheterisation. Asymptomatic catheter UTI should not be treated. If infection is symptomatic, it is unlikely to be eradicated by antibiotics whilst the catheter remains *in situ*. Try to remove the catheter, begin treatment and then recatheterise if necessary. Antiseptic or antibiotic irrigation is of no benefit.

Acute urethral syndrome (AUS)

This describes acute dysuria and frequency in women whose MSU is sterile or contains only low bacterial counts. Vaginitis and sexually transmitted causes of urethritis should be excluded. Most women with this syndrome have acute bacterial urethrocystitis, and are treated with antibiotics as above.

Recurrent UTI

Many women have occasional attacks of cystitis, but some have frequent recurrences (e.g. more than twice/year). Patients with recurrent UTI require urological evaluation for UT abnormality, but in the majority none will be found. Risk factors such as diaphragm and spermicide use should be avoided, and patients should void after sexual intercourse. Successful regimens for antibiotic prophylaxis include continuous low-dose therapy (e.g. trimethoprim 100 mg 24-hly, co-trimoxazole 460 mg 24-hly, cephalexin 250 mg 24-hly or norfloxacin 400 mg 24-hly), self-administered single-dose therapy or post-coital single-dose prophylaxis.

Acute bacterial prostatitis

Risk factors: Usually none; may follow urethral instrumentation or surgery.

Clinical features: Fever, perineal pain, symptoms of UTI. Rectal examination reveals a swollen, tender prostate. Patients are often very unwell, with bacteraemia and Gram-negative sepsis.

Organisms: Coliforms including *Escherichia coli* (25%), less often *Pseudomonas aeruginosa*, *Enterococcus* spp.

Microbiological investigations: MSU: pyuria and bacteriuria are usually present. Blood cultures if unwell. Results of urine culture should guide antibiotic therapy; prostatic massage is **not** required.

Antibiotic   management: Trimethoprim   or ciprofloxacin. Parenteral or broad-spectrum cephalosporin (e.g. cefotaxime) or ciprofloxacin if bacteraemic. Antibiotics should be given for 4 weeks to prevent relapse.

Complications: Prostatic abscess which may rupture spontaneously into the urethra or more rarely the rectum. Urological advice should be sought at the onset of treatment ☎.

Chronic prostatitis

This is a difficult diagnosis to make; urological opinion should be sought. The prostate may serve as a reservoir of infection resulting in recurrent UTI. **Prostatic localisation studies** involve collecting urine samples before and after prostatic massage. Expressed prostatic secretions are also collected and quantitative bacterial culture is used to determine the likelihood of persistent bacterial prostatitis. There is rarely a history of acute prostatitis. Some patients complain of perineal or low back pain and may have difficulty voiding. The prostate is sometimes tender on palpation. Chronic prostatitis may follow chlamydial urethritis (➤66) and treatment with doxycycline for 4 weeks helps some patients.

Epididymitis

Inflammation of the epididymis is acquired via ascending infection from the urethra, particularly if the urethra is instrumented in the presence of bacteriuria. Pain, fever and swelling of the epididymis are present sometimes with symptoms of concurrent UTI or urethritis. In sexually active men, infection follows urethritis due to chlamydiae or *Neisseria gonorrhoeas*, which should be treated appropriately (➤65). Non-sexually transmitted epididymitis is caused by coliforms, *Enterococcus* spp. and occasionally *Staphylococcus* spp. or *Streptococcus* spp. Non-sexually acquired infection should be treated with trimethoprim or norfloxacin for 2 weeks.

Orchitis

Orchitis is usually viral, associated in particular with mumps (➤102). Pyogenic orchitis usually arises as a complication of epididymitis, due to the same organisms. Parenteral antibiotics are required and urgent urological advice should be sought, in particular to exclude testicular torsion.

Intrarenal and perinephric abscess

Risk factors: Renal cortical abscesses: haematogenous spread of (most commonly) *Staphylococcus aureus*, usually from a skin infection. IVDU, diabetes mellitus and haemodialysis predispose. **Corticomedullary abscesses:** ascending infection usually secondary to UT abnormality, especially calculi and obstruction in adults and vesicoureteric reflux in children.

Clinical features: Onset is characteristically insidious. Fever, rigors and flank pain. There may be renal angle tenderness with a flank bulge or kyphosis. Corticomedullary abscess is usually associated with nausea and vomiting and urinary symptoms, but these are usually absent in cortical abscess, which rarely communicates with the lower UT.

Organisms: *Staphylococcus aureus* (cortical abscess); coliforms, in particular *Escherichia coli* and *Proteus* spp. (corticomedullary abscess).

Microbiological investigations: MSU (often normal in cortical abscess). Blood culture. Culture of aspirated pus.

Other investigations: Ultrasound and/or CT scan are required to localise the abscess, and may be used to guide aspiration or percutaneous drain insertion.

Differential diagnosis: Renal carcinoma.

Antibiotic management: For staphylococcal cortical abscess, high-dose flucloxacillin (2 g 6-hly, iv) for 2 weeks (± iv gentamicin or oral fucidin), followed by 2 weeks of oral flucloxacillin. For corticomedullary abscess, benzylpenicillin + gentamicin initially. Guided thereafter by the results of cultures.

Supportive management: Smaller abscesses are treated with antibiotics alone, but large abscesses or those that fail to respond after 2–4

days' therapy with appropriate antibiotics will require drainage (often percutaneous). Obstruction should be relieved if present.

Complications: Rupture through the renal capsule leads to **perinephric abscess.** Onset is often insidious with symptoms as above; extension towards the diaphragm causes pleuritic pain and raised fixed hemidiaphragm with pleural effusion. There may be signs of psoas irritation with scoliosis and pain on hip flexion. Drainage is always required.

Prolonged severe infection, particularly with *Proteus* spp., and obstruction may lead to **xanthogranulomatous pyelonephritis.** The renal pelvis is dilated, often with a staghorn calculus. There may be an abscess cavity, and the surrounding tissue is replaced by a yellow zone, histology of which shows macrophages laden with cholesterol and lipid material. Nephrectomy is usually required.

> **Practice point:** Urine culture positive for *Staphylococcus aureus* in patients who have not been catheterised suggests previous staphylococcal bacteraemia and possible secondary renal abscess.

Gynaecological and obstetric infections

Normal flora of the vagina and cervix include non-sporing anaerobes (not *Bacteroides fragilis* group), lactobacilli, *Staphylococcus epidermidis*, diphtheroids and less commonly coliforms, *Enterococcus* spp., *Candida* spp., Gp B β-haemolytic streptococci and *Staphylococcus aureus*. The composition of this flora changes before and after puberty and the menopause, and during the menstrual cycle. Use of antibiotics favours an increase in coliforms and *Candida* spp. and a decrease in lactobacilli.

Vulvovaginal candidiasis

Risk factors: Pregnancy, diabetes mellitus, oral contraceptive pill, antibiotics, immunosupression (e.g. therapeutic or HIV-related ➤121).

Clinical features: Pruritus, 'external' dysuria and

dyspareunia, vaginal discharge. On examination, vulval erythema and excoriation and a thick white cheesy discharge.

Organisms: *Candida albicans* (➤291), rarely other *Candida* spp.

Microbiological investigations: Gram stain and culture of high vaginal swab (HVS). As *Candida albicans* is a frequent commensal (10% of asymptomatic women), diagnosis depends on the association of positive culture result with appropriate history and clinical findings.

Differential diagnosis: Trichomoniasis (➤70), bacterial vaginosis (➤70).

Antibiotic management: Clotrimazole, econazole and miconazole are all available in a variety of topical preparations, including single-dose pessaries. Nystatin is an alternative. In severe cases or in the immunocompromised, oral fluconazole is required.

Comments: Chronic recurrent candidiasis is probably due to failure of eradication of infection during treatment of acute attacks. Recurrences should be treated for longer than usual or with a course of oral fluconazole, to abolish gut colonisation, which may act as a reservoir. Reinfection from a partner is likely—20% of male partners have penile colonisation and topical therapy is recommended. Rarely prolonged suppressive therapy with ketoconazole (100 mg 24-hly) is necessary.

Practice point: Some topical vaginal preparations may damage condoms and diaphragms. Up-to-date information is available in manafacturer's data sheets or the BNF.

Puerperal infection

Endometrial infection following delivery.

Risk factors: Caesarean section is associated with a greatly increased risk. Other factors include prolonged labour and prolonged rupture of membranes.

Clinical features: Fever, uterine tenderness, foul lochia, leucocytosis. Malaise, abdominal pain and rigors.

Organisms: Mixed aerobic and anaerobic genital flora including coliforms, *Streptococcus*

'milleri', *Enterococcus* spp., Gp B β-haemolytic streptococci, anaerobic streptococci, *Bacteroides* spp., *Gardnerella vaginalis*, genital *Mycoplasma* spp., *Clostridium* spp.

Microbiological investigations: Culture of lochia and blood.

Differential diagnosis: Pyelonephritis, UTI, wound infection.

Antibiotic management: Benzylpenicillin + gentamicin + metronidazole **or** cefotaxime + metronidazole **or** oral co-amoxiclav.

Complications: Pelvic abscess formation. Sepsis syndrome (➤158). **Septic pelvic thrombophlebitis** is an uncommon but important complication. It is due to mixed aerobic and anaerobic flora, but in particular *Bacteroides* spp. It presents in two ways. Ovarian vein thrombosis presents with acute onset of severe abdominal pain and signs of peritonism. There is a palpable abdominal mass in 50% of cases. In other patients onset is gradual, with spiking fevers that are unresponsive to antibiotics. Septic pulmonary embolism (➤28) is a rare serious complication. Venography and CT scanning are required. Treatment comprises antibiotic therapy as above, with heparinization and consideration of surgical intervention.

Infected abortion

Infection is associated with illegal and occasionally therapeutic abortion. The history of illegal or attempted abortion may not be obtained and the diagnosis should be considered in any febrile woman with vaginal bleeding during the first half of pregnancy.

Risk factors: Incomplete removal of the products of conception. Uterine perforation. Pre-existing untreated infection with *Neisseria gonorrhoeae* or *Chlamydia trachomatis*.

Clinical features: Fever, rigors, abdominal pain, pelvic tenderness, history of passage of products of conception. On examination there may be a tender enlarged uterus, foul cervical discharge and open os with evidence of passage of products of conception or instrumentation. Uterine perforation with pelvic abscess or peritonitis are now uncommon.

Organisms: As for puerperal infection. Clostridial infection ('uterine gas gangrene') may sometimes cause full-blown clostridial septicaemia with haemolysis, jaundice, shock, renal failure and disseminated intravascular coagulation (➤159).

Microbiological investigations: Gram stain and culture of discharge. Blood cultures.

Other investigations: Imaging, usually ultrasound, to define pelvic abscess.

Antibiotic management: Benzylpenicillin + gentamicin + metronidazole **or** cefotaxime + metronidazole **or** oral co-amoxiclav.

Supportive management: Removal of remaining products of conception and exclusion of uterine perforation.

Complications: See puerperal infection (➤62).

Intra-amniotic infection

Amniotic fluid infection usually follows rupture of the membranes, although it also occurs as a complication of instrumentation, e.g. amniocentesis.

Clinical features: Fever, maternal and foetal tachycardia, uterine tenderness, malodorous amniotic fluid.

Organisms: As for puerperal infection.

Microbiological investigations: Culture of amniotic fluid and blood.

Antibiotic management: Benzylpenicillin + gentamicin + metronidazole **or** cefotaxime + metronidazole.

Supportive management: Prompt delivery is required. Antibiotics should be given immediately the clinical diagnosis is made.

> **Practice point:** Certain vaginal infections are suspected of causing premature rupture of membranes (e.g. bacterial vaginosis ➤70, heavy colonisation with Gp B β-haemolytic streptococci ➤173); appropriate treatment may prevent this complication.

Bartholinitis

Infection of Bartholin's glands presents as a localised abscess or as cellulitis of the surrounding skin. Infection is usually due to mixed genital flora (➤61); *Neisseria gonorrhoeae* is a rarer

cause which must be excluded by Gram stain and culture (including endocervical, rectal and throat swabs). For localised abscess, surgical incision and drainage is required. For cellulitis, co-amoxiclav **or** amoxycillin + metronidazole is given. For severe infection give benzylpenicillin + gentamicin + metronidazole **or** cefotaxime + metronidazole.

Toxic shock syndrome (TSS)

TSS is caused by toxic shock syndrome toxin-1 (TSST-1) produced by some strains of *Staphylococcus aureus*.

Risk factors: Most cases are associated with tampon use in menstruating women, but TSS can complicate any focal staphylococcal infection. Menstrual cases have been reported in women who have not used tampons; non-menstrual cases have occurred secondary to surgical wound infection, nasal packing, postpartum, due to infection of intrauterine contraceptive devices and in association with postinfluenzal staphylococcal pneumonia (➤25). The incidence of menstrual cases has fallen dramatically since the withdrawal of high-absorbency tampons. Σ ~18.

Clinical features: Diagnosis is clinical, since *Staphylococcus aureus* is not always isolated. Diagnostic criteria have been established to allow recognition and surveillance. Patients should have **all** of the following: fever (≥38.9°C); diffuse macular rash, which should desquamate 1–2 weeks after the onset of illness; hypotension (SBP ≤90 mmHg); **plus** at least **three** of the following categories of multiorgan involvement: (i) vomiting or diarrhoea; (ii) severe myalgia with elevated creatine phosphokinase (≥2 × normal); (iii) mucous hyperaemia affecting vagina, oropharynx or conjunctiva; (iv) renal failure (creatinine ≥2 × normal) or pyuria in the absence of UTI; (v) abnormal liver function tests; (vi) thrombocytopenia (≤100 × 10⁹/l); (vii) disorientation or altered conscious level without focal neurological signs.

Organisms: *Staphylococcus aureus*. A similar illness is rarely caused by exotoxin-producing β-haemolytic streptococci.

Microbiological investigations: Culture of blood,

vagina, nose, urine and, if there is doubt about the diagnosis, CSF are required, in particular to exclude other infections such as meningococcaemia (➤74).

Differential diagnosis: Meningococcaemia, scarlet fever (➤108), Gram-negative bacteraemia (➤158), Kawasaki's disease (➤154).

Antibiotic management: Antibiotics do not modify the course of the illness, which is toxin-mediated, but they prevent relapse. Supportive management is most important. Flucloxacillin (1 g 6-hly) should be given iv for a week, then orally for another week. If meningococcaemia cannot be excluded, then give cefotaxime instead.

Supportive management: Fluid replacement and monitoring, pressor agents and other intensive care therapies may be required (➤160).

6: Sexually Transmitted Diseases (STDs)

Sexual contact is critical to the transmission of all the conditions described in this section, although it is not necessarily the only route of acquisition. There are certain important concepts unique to management of STDs.

• STDs are diseases of lifestyle. The risk of transmission is related primarily to number of partners, and the same risk factors apply for most STDs. These include frequency of partner change, lower socio-economic status and non-barrier contraception.

• Patients with one STD are therefore likely to have others. All patients should be evaluated for multiple STDs including urethritis and syphilis. It may also be appropriate to discuss the need for serological testing for HIV infection.

• Contact tracing is very important. Since many STDs are asymptomatic and/or difficult to exclude clinically, it is often appropriate to treat asymptomatic contacts presumptively.

• Patients attending STD clinics are drawn predominantly from less advantaged socio-economic groups, and frequently reattend with newly acquired infections. Clinic attendance is an opportunity for discussion and education about risk reduction, contraception and other matters of sexual health, and allows provision of services such as cervical smear testing to groups who are otherwise unlikely to have contact with health services.

Gonorrhoea

Epidemiology: Common worldwide. Risk factors as above. Σ 61 per 100 000 population (1990). Σ 300 β-lactamase-producing isolates.

Clinical features: *Neisseria gonorrhoeae* causes mucosal infection of the urethra, cervix, rectum, conjunctiva and pharynx. Asymptomatic infection is common at all sites. Symptomatic infection in males causes urethritis with copious purulent urethral discharge and dysuria, after an incubation period of 2–5 days. Local complications include epididymitis (➤60) and rarely periurethral abscess. Infection in women is usually a cervicitis, which can be asymptomatic or cause discharge, dysuria and itching. Concurrent urethritis and proctitis is usual. Infection of Bartholin and Skene glands may occur (➤63). Infection of the vaginal epithelium occurs in prepubertal girls. Anorectal infection occurs in women and especially in homosexual men, but is unusual in heterosexual males. It is usually asymptomatic, but if not there is discharge, pain and tenesmus. Ophthalmia neonatorum (➤83) and disseminated infection both occur in neonates.

Organisms: *Neisseria gonorrhoeae* (➤206).

Microbiological investigations: Gram stain and culture of material from urethra, endocervix, rectum or pharynx. Organisms appear as Gram-negative intracellular diplococci. Sensitivity to penicillin should always be tested, as penicillinase-producing *Neisseria gonorrhoeae* remain prevalent. Screening for other STDs, in particular syphilis, is routine.

Differential diagnosis: Chlamydial and other causes of non-specific urethritis (NSU). Vaginal candidiasis, trichomoniasis and bacterial vaginosis.

Antibiotic management: β-Lactamase-producing strains appeared in 1976, and remain largely associated with contacts from the Far East and Africa. **Drugs of choice in the UK** remain single-dose oral ampicillin (3.5 g) or amoxycillin (3.0 g) **plus** probenecid (1 g). For known or suspected resistance or in penicillin allergy, use **single-dose oral** ciprofloxacin, cefuroxime axetil + probenecid, or **parenteral** cefotaxime, ceftriaxone (single-dose 250 mg im) or spectinomycin. Oral ampicillin/amoxycillin is less effective for pharyngeal or rectal gonorrhoea, for which ciprofloxacin or a parenteral or broad-spectrum cephalosporin should be given. Many physicians treat all patients with gonorrhoea for possible concomitant chlamydial infection (e.g. ceftriaxone, single dose, plus doxycycline for 1 week). Screening/treatment of sexual partners is essential.

Complications: Pelvic inflammatory disease (>71). **Disseminated gonococcal infection (DGI)** occurs in 1–2% of untreated cases, causing bacteraemia with a pustular rash and asymmetrical polyarthritis affecting mainly hands, wrists, ankles and knees (>95). Endocarditis and meningitis occur very rarely.

Chlamydial infections

Epidemiology: Very common worldwide. Risk factors as other STDs (>65). Σ 30 000 lab reports of genital chlamydial infection; 80 000 cases of non-gonococcal urethritis.

Clinical features: Infection is very commonly asymptomatic, particularly in women (≤ 70%). Untreated infection can persist for many years. Symptomatic infection in men causes urethritis with dysuria and mucopurulent discharge, usually less copious than in gonorrhoea. Epididymitis may follow. In women, mucopurulent cervicitis with discharge and associated urethritis. Proctitis and pharyngitis occur in either sex. Chlamydial urethritis can be prolonged or present as apparent treatment failure after confirmed gonorrhoea ('postgonococcal urethritis'). Conjunctivitis (>83) and pneumonia (>113) occur in infants born to infected mothers.

Organisms: *Chlamydia trachomatis*, trachoma biovar, serovars D–K (>233).

Microbiological investigations: Culture is difficult and diagnosis depends on indirect evidence such as the presence of pus cells on Gram stain of urethral smear, or purulent exudate in first-catch urine ('two-glass test'), or on direct evidence from rapid diagnostic tests (e.g. immunofluorescence or ELISA) which demonstrate the presence of chlamydial antigens in genital secretions.

Differential diagnosis: Gonococcal urethritis (>65). Non-specific urethritis may also be caused by *Ureaplasma urealyticum* (>233). Genital Herpes simplex (see below) may cause urethritis, with severe dysuria but little discharge. *Trichomonas vaginalis* (>70) infection in men may cause urethritis, but is usually asymptomatic.

Antibiotic management: Tetracycline **or** erythromycin for 1 week. Longer duration of therapy is required for conjunctivitis and for pneumonia in infants. In contrast to tetracycline, erythromycin is safe in pregnancy, and is effective against *Ureaplasma urealyticum*. Azithromycin (single 1 g dose) is also effective.

Complications: Pelvic inflammatory disease (>71). Reiter's disease (>96). Perihepatitis (Fitz-Hugh–Curtis syndrome). Conjunctivitis (>83).

Comments: Recurrent disease is usually due to reinfection, often because of inadequate treatment of sexual partners. Since infection in women is usually asymptomatic, female partners of men with NSU should be treated whether or not there is clinical evidence of infection. Failure to respond to tetracycline suggests infection with *Ureaplasma urealyticum* or *Trichomonas vaginalis*, and metronidazole and erythromycin may be required. In male patients it is common to see an initial response to therapy followed by symptomatic relapse, in the absence of persistent polymorphonuclear exudate in the urethral smear. Many such patients benefit from prolonged (3–6 weeks) therapy with tetracycline or even long-term suppressive therapy, but complications and infection of sexual partners are rare in this context.

Genital herpes

Primary Herpes simplex virus (HSV) infection is followed by latent infection of sacral ganglia, and subsequent reactivation, which is either subclinical or symptomatic.

Epidemiology: Infection is common worldwide. The incidence has increased in recent decades in the UK, as a result of changes in sexual behaviour and a reduction in childhood infection by HSV-1. Severity of HSV-2 infection is reduced by prior exposure to HSV-1 and vice versa.

Clinical features: The incubation period is 3–7 days (range 1–14 or more days), although ≥ 60% of primary infections are asymptomatic. Subclinical reactivation and viral shedding occur more frequently than overt recurrent disease. The **first clinical attack of genital herpes** may therefore be due to primary infection, or may represent a first reactivation episode ('initial non-primary herpes'). First attacks, whether primary or initial non-primary, are more severe than recurrences. Local burning and tenderness are followed by a vesicular eruption, usually bilateral. In moist areas the vesicles rupture, leaving shallow, very tender ulcers. In drier areas vesicles often remain intact to develop into pustules and scabs. New lesions continue to appear for about 1 week. In men the glans penis, prepuce and shaft of the penis are usually involved. Lesions occur less frequently on the scrotum and thighs. In women lesions form initially on the external genitalia and vulva, but the cervix is usually subsequently involved and there is usually a watery vaginal discharge. Urethritis and dysuria occur in both sexes. Constitutional symptoms and local lymphadenopathy are usual. Resolution occurs over 1–3 weeks. Herpetic proctitis, with rectal discharge, pain, tenesmus and sometimes urinary retention, occurs in both sexes.

One or more **recurrent attacks** are experienced by 60–80% of patients during the first year after the first episode. Recurrences are less severe and of shorter duration, and constitutional symptoms, lymphadenopathy and urethritis are unusual. Frequent and severe recurrent infection occurs in immuno-compromised patients (➤131). HIV patients may develop chronic anal ulceration (➤121).

Organisms: Herpes simplex virus type 2, and, less often, type 1 (➤241).

Microbiological investigations: Culture of virus from lesions. Serology is often unhelpful, as it does not reliably distinguish between types 1 and 2. Rapid diagnostic methods for demonstration of viral antigens are available.

Differential diagnosis: Other causes of genital ulceration, in particular syphilis and, in the tropics, chancroid, lymphogranuloma venereum and granuloma inguinale (➤71). Dark-ground examination of material from lesions may be indicated. Less common causes of genital ulceration include Behçet's disease, Herpes zoster, candidiasis and impetigo.

Specific management: Systemic (oral or iv) acyclovir (ACV) effectively shortens the duration of first attacks. Treatment should commence as soon as possible for maximum benefit. Systemic ACV is of marginal benefit in recurrent attacks, and topical ACV is not effective. ACV is effective in the treatment and prophylaxis of herpes infection in immunocompromised patients (➤242), and in immunocompetent individuals with very frequent recurrences (e.g. 400 mg 12-hly). Intravenous ACV is indicated for severe, disseminated or neonatal infection (➤242). ACV does not prevent the establishment of latent infection.

Complications: Neonatal infection (➤242). Bacterial and candidal superinfection occur rarely. Herpetic whitlow (➤93). Viral meningitis may complicate first attacks of genital herpes (➤77). Severe disseminated infection occurs rarely in the immunocompetent (➤242).

Syphilis

Risk factors: As for other STDs (➤65).

Epidemiology: Common worldwide. Concurrent HIV infection alters the course of infection, with more frequent and rapid onset of neurological disease, and treatment failures with standard antibiotic regimens.

Transmission: By sexual contact and vertically. Very rarely by blood transfusion. *Treponema pallidum* cannot penetrate intact skin, but infection may occur through macroscopically invisible cuts and abrasions.

Clinical features: Primary syphilis: 14–20 days (range 10–90) after inoculation a red painless **papule** develops and ulcerates to form a **chancre**, usually 0.5–2 cm in diameter, painless with a clean base and an indurated edge. Moderate bilateral local lymphadenopathy is usual. Chancres are usually located on penis, fourchette or cervix, but may be anywhere, e.g. mouth, hands, anus and rectum. Multiple chancres are sometimes seen. Spontaneous resolution occurs after 3–8 weeks.

Secondary syphilis follows systemic dissemination of organisms from the chancre. A generalised symmetrical scaly papular **rash** develops 4–10 weeks after the development of the chancre. This involves trunk and extremities including palms and soles. The papules may be smooth, pustular or itchy. Mucosal ulcers are common. **Condylomata lata** are raised grey-white lesions found in warm moist areas. Unlike the rash, they are highly contagious. Malaise, fever, sore throat, lymphadenopathy and myalgia are common, sometimes with subclinical hepatitis and periostitis. **Neurological disease** may rarely present during the secondary stage ('early neurosyphilis') with meningitis, headache, cranial nerve lesions, intranuclear ophthalmoplegia, cerebrovascular accident or signs of spinal cord involvement. Early neurosyphilis is more common in patients coinfected with HIV. Iritis, arthritis and glomerulonephritis occur infrequently. Spontaneous resolution occurs after 3–12 weeks, after which patients are said to have entered **latency**. Without treatment, 25% have recrudescence of secondary disease during the first year of latency.

After a variable latent period (2–20 years) **tertiary syphilis** (late benign syphilis, visceral syphilis, cardiovascular syphilis or neurosyphilis) develops in a minority of patients. **Late benign syphilis** describes the development of large granulomatous lesions ('gummata'), in skin and soft tissues, particularly on the head, neck and arms. Gummata may be indurated, nodular or ulcerated. **Visceral syphilis** describes the development of gummata in the viscera and bones. Lesions affecting the palate, pharynx, nasal septum or tongue can be locally destructive. Bony lesions are particularly painful. Other organs that can be involved include liver, testis, eye, stomach and, rarely, lungs. **Cardiovascular syphilis** affects the aorta and is due to endarteritis of the vasa vasorum. Aortic regurgitation occurs more commonly than aneurysm and presents with angina and dyspnoea secondary to left ventricular failure. Aneurysm typically affects the ascending aorta, and may involve the ostia of the coronary arteries. The arch and descending aorta are less frequently affected. VDRL may be negative, suggesting that development of aneurysm is due to ongoing mechanical damage in a previously inflamed aorta. **Neurosyphilis** includes asymptomatic latent syphilis, in which the CSF is found to be abnormal, mening-ovascular syphilis, general paralysis of the insane (GPI) and tabes dorsalis. *Meningovascular syphilis* presents approximately 5 years after primary infection, either as a cerebral pachymeningitis with headaches, fits and limb paralysis, or more commonly as a chronic diffuse basal meningitis, causing headaches and isolated cranial nerve palsies. Mental changes, with memory impairment and poor concentration follow and in severe cases there are multiple cranial nerve palsies and severe mental deterioration, leading to stupor. Cerebral artery thrombosis can occur, leading to stroke. Meningovascular syphilis also affects the spinal cord, causing cervical myelopathy or hemiplegia. *GPI* describes severe cerebral atrophy developing 10–20 years after primary infection, with gradual onset of confusion, hallucinations, delusions, fits and severe cognitive deficit. On examination there are coarse tremors of the lips and tongue, brisk tendon reflexes and extensor plantars. *Tabes dorsalis* develops 15–35 years after primary infection. There is atrophy of the dorsal columns of the spinal cord below the cervical region, with autonomic neuropathy and cranial nerve lesions. Patients present with ataxia, sensory loss, lightning pains and sphincter disturbance. Classical signs on examination include sensory loss, areflexia and Argyll–Robertson pupils (irregular pupils that may constrict to accommodation but do not react to light).

Organisms: *Treponema pallidum* (➤223).

Microbiological investigations: Diagnosis of primary syphilis is confirmed by **dark-ground microscope examination** of material from the base of the chancre for spirochaetes. Two types of **serological tests** are used (Table 21). *Non-specific tests* include VDRL (Venereal Disease Reference Laboratory) and RPR (rapid plasma reagin). These tests are based on the original Wassermann reaction (WR) and detect antibodies against cardiolipin, which is found in mammalian cell membranes and is incorporated by the spirochaete into its outer membrane. False positive non-specific tests occur in a large number of conditions, including acute viral infections, connective tissue diseases, pregnancy and leprosy. The

Table 21 Serological tests for syphilis

Clinical situation	Non-specific serology (VDRL)	Specific serology (TPHA)
Primary syphilis*	Positive in ~75%	Positive in ~90%
Secondary syphilis	Positive at high titre in ~100%	Positive in ~100%
Latent infection	May remain positive. Titre falls with time and after treatment. Rise in titre suggests reinfection	Remains positive
Late benign syphilis	Usually strongly positive	Remains positive
Syphilitic aortitis	Positive in only 60% of cases	Remains positive
Late neurosyphilis†	May be negative or weakly positive	Remains positive

* Definitive diagnosis by dark-ground examination of chancre.
† CSF may show pleocytosis with raised protein and positive VDRL.

value of non-specific tests is that they fall in titre after successful treatment of syphilis. A reappearance or fourfold rise in titre of VDRL is regarded as evidence of relapse or reinfection. *Specific tests,* including fluorescent treponemal antigen tests (FTA and FTA-ABS) and *Treponema pallidum* haemagglutination assay (TPHA), use *Treponema pallidum* antigens as targets. They are specific for syphilis, but remain positive for life and are not useful for assessing success of treatment. Their value lies in confirming the diagnosis of primary syphilis, as they become positive before VDRL in this situation, and excluding syphilis in suspected secondary and tertiary disease. False positive reactions occur in Lyme disease (≻224) and other spirochaetal infections (≻223). Particular difficulty may be encountered in making the diagnosis of syphilis in patients with HIV (≻127).

Antibiotic management: Penicillin is the drug of choice. Procaine penicillin by daily im injection for 10 days, extended to 3 weeks if neurosyphilis is suspected on the basis of clinical signs or positive findings in CSF.

Complications: Jarisch–Herxheimer reaction is a hypersensitivity reaction precipitated by lysis of organisms. It occurs 1–6 hours after initiating treatment in many patients and comprises fever, rash, lymphadenopathy and hypotension.

Genital warts
(syn. condylomata acuminata)

Clinical features: After an incubation period of about 4–6 weeks, warts develop as small irregular papules around the external genitalia, in the perianal region and, less often, in the vagina, in the urethra and on the cervix. Subclinical infection of surrounding epithelium is the rule. On the cervix the presence of infected epithelium is demonstrated by the application of acetic acid, which turns infected areas white. Biopsy of aceto-white areas is indicated to confirm infection and exclude intraepithelial neoplasia.

Organisms: Infection by human papillomavirus (HPV) types 6 and 11 is associated with genital warts, whereas types 16, 18, 31, 33, 35 and others are associated with the development of cervical cancer (≻246).

Microbiological investigations: Viral culture is not possible. DNA hybridisation kits are available for determining which HPV type is present.

Differential diagnosis: Moles and skin tags. Syphilis (condylomata lata) (≻67), molluscum contagiosum (≻94).

Management: Specific antiviral therapy is not available; therapy is directed towards removal of warts and relief of symptoms. Caustic agents such as podophyllin or trichloracetic acid are effective in ~50% of cases but have a high rate of recurrence. Podophyllin is very irritant and excess topical application can lead to systemic toxicity with nausea, vomiting, lethargy and neuropathy. It is antimitotic and contraindicated in pregnancy and infancy. 5-Fluorouracil has a higher success rate but can be extremely irritating. Intralesional interferon is effective but is not yet in widespread use, not least due to its cost. Cryotherapy is widely used. Laser therapy is particularly useful for cervical lesions. If external warts are very numerous, surgical removal may be necessary.

Complications: Juvenile-onset respiratory papillomata are due to infection with HPVs causing mucosal warts, probably acquired intrapartum from the maternal genital tract.

Trichomoniasis

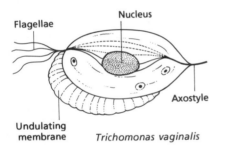

Trichomonas vaginalis

Labels: Flagellae, Nucleus, Axostyle, Undulating membrane

Transmission occurs by sexual contact. Although *Trichomonas vaginalis* can survive in urine on towels or clothing for several hours, non-sexual transmission is believed to be very rare. Symptoms are more likely to occur during pregnancy or menstruation when the vaginal pH is highest, as this favours parasite replication. $\Sigma > 6000$.

Clinical features: Infection in men is usually asymptomatic; there may be mild dysuria. Up to 50% of infected women are asymptomatic. Symptoms may develop after an incubation period of 1–4 weeks, with yellow vaginal discharge, frequently copious, frothy and offensive. Dysuria, dyspareunia, lower abdominal pain and vulval itching also occur. On examination there is erythema of the vaginal walls and cervix, which may be friable with punctate haemorrhages ('strawberry cervix').

Organisms: *Trichomonas vaginalis* (➤262).

Microbiological investigations: Microscopy (phase-contrast or dark-ground best) of wet preparation of vaginal discharge shows motile flagellated protozoa. Culture is also possible in liquid medium (Feinberg's). Organisms are also seen on fixed cervical smears examined cytologically.

Antibiotic management: Metronidazole (2 g single dose). Sexual partners should be treated. Asymptomatic patients should be treated, except during pregnancy, when metronidazole is relatively contraindicated. It may be given after the first trimester if symptoms are severe.

Differential diagnosis: Candidiasis (➤61), bacterial vaginosis, gonorrhoea (➤65), non-specific cervicitis (➤66).

Bacterial vaginosis

Gardnerella vaginalis is a vaginal commensal organism. Under certain circumstances it acts in synergy with commensal anaerobes to multiply and inhibit the growth of lactobacilli and other vaginal flora.

Clinical features: Many patients are asymptomatic. Mild vaginal discharge with a fishy odour and pruritis may occur. On examination there is little or no vaginal inflammation. Discharge is thin, grey and homogeneous. When potassium hydroxide is added a fishy odour is liberated ('whiff test').

Organisms: *Gardnerella vaginalis* is a vaginal commensal organism, so isolation by culture is not significant. Quantification and culture for anaerobes is not routinely practicable.

Microbiological investigations: Gram-stained microscopy of wet preparation characteristically shows 'clue cells'—squamous epithelial cells studded with *Gardnerella*. Diagnosis depends on the presence of three out of four of the following—positive whiff test, clue cells, characteristic vaginal discharge and vaginal pH > 5.0.

Differential diagnosis: Candidiasis (➤61), trichomoniasis (➤70), gonorrhoea (➤65), non-specific cervicitis (➤66).

Antibiotic management: Metronidazole (400 mg 8-hly for 1 week). Metronidazole is relatively contraindicated during pregnancy. Ampicillin is effective in some cases.

Complications: Bacterial vaginosis is associated with increased risk of premature labour, chorioamnionitis and puerperal sepsis. The value of treating asymptomatic pregnant women remains to be established.

Pelvic inflammatory disease (PID)
(syn. salpingitis)

PID complicates 10–15% of cases of gonococcal and chlamydial cervicitis. Damage caused by these organisms also facilitates entry of aerobic and anaerobic vaginal flora (➤61) into the Fallopian tube, so that many infections are polymicrobial.

Risk factors: Commonest in teenage girls with multiple sexual partners and non-barrier methods of contraception, especially intra-uterine device (IUD). Previous PID predisposes to further episodes.

Clinical features: Fever, pelvic pain, abdominal tenderness, adnexal and cervical tenderness, vaginal discharge. Symptoms do not correlate well with the presence of infection and the likelihood of subsequent complications

Organisms: *Neisseria gonorrhoeae*, *Chlamydia trachomatis*. Infection is often polymicrobial with mixed aerobic and anaerobic genital flora, including *Bacteroides* spp., *Escherichia coli*, *Gardnerella vaginalis*. *Mycoplasma hominis* and *Ureaplasma urealyticum* have also been implicated in PID.

Microbiological investigations: Microscopy and culture of endocervical swab is routine but, with the exception of *Neisseria gonorrhoea*, do not accurately reflect contents of Fallopian tube. Material from peritoneal cavity and tube obtained by laparoscopy is cultured if available.

Other investigations: In view of difficulty of diagnosis, leucocytosis and raised ESR may be helpful indicators of ongoing infection. Laparoscopy is frequently used to confirm diagnosis. Ultrasound is performed to examine for tubo-ovarian abscess.

Differential diagnosis: Ectopic pregnancy, appendicitis, ruptured or haemorrhagic ovarian cyst, endometriosis.

Antibiotic management: Admission for intravenous therapy is often required. Cover for aerobic and anaerobic organisms is recommended. Doxycycline + metronidazole **or** doxycycline + co-amoxiclav **or** cefotaxime + doxycycline are all effective. IUD should be removed after antibiotic therapy has commenced.

Complications: Infertility, chronic pelvic pain. **Tubo-ovarian abscess** (TOA) presents with similar symptoms to uncomplicated PID, and should be excluded by ultrasound (or CT) scan if patient is unwell or if symptoms fail to settle. Early gynaecological referral is essential as a ruptured TOA requires immediate surgery. Intravenous antibiotics should be given. Surgery may be required if there is no response after 72 hours or if clinical features suggest rupture. An adnexal mass > 8 cm in diameter is unlikely to respond to antibiotic therapy alone. Percutaneous laparoscopic drainage is sometimes employed as an alternative to laparotomy.

Tropical genital ulceration

The prevalence of genital ulceration in patients presenting with STDs is much higher in the developing world than in the UK. Whereas syphilis and herpes account for most genital ulcers in the developed world, chancroid is responsible for most tropical genital ulceration. This has recently acquired greater significance as it is now believed that genital ulceration is an important factor in the heterosexual transmission of HIV in Africa and Asia.

Chancroid (syn. soft sore)
Common throughout the tropics and subtropics.
Clinical features: Incubation period is ~1 week. Painful papules develop on external genitalia of both sexes and rapidly ulcerate. Ulcer is typically sloughy, irregular, painful, non-indurated and haemorrhagic. 'Kissing' lesions develop on adjacent skin surfaces such as scrotum or thigh. Cervical and vaginal wall ulcers are rare. Suppurative local lymphadenopathy is common, progressing to bubo and sinus formation. Local complications include phimosis and urethral stricture.

Organisms: *Haemophilus ducreyi* (➤205).
Microbiological investigations: Gram stain ('shoal of fish' appearance) and culture of material obtained from ulcer or aspirated from lymph nodes. Concurrent syphilis and gonorrhoea should be excluded.
Antibiotic management: Erythromycin **or** co-amoxiclav **or** ciprofloxacin for 1 week.
Supportive management: Aspiration of bubo.

Lymphogranuloma venereum (LGV)
LGV causes inconspicuous genital ulceration, followed by severe local sequelae. Clinical infection is much commoner in men than women. Asymptomatic infection in women serves as a reservoir. LGV occurs throughout the tropics.
Clinical features: Incubation period is 5–21 days. Primary lesion is an inconspicuous transient painless genital ulcer which heals without scarring and is recalled by ~20% of patients. Cervicitis is a common primary site. Extremely tender local lymphadenopathy then develops, with fever, headache, weight loss and sometimes meningoencephalitis, pneumonia, arthritis and erythema nodosum. Lymphadenopathy may be very marked, with cleavage of the inflammatory mass by the inguinal ligament (the 'groove' sign). Multiple abscesses with sinus formation followed by fibrosis of the sacral and iliac lymphatics leading to lymphoedema of the perineum. Other features include haemorrhagic proctitis with perirectal abscess, rectal stricture and fistula formation.
Organisms: *Chlamydia trachomatis* serovars L1, L2 and L3 (➤233).
Microbiological investigations: Diagnosis is based on clinical features. Serology for antichlamydial antibodies is also helpful. Immunofluorescent and ELISA antigen capture assays for chlamydial antigens are available but are not specific for LGV serovars. Culture is possible but not widely available in the countries where LGV occurs.
Antibiotic management: Tetracycline **or** erythromycin for 3 weeks.
Supportive management: Aspiration of lymph nodes may be required to avert sinus forma-tion but surgical debridement should be avoided.

Granuloma inguinale (syn. Donovaniasis)
Endemic in South India, Papua New Guinea and certain Caribbean islands. Non-sexual transmission also occurs; infection is common in children in endemic areas.
Clinical features: Painless, non-purulent, 'beefy-red' ulcer progressively enlarging over months to 5 cm or more in diameter, commonly on the prepuce or labia. Local extension, healing and fibrosis may all occur simultaneously. Secondary infection causes increased purulence and necrosis. Other cutaneous sites may be involved, often in patients who also have genital disease. Metastatic haematogenous spread to bones, joints and liver has been reported very rarely. Regional lymphadenopathy is rare.
Organisms: *Calymmatobacterium granulomatis* (➤203).
Microbiological investigations: Microscopy of Giemsa-stained material from ulcers shows bipolar intracellular bacteria, visible as 'Donovan bodies' with characteristic safety-pin appearance. Culture and serology are not available.
Antibiotic management: Tetracycline **or** erythromycin **or** co-trimoxazole for 3 weeks. Clinical resistance to tetracycline has been reported and if there is no response after 2 weeks' treatment an alternative agent should be given.

Pubic lice

Clinical features: Severe pruritus. One to 2 mm grey-brown lice and 0.5 mm ovoid nits attached to hair shafts may be visible. Tiny red dots on affected skin are due to louse excreta. Pubic, axillary, chest and abdominal hair and eyelashes may be infested (➤81).
Organisms: *Pthirus pubis.*
Management: Preparations containing lindane, carbaryl and malathion are effective. Lindane is contraindicated in pregnancy and childhood and in patients with low body weight or epilepsy. All hairy parts of the body should be

treated. Retreatment after 1 week is recommended.

Scabies ①

Scabies is acquired by any close contact, including household contact, as well as sexually.

Risk factors: Poor hygiene. Crowded housing. Sexual contact.

Clinical features: Incubation period is approximately 4 weeks. Severe pruritus. Infestation is usually confined to the interdigital areas and the flexor surfaces of the wrists, where papulovesicular lesions and scaly plaques may be seen. Classical linear burrows are often very difficult to see. Excoriation is usual. Other areas, including the genitalia, buttocks, thighs, breasts, belt line, umbilicus, feet, ankles, elbows and axillae, are often infested.

Organisms: *Sarcoptes scabiei.*

Microbiological investigations: Diagnosis is clinical, confirmed by microscopical demonstration of mites or eggs in skin scrapings.

Management: Lindane, malathion or permethrin preparations are effective. The whole body below the chin must be treated, paying particular attention to the finger webs and under the edges of the fingernails. Lindane is contraindicated in pregnancy and childhood and in patients with low body weight or epilepsy.

Complications: In immunosuppressed patients Norwegian scabies may develop. This is characterised by very heavy infestation with little or no itching. There is widespread keratosis and erythema, and these patients are highly infectious. Patients with HIV infection develop papulosquamous lesions along lines of skin cleavage.

7: CNS Infections

Bacterial meningitis ⊠

Infection and inflammation of the arachnoid and pia mater and the cerebrospinal fluid (CSF).
Risk factors and organisms: Most cases are caused by *Neisseria meningitidis*, *Streptococcus pneumoniae* and *Haemophilus influenzae* type b. Likely organisms vary depending on the age of the patient and a large number of risk factors.

Commonest organisms by **age-group:** **<1 month:** Gram-negative bacilli, Gp B β-haemolytic streptococci, *Listeria monocytogenes*; **1 month–5 years:** *Streptococcus pneumoniae*, *Neisseria meningitidis*, *Haemophilus influenzae* type b (becoming rarer since the introduction of Hib vaccine); **6–59 years:** *Streptococcus pneumoniae*, *Neisseria meningitidis*; **>59 years:** *Streptococcus pneumoniae*, Gram-negative bacilli, *Listeria monocytogenes*.

Other **specific risk factors** include the following. **Open cranial trauma:** coliforms, *Staphylococcus aureus*, pseudomonads. **Closed trauma** (e.g. with fracture into sinuses): *Streptococcus pneumoniae*, *Haemophilus influenzae* type b, polymicrobial meningitis, with coliforms and non-sporing anaerobes. **Meningitis following neurosurgery** may involve typical surgical pathogens such as *Staphylococcus aureus*, *Staphylococcus epidermidis* and coryneforms (often in association with shunts and prosthetic material), wet-source environmental organisms such as coliforms and pseudomonads, or nasopharyngeal flora such as staphylococci, streptococci, *Neisseria meningitidis* and coliforms (often after fracture or transmucosal pharyngeal operative approaches). **Otitis media and sinusitis:** *Streptococcus pneumoniae*, *Haemophilus influenzae* type b, coliforms, non-sporing anaerobes, other streptococci. **Complement deficiency:** recurrent infection with *Haemophilus influenzae* type b, *Streptococcus pneumoniae*, *Neisseria meningitidis*. **Immunosuppressed patients:** fungal meningitis (≻77) and *Listeria monocytogenes* (≻178), as well as all bacteria listed. **Neonatal ICUs** may have outbreaks of meningitis due to *Citrobacter koseri*, *Campylobacter jejuni*, *Klebsiella* spp. and *Serratia* spp.

Very rare causes include *Leptospira interrogans*, *Nocardia asteroides*, *Treponema pallidum*, *Borrelia burgdorferi*, *Brucella* spp., *Francisella tularensis*. A few (1%) are polymicrobial, usually associated with CSF leak or invasive tumour.

Salmonella **spp.** are common in neonates worldwide. In China and Hong Kong the commonest cause of meningitis is *Streptococcus suis* (Gp R) acquired from pigs (also recognised as an industrial disease of butchers). **Eosinophilic meningitis** in tropical areas may be caused by a number of helminths including *Gnathostoma* spp. and *Angiostrongylus* spp. (≻285).

Exposure history is particularly relevant to *Neisseria meningitidis*, which may cause epidemics in institutions such as barracks and schools. Asymptomatic nasal carriage rate is typically 15% for UK adults. Meningococcal meningitis is endemic in the developing world; in sub-Saharan Africa, periodic epidemics occur in the 'meningitis belt' (≻142 advice to travellers).

Clinical features: Onset ranges from very rapid (<1 day) to subacute (1–3 days), frequently with symptoms of URTI. **Headache, fever, photophobia** and **neck stiffness**. Patients may be fully alert, confused or unconscious. To demonstrate **Kernig's sign**, flex the hip and the knee, and then attempt to extend the knee. Muscle spasm in the hamstrings prevents knee extension if there is meningeal irritation. Brudzinski's sign is used in children; when the neck is flexed, the knees and hips also flex. Focal neurological signs (10–20%), fits (15–30%). Meningococcal septicaemia is associated with a characteristic **petechial or purpuric rash**; similar rashes occur rarely in

Table 22 Interpretation of CSF findings

Infection	Cells/μl	Cell type	Appearance	Protein	Glucose
Meningitis					
Bacterial	500–10 000	PMN	Turbid	↑ or ↑↑	↓ or ↓↓
Viral	50–1000	Monocytes	Clear	N or ↑	N
TB	50–1000	Monocytes	Opalescent	↑	↓
Brain abscess	5–100	PMN, monocytes	Clear	↑ or ↑↑	N
Viral encephalitis	5–100	Monocytes	Clear	N or ↑	N
Parameningeal abscess	5–100	PMN, monocytes	Clear	↑ or ↑↑	N

↑ = raised, ↓ = low, N = normal, PMN = neutrophils. CSF glucose should be > 0.5 × blood glucose. Normal protein concentration is ≤ 0.4 g/l. CSF lactate and LDH levels are not specific enough to be useful in routine clinical practice. Always collect CSF in three bottles and number them. This allows differentiation between uniformly bloody CSF of subarachnoid haemorrhage, and sequentially falling RBC count of traumatic tap. Cell counts are at best approximate guides to the most likely organisms.

other septicaemias (e.g. *Staphylococcus aureus*). **Raised intracranial pressure** (ICP) may lead to coma, hypertension and bradycardia. Presentation in infants is non-specific, with fever, vomiting, behavioural change. Neck stiffness is not usually present. Bulging fontanelle may be present late in disease.

Microbiological investigations: If meningitis is suspected, start empirical treatment before performing lumbar puncture (LP) (see Table 24). Lumbar puncture is performed as soon as possible (Table 22). Relative contraindications to LP include suspected raised ICP or intracranial space-occupying lesion, coagulopathy, severe cutaneous sepsis in the lumbar region.

CSF Gram stain may be diagnostic, allowing definitive narrow-spectrum antibiotic therapy. In immunosuppressed patients, request India ink staining for fungi, and send serum and CSF for cryptococcal antigen (➤292). Fungal and viral culture should be requested if appropriate. Mycobacterial stain and culture requires larger volume of CSF (≥10ml). CSF should be sent for cytology if malignancy is considered possible.

Raised opening pressure: Normal < 18cmH$_2$O. If pressure is greater than 45cmH$_2$O, remove only the CSF in the manometer and give iv 20% mannitol (1 g/kg by rapid infusion) and dexamethasone (1 mg 6-hly). Be prepared to repeat the mannitol. Intubation and hyperventilation may be required if signs of cerebral herniation develop.

Equivocal CSF results: Very rarely, CSF is normal in early bacterial meningitis. In early viral meningitis, low/moderate cell counts with PMN and monocytes may be seen. Prior treatment with antibiotics inadequate to cure meningitis may cause low cell count, lymphocyte predominance, negative CSF and blood culture and abnormal Gram stain appearances. In these situations, it may be appropriate to observe, repeat the LP after a few hours, or commence treatment. If in doubt, treat.

Blood cultures are often positive in untreated meningitis and often negative in partially treated cases. Culture of *Neisseria meningitidis* by some laboratories requires special medium ('meningitis bottle' ➤206). If **rash** is present, it can be scarified gently with a needle, and an impression smear made for Gram stain to show *Neisseria meningitidis* or *Staphylococcus aureus*. Nose and throat swabs are usually unhelpful unless there is CSF leak.

Other investigations: If diagnosis is not

clear-cut, chest X-ray and CT head scan are needed. Peripheral blood leucocytosis occurs in both viral and bacterial meningitis.

Differential diagnosis: Bacteraemia due to *Staphylococcus aureus* or coliforms. Meningism commonly accompanies community-acquired *Staphylococcus aureus* endocarditis. Viral and fungal meningitis. Subarachnoid haemorrhage. Meningism occurs rarely in Behçet's disease and familial Mediterranean fever.

Antibiotic management: Antibiotics should be given intravenously in high dose as soon as diagnosis is suspected. Early treatment improves prognosis in all cases. If LP is delayed or diagnosis is unclear, treat empirically for most likely pathogens. Once an organism is isolated or identified on Gram stain, therapy can be targeted appropriately. See Tables 23 & 24.

Practice point: Give benzylpenicillin as a single iv dose as soon as the diagnosis of meningitis is suspected, before admission to hospital. GPs should carry this antibiotic routinely on house calls.

Supportive management: Steroids have been shown to reduce the incidence of neurological sequelae in children and should now be used routinely. Dexamethasone 0.4 mg/kg 12-hly for 2 days, starting with the first dose of anti-

Table 23 Intravenous therapy of meningitis when organism is known

Organism	Duration (days)	
Streptococcus pneumoniae,	10–14	Benzylpenicillin **or** cefotaxime
Neisseria meningitidis,	7–10	**or** chloramphenicol
Streptococcus spp.	10–14	
Haemophilus influenzae type b	7–10	Cefotaxime, **or** chloramphenicol + ampicillin
Staphylococcus aureus	28	Flucloxacillin, **or** cefotaxime + (fusidic acid or rifampicin)
Listeria monocytogenes	21–28	Ampicillin **or** benzylpenicillin, + gentamicin
Gram-negative bacilli	10–14 after negative CSF culture	Cefotaxime + gentamicin initially, then guided by microbiology

Table 24 Empirical therapy for bacterial meningitis before pathogen identified

Clinical situation	Antibiotic regimen
Neonate <1 month old	Ampicillin + gentamicin, **or** cefotaxime + gentamicin
Child with community-acquired meningitis	Cefotaxime, **or** chloramphenicol + ampicillin
Adult with community-acquired meningitis or closed head trauma	Benzylpenicillin **or** cefotaxime
Open head trauma, postneurosurgical patient	Cefotaxime (or ceftazidime) + gentamicin ± metronidazole initially, then guided by microbiology

biotic. Their use in adults remains controversial. Patients with sepsis syndrome require full supportive therapy (➤160). Very ill patients may require intubation and ventilation.

Complications: Cranial nerve palsy (III, VI, VIII). Fits and focal neurological deficit (e.g. hemiparesis). Shock and sepsis syndrome (➤158). Ten per cent of patients with *Neisseria meningitidis* develop serum-sickness-like illness at 4–10 days, with arthritis, fever and pericarditis, which must be distinguished from persisting metastatic infection.

Comments: *Haemophilus influenzae* meningitis is very rare in adults—cranial trauma with CSF leak, otitis media, sinusitis and underlying immunodeficiency should be excluded. The same factors should be excluded in **recurrent meningitis.** Mollaret's meningitis describes a rare condition of recurrent brief episodes of meningitis alternating with asymptomatic intervals. CSF shows pleocytosis and characteristic epithelial cells. No infectious cause is found and the prognosis is good.

Prophylaxis: This must be given quickly to be effective and involves liaison between hospital clinicians, GPs, CCDC and microbiologists. *Neisseria meningitidis.* household and intimate contacts should receive rifampicin 600 mg 12-hly for 2 days (children: >1 month old, 10 mg/kg up to 600 mg 12-hly; <1 month old, 5 mg/kg 12-hly). Alternatives include ciprofloxacin and ceftriaxone ☎. Taking nose swabs from contacts is not helpful as 15% of normal population are carriers. **Patients** should also receive rifampicin as treatment regimens may not eradicate nasal carriage. **Hospital staff** only need prophylaxis if they have performed mouth-to-mouth resuscitation or had other mucosal contamination. **Meningococcal vaccine** protects against groups A and C, and some recommend its use for contacts of patients with these serogroups. Vaccination may be helpful in outbreaks within closed communities such as boarding-schools and is also recommended for travellers to the 'meningitis belt' of sub-Saharan Africa and for pilgrims to Mecca (➤142). *Haemophilus influenzae* **type b:** prophylaxis is given to **all** household contacts of cases if

there is an unvaccinated sibling under 4 years. Recommended prophylactic regimen is rifampicin 600 mg 24-hly for 4 days (children's doses as above).

Viral meningitis

'Aseptic' meningitis indicates that no bacterial cause can be found. The majority are viral. A large number of viruses have been implicated, and, depending on the agent, incubation periods, modes of transmission and associated clinical features vary. Viral meningitis is commonest in children and adolescents, and is a common cause of hospital admission in the UK. It is essential to exclude bacterial meningitis.

Clinical features: Headache, fever, neck stiffness, photophobia, irritability. There are often signs of underlying associated virus infection such as parotitis (mumps), pharyngitis, GI disturbance or rash.

Organisms: Enteroviruses (Coxsackie A and B, echoviruses, polioviruses ➤249), herpesviruses (HSV-1 and HSV 2, EDV, VZV ➤241), mumps (➤102), measles (➤100), arenaviruses (lymphocytic choriomeningitis ➤256), adenoviruses (➤240)

Microbiological investigations: CSF changes are discussed above. Attempt virus culture from CSF, throat swab and stools. Many patients have a peripheral blood leucocytosis.

Differential diagnosis: Essential to consider and exclude bacterial, mycobacterial and fungal meningitis. Other very rare causes of aseptic meningitis include syphilis (➤67), leptospirosis (➤226), Lyme disease (➤224) and eosinophilic meningitis (➤285).

Fungal meningitis

Fungal meningitis is associated with immunodeficiency such as HIV infection, when the commonest cause is *Cryptococcus neoformans* (➤292). Diagnosis is made by India ink staining of CSF and antigen detection in CSF and serum. Other fungal meningitides are rare in the UK; fungal infections that cause invasive disease in the immunocompetent host such as *Histoplasma capsulatum*, *Blastomyces dermatitidis* and *Coccidioides immitis* are geographically restricted in their distribution (➤293). They should be considered if there is an appropriate travel history. *Candida* spp. (➤291) are associated with meningitis in neonates and in patients with CSF shunts.

CSF shunt infections

CSF shunt infections occur in up to 50% depending on the patient group studied, the duration of follow-up and the device used. The majority present within 2 months of surgery and are due to skin flora, suggesting contamination at the time of operation. *Staphylococcus epidermidis*, *Staphylococcus aureus*, coryneforms, *Enterococcus* spp. and coliforms are most often isolated, but a large range of other organisms have been reported. Signs of infection can be subtle and non-specific: fever, erythema over the course of the catheter or malfunctioning of the shunt. A minority of patients have symptoms of meningitis. An infected ventriculoperitoneal shunt may present with abdominal pain. Treatment comprises removal of all or part of the shunt, culture of blood and CSF and prolonged administration of antibiotics, often including intrathecal injection of antibiotics via the externalised shunt.

Chronic meningitis

Symptoms and signs of meningeal irritation lasting longer than 4 weeks with CSF pleocytosis. Tuberculosis is the commonest infectious cause and must be vigorously pursued (➤30). Other infectious causes include syphilis (➤67), Lyme disease (➤224), listeriosis (➤179), fungal meningitis (➤77), brucellosis (➤209), and helminth infections such as schistosomiasis, cysticercosis and hydatid disease (➤281). Non-infectious causes are common and include carcinomatous meningitis, lymphoma, sarcoid and connective tissue diseases such as systemic lupus erythematosus.

Herpes simplex encephalitis (HSE) ⊠

Encephalitis implies infection of the brain parenchyma. The commonest, and treatable, cause of viral encephalitis in the developed world is Herpes simplex virus (HSV).

Risk factors: HSE occurs in otherwise healthy individuals, but the incidence is higher in the immunocompromised, such as HIV-infected patients. Most episodes are believed to result from reactivation of latent virus rather than primary infection.

Clinical features: Onset varies from abrupt (hours) to insidious (1–3 days). There is often a brief prodrome with headache, fever, lethargy, behavioural change and somnolence, followed by rapid progression to severe CNS dysfunction, often with focal (usually temporal lobe) signs, seizures and coma. Patients do not usually have concurrent cold sores or genital herpes. Mortality is 60–80% untreated.

Organisms: HSV-1 (encephalitis in adults), HSV-2 (meningitis in adults, encephalitis in neonates).

Microbiological investigations: LP to exclude bacterial, fungal and mycobacterial meningitis (➤75). PCR for HSV in CSF is sensitive and specific and is now available at several centres ☎. Serum/CSF serological titres against HSV rise during infection but in general this occurs too late, and the results are insufficiently sensitive, for them to be clinically useful except in retrospect. Brain biopsy for histology and viral culture is required for definitive diagnosis; need for early biopsy in all cases remains controversial. Most physicians treat on the basis of CT, EEG and clinical signs and observe response to acyclovir.

Other investigations: CT scan shows low-density lesions with ring enhancement, particularly in the temporal lobe. EEG may show focal temporal lobe abnormality. Both CT and EEG may be normal early in the illness, and, if HSE is strongly suspected, they should be repeated after 48 h.

Differential diagnosis: Meningitis, brain abscess, cerebrovascular accident and tumour. Other viral encephalitides include rabies and the arthropod-borne flaviviruses, togaviruses and bunyaviruses. These are geographically restricted and should be considered if there is an appropriate travel history (see Table 25).

Table 25 Viruses associated with encephalitis ⊠

Disease	Geographical distribution	Vector	Months of greatest risk	Usual incubation (days)
Herpesviruses (➤241)				
Herpes simplex	Worldwide	–	Any	Variable
Togaviruses (➤253)				
Western equine encephalitis	Western North America, South America	M	JJAS	5–15
Eastern equine encephalitis	Eastern USA	M	JJA	5–15
Venezuelan equine encephalitis	South America	M	Rainy months	2–6
Flaviviruses (➤253)				
St Louis encephalitis	USA	M	JJA	5–15
Japanese B encephalitis	SE Asia	M	MJJAS	5–15
Murray Valley encephalitis	South Australia	M	JFMAM	5–15
West Nile encephalitis	N Africa, SE Asia	M	JJAS	3–12
Tick-borne encephalitis	Central Europe, Asia	T	JJA	7–14
Powassan encephalitis	Northern USA, southern Canada	T	JJAS	7–14
Rocio	Brazil	M	FMAMJJ	5–15
Bunyaviruses (➤255)				
California encephalitis	Western USA	M	JJASO	5–15
La Crosse	Midwestern USA	M	JJAS	5–15

M = mosquito, T = tick.

Enteroviruses and mumps, which more often produce meningitis, may cause a mild self-limiting encephalitis.

Antibiotic management: Acyclovir 10 mg/kg iv 8-hly for 10 days. Treatment reduces the mortality to ~25%.

Supportive management: Anticonvulsants, intubation and ventilation may all be required. There may be long-term neurological sequelae in survivors.

> **Practice point:** Start antiviral treatment whenever the diagnosis of HSE is suspected, even in the absence of typical CT appearances.

Cerebral abscess

Localised collection of pus within the brain parenchyma.

Risk factors: Up to 80% have an identifiable predisposing cause including recent neurosurgery, contiguous parameningeal infection (sinusitis, otitis, mastoiditis, dental abscess), distant infection with metastatic spread (lung abscess, empyema, endocarditis), or cranial trauma. Congenital heart disease with right-to-left shunt greatly increases risk.

Clinical features: Symptoms and signs of intracranial mass with focal signs and evidence of raised intracranial pressure. Headache, fever, changes in mental status, nausea and vomiting, fits. Onset usually occurs over

1–4 weeks, but may be slower. There may be signs of primary infection elsewhere.

Organisms: Mixed infections occur in 50%. *Staphylococcus aureus*, *Streptococcus pneumoniae*, *Streptococcus 'milleri'*, coliforms, *Haemophilus influenzae* and other fastidious Gram-negative rods, *Pseudomonas aeruginosa*, non-sporing anaerobes. Aspirated material is sterile in up to 15% of cases, usually after antibiotic therapy.

Microbiological investigations: If cerebral abscess is suspected, LP is **contraindicated**, even in the absence of papilloedema, due to the risk of neurological deterioration and the fact that CSF findings are rarely helpful (➤75). If signs suggest possible cerebral abscess or meningitis, treatment for the latter should be started whilst a CT scan is obtained. Cultures of blood and any other infected sites such as empyema, sinus aspirate.

Other investigations: Leucocytosis is common. CT head scan shows ring-enhancing lesion with surrounding oedema. In early disease CT may be normal or show low-density lesion only.

Differential diagnosis: Meningitis (including mycobacterial and fungal). Cerebrovascular accident, tumour, viral encephalitis. Tuberculoma, cryptococcoma or toxoplasma encephalitis in the immunocompromised patient. Rarely cysticercosis, hydatid disease.

Antibiotic management: Cefotaxime + metronidazole initially, guided thereafter by the results of aspiration, microscopy and culture of abscess contents.

Supportive management: The optimum timing of aspiration and/or open drainage are matters for expert neurosurgical opinion ☎. Small abscesses in otherwise healthy people have been treated with antibiotic therapy alone. Anticonvulsants, careful attention to fluid balance and nutrition, intubation and ventilation may all be required. Dexamethasone and mannitol may be used to control cerebral oedema, but steroids should not be given routinely as animal studies suggest they delay resolution.

Complications: Rupture into CSF, recurrence, residual neurological deficit, epilepsy.

8: Eye Infections

Topical antibiotics for ophthalmic use

Chloramphenicol is widely used, although agranulocytosis after ophthalmic use has been reported very rarely. Fusidic acid preparations allow twice-daily instillation of drops but are expensive. Gentamicin, neomycin, ciprofloxacin and ofloxacin are also available. Tetracycline drops are available for *Chlamydia trachomatis* infection, but systemic treatment is also required in this situation. Severe ophthalmic infections are treated by combinations of antibiotics given topically, subconjunctivally, intravitreally and/ or systemically: ophthalmological and micro-biological opinion should be sought ☎.

Stye ('hordeolum') and chalazion

Acute bacterial infection of one of the glands of Zeiss, adjacent to the eyelash follicles. Infection of the Meibomian glands presents either acutely as an 'internal stye' or as a chronic painless cyst known as a chalazion.

Clinical features: Painful, red, localised swelling at the lid margin with surrounding erythema. The Meibomian glands are located deeper in the tarsal plate, and infection there tends to produce more pain and swelling, usually visible on the conjunctival surface of the lid. Rarely infection spreads from an internal stye to cause preseptal cellulitis (➤85).

Organisms: Usually *Staphylococcus aureus* or culture-negative.

Microbiological investigations: Not usually indicated. Gram stain and culture of expressed material for serious infection.

Antibiotic management: Local antibiotic ointment/drops.

Supportive management: Warm compresses may give symptomatic relief. Incision and drainage may be required, particularly for chalazia.

Blepharitis

Diffuse inflammation of the eyelids or their margins.

Risk factors: Blepharitis is usually associated with seborrhoeic dermatitis, which causes scalp irritation and dandruff. It is also associated with acne rosacea, or with pubic lice, which infest the scalp, axillae and eye-lashes of sexually active adults, and of children, who may acquire the infection by non-venereal contact.

Clinical features: Chronic bilateral irritation and hyperaemia of the lid margins, with scaling of the skin, flakes of epithelium clinging to the lashes and destruction of lash follicles. There may be superficial ulceration of the lid margins. The roots of the lashes should be examined carefully to exclude the presence of lice and their eggs (nits).

Organisms: *Staphylococcus aureus* is often isolated, and is believed to play a role in pathogenesis although asymptomatic ocular carriage of *Staphylococcus aureus* is also common.

Antibiotic management: Long-term treatment with topical antibiotic ointment/drops. If associated with acne rosacea, oral tetracycline for 2–4 weeks is effective. Lice should be treated by topical application of lindane-containing shampoo to scalp, axillae and pubic areas (➤72). Eyelid infestation is treated by coating with vaseline for 3–4 days, although cutting back of the lashes to remove nits may also be required.

Supportive management: Regular careful cleaning of the eyelids and removal of scaling with plain water and cotton wool buds. Treatment of seborrhoeic dermatitis (➤92) with topical miconazole/hydrocortisone ointment and ketoconazole shampoo.

Conjunctivitis

Conjunctivitis may be bacterial, chlamydial,

viral or allergic. Some chlamydial and viral agents, such as *Chlamydia trachomatis*, cause specific characteristic syndromes; other causes of bacterial and viral conjunctivitis are not clinically distinguishable. Conjunctivitis is also seen as a minor part of systemic infections such as influenza, leptospirosis, rubella or measles. The major clinical features of conjunctivitis are itching and burning of the eyes, with a serous or purulent discharge. Pain is mild, photophobia and lacrimation are usually absent and there is no impairment of vision, unless infection progresses to keratitis and corneal ulceration, which are discussed separately below. There is erythema of both tarsal and bulbar conjunctivae; in viral infection this is 'follicular', with tiny translucent follicles of lymphoid hyperplasia over the conjunctival surface.

Differential diagnosis of acute conjunctivitis: A number of clinical features help to differentiate acute conjunctivitis, which may usually be treated by the non-specialist, from other causes of acute red eye which require urgent ophthalmic referral. Conjunctivitis is rarely painful. Grittiness and irritation are common, but real pain suggests corneal involvement or intraocular disease. Visual acuity is normal; sometimes vision is impaired by a film of mucopus over the cornea but this can be removed by blinking. Vasodilatation and redness is spread all over the conjunctivae or is most obvious nearest the fornices. Conjunctival vasodilatation found only around the limbus strongly suggests corneal or intraocular disease. The cornea should be clear and give a sharp bright reflection. Keratitis causes dulling of the corneal reflection.

Bacterial conjunctivitis
Much less common than viral conjunctivitis.
Clinical features: Infection is usually unilateral initially, spreading to the other eye within a few days. The discharge is usually thick and purulent.
Organisms: *Staphylococcus aureus*, Gp A β-haemolytic streptococci, *Streptococcus pneumoniae, Haemophilus influenzae. Staphylococcus aureus* and coliforms may occasionally cause chronic low-grade conjunctivitis. Rarely, *Neisseria gonorrhoeae, Neisseria meningitidis, Moraxella lacunata, Corynebacterium diphtheriae.*

Microbiological investigations: Gram stain and culture of discharge. Fluorescence microscopy for chlamydial inclusion bodies. Viral culture.
Other investigations: Fluorescent staining to rule out corneal ulcer and abrasion should always be performed.
Differential diagnosis: Keratitis. Subconjunctival haematoma. Allergic, viral or chlamydial conjunctivitis.
Antibiotic management: Local antibiotic ointment/drops.
Supportive management: Topical steroids should not be given because of the possibility of herpetic dendritic ulcer (➤84). Do not apply an eye-patch.
Complications: More virulent organisms such as *Neisseria gonorrhoeae, Pseudomonas aeruginosa, Moraxella lacunata* and *Streptococcus pneumoniae* can cause corneal ulceration. Infection by these organisms and *Neisseria meningitidis* and Gp A β-haemolytic streptococci may require systemic antibiotic therapy.

Viral conjunctivitis
Many viruses cause conjunctivitis as part of systemic or upper respiratory infection. Certain specific agents cause more severe disease—see below.
Clinical features: As for bacterial conjunctivitis. The discharge is thinner and more watery, and the conjunctivitis is follicular and less florid. There is often local lymphadenopathy. Purulent discharge suggests bacterial superinfection.
Microbiological investigations, differential diagnosis: As for bacterial conjunctivitis.
Antibiotic management: Local antibiotic ointment/drops to prevent bacterial superinfection, as well as specific antiviral medication if appropriate (see below).

Specific forms of conjunctivitis
ADENOVIRUS CONJUNCTIVITIS
Risk factors: Exposure to other infected

children, hence 'swimming-pool conjunctivitis'.

Clinical features: Severe conjunctivitis with fever, sore throat and preauricular lymphadenopathy. There may be punctate keratitis, progressing to corneal ulceration, which can persist for months.

Organisms: Adenovirus, particularly types 8, 10 and 19.

Practice points: Adenovirus infection is highly contagious and careful hand-washing by patient and physician and disinfection of medical equipment is required to avoid spread.

ACUTE HAEMORRHAGIC CONJUNCTIVITIS

Risk factors: Crowding and poor hygiene, particularly in the developing world.

Clinical features: Severe eyelid oedema and irritation, conjunctivitis and subconjunctival haemorrhage, typically lasting a week to 10 days. Punctate keratitis may develop and there may be signs of systemic viral infection.

Organisms: Enterovirus type 70, Coxsackievirus A24, adenovirus 11.

HERPES SIMPLEX CONJUNCTIVITIS

Primary infection by HSV is a rare cause of conjunctivitis. Herpetic vesicles are seen on the eyelids. The majority of patients with HSV conjunctivitis develop corneal lesions, usually after 7–10 days. Recurrent HSV usually causes HSV keratoconjunctivitis (see below).

CHLAMYDIA TRACHOMATIS INFECTIONS

Chlamydia trachomatis (➤233) causes two distinct ocular syndromes – adult inclusion conjunctivitis (IC), which is a sexually transmitted infection due to serotypes D–K, and trachoma, a chronic follicular keratoconjunctivitis caused by serotypes A, B and C, which leads over years to corneal scarring and opacity. Trachoma is a major cause of blindness in the developing world. *Chlamydia trachomatis* is also an important cause of ophthalmia neonatorum.

Risk factors: IC predominantly affects sexually active young adults. Trachoma is a disease of poverty, related to frequent reinfection spread by flies, fomites and person to person.

Clinical features: IC presents as follicular conjunctivitis, which may persist for months untreated. The lower lid is preferentially affected. In trachoma, follicular conjunctivitis is followed by keratitis, corneal vascularisation, scarring and scar retraction. Much of the corneal damage is secondary to distortion of the eyelids by scarring and secondary bacterial keratitis.

Microbiological investigations: Diagnosis is confirmed by demonstrating basophilic cytoplasmic inclusion bodies on Giemsa stain or immunofluorescence microscopy of conjunctival scrapings.

Differential diagnosis: Viral conjunctivitis, Herpes simplex keratitis.

Antibiotic management: Oral erythromycin **or** tetracycline, for 3 weeks in IC and for 3–6 weeks in trachoma. In trachoma-endemic areas reinfection is common and public health measures aimed at reducing transmission rates are of major importance.

Complications: Trachoma if untreated.

OPHTHALMIA NEONATORUM ✉

Infectious conjunctivitis in the neonatal period. Infection is acquired during passage through the birth canal, and may be due to *Neisseria gonorrhoeae*, *Chlamydia trachomatis*, *Staphylococcus aureus*, *Streptococcus pneumoniae* and rarely HSV. Treatment depends on the infecting organism. *Neisseria gonorrhoeae* infection merits systemic treatment with benzylpenicillin, unless penicillinase-producing organisms are isolated or locally prevalent. Chlamydial conjunctivitis requires topical tetracycline and systemic erythromycin to prevent respiratory infection. Other bacterial causes are treated topically. HSV requires topical acyclovir.

PHLYCTENULAR CONJUNCTIVITIS

A localised hypersensitivity reaction, usually secondary to pulmonary tuberculosis (TB ➤29). A raised pinkish nodule (the 'phlycten') appears on the bulbar conjunctiva, close to the limbus. It subsequently ulcerates and heals with minimal or no scarring. This process takes about 2 weeks. Symptoms are few, unless the phlycten encroaches on the cornea, where it causes pain, photophobia and visual loss associated with scarring. Topical steroids accelerate healing and minimise scarring. Patients must be fully assessed for intercurrent pulmonary TB.

MOLLUSCUM CONTAGIOSUM (➤94)
Infection with the poxvirus that causes molluscum contagiosum may involve the eyelid margins to cause follicular conjunctivitis. Careful examination is required to exclude the presence of characteristic umbilicated papules, which hide close to the eyelash roots. Treatment is by excision, cryotherapy or curettage.

Keratitis

Infectious inflammation of the cornea ☞. Keratitis merits urgent referral to an ophthalmologist, since visual impairment may develop rapidly.

Risk factors: Bacterial keratitis usually follows trauma (which may be minor). Soft contact lenses are a particular risk factor for *Pseudomonas aeruginosa* and *Acanthamoeba* infection, following contamination of lens solutions.

Clinical features: Unilateral red eye with moderate to severe pain, photophobia, lacrimation and **impaired vision**. There is usually no exudate. Fluoroscein staining reveals defects in the corneal epithelium. Herpes simplex virus (HSV) causes a characteristic dendritic ulcer. Herpes zoster (➤105) affecting the ophthalmic division of the trigeminal nerve causes keratitis in 75% of cases. Vesicles on the tip of the nose imply involvement of the nasociliary nerve, and this increases the likelihood of corneal involvement.

Organisms: HSV. Varicella zoster virus. *Staphylococcus aureus, Staphylococcus epidermidis, Bacillus cereus,* Gp A β-haemolytic streptococci, *Streptococcus pneumoniae, Moraxella lacunata,* pseudomonads. Rarely fungi (commoner in the tropics, esp. *Fusarium* spp.) and *Acanthamoeba* spp. (➤264).

Microbiological investigations: Bacterial fungal and viral culture of conjunctival scrapings. Fluorescent antibody stains and special culture techniques are needed to demonstrate

Acanthamoeba ➤. Corneal biopsy may be required to diagnose fungal keratitis.

Antibiotic management: Ophthalmological referral and specialist management are essential. Debridement is often performed. For HSV and zoster, topical and systemic acyclovir are given. Topical steroids may be required, but should only be given under experienced ophthalmological supervision. Bacterial keratitis is treated with very frequent instillation of antibiotic drops, plus parenteral antibiotics in severe cases. Fungal keratitis responds to topical amphotericin, miconazole and econazole. *Acanthamoeba* keratitis is treated with topical dibromopropamidine and neomycin.

Comments: If keratitis is related to contact lens use, it is essential to ensure adequate and regular disinfection of lenses and equipment to avoid recurrence.

> **Practice point:** If patients with red eye have reduced visual acuity they should always be referred for immediate ophthalmological opinion.

Uveitis

Anterior uveitis (syn. iridocyclitis)
Inflammation of iris and ciliary body.

Clinical features: Unilateral red eye, deep ocular pain with a tender eyeball, irregular or constricted pupil, photophobia and tearing.

Organisms: Anterior uveitis is a minor feature of a number of infections, including mumps (➤102), rubella (➤101), measles (➤100), HSV (➤241), Herpes zoster (➤105) and secondary syphilis (➤67), and, more rarely, *Neisseria gonorrhoeae* (➤65), leptospirosis (➤226), brucellosis (➤209) and Lyme disease (➤224). It is also a feature of Reiter's syndrome (➤96), but it is more commonly seen as a complication of non-infectious diseases, including connective tissue diseases, inflammatory bowel disease, Behçet's disease and sarcoidosis.

Differential diagnosis: Acute glaucoma causes a cloudy cornea and a dilated pupil. Conjunctivitis (➤81).

Posterior uveitis (syn. chorioretinitis)
Indicates inflammation of the choroid, usually with extension to the adjacent retina.
Clinical features: Gradual onset of painless visual loss. Ophthalmoscopy reveals retinal scarring.
Organisms: *Toxoplasma gondii* (➤264), *Toxocara* spp. (➤279), *Mycobacterium tuberculosis*, usually associated with miliary TB (➤30), very rarely *Histoplasma capsulatum*, if there is an appropriate travel history (➤293). HSV (➤241) and CMV (➤243). VZV may cause chorioretinitis, particularly after an attack of herpes zoster (➤105). In the immunocompromised, *Cryptococcus neoformans* (➤292), CMV (➤128), *Pneumocystis carinii*–for example, in HIV patients treated with aerosolised pentamidine as prophylaxis against pulmonary pneumocystis.
Microbiological investigations: Depending on the clinical situation, appropriate tests to look for extraocular infection by pathogens mentioned include staining, culture and antigen detection in aspirated material. Serological testing may be helpful. The ophthalmoscopic appearances may be sufficiently characteristic to allow an informed guess.
Comments: Urgent ophthalmological referral is required for both forms of uveitis. Aspiration of aqueous or vitreous humour may allow identification of the causative organism.

Endophthalmitis

Suppurative infection of the vitreous leading to abscess formation.
Risk factors: Exogenous infection secondary to trauma, surgery, penetrating corneal ulcer. Endogenous metastatic infection during bacteraemia or fungaemia.
Clinical features: Pain, photophobia, headache and reduced visual acuity. Conjunctival injection, eyelid swelling, hypopyon and reduced red reflex.
Organisms: Following surgery: *Staphylococcus epidermidis*, coryneforms, *Staphylococcus aureus*. **Following trauma:** *Staphylococcus aureus*, Gp A β-haemolytic streptococci, coliforms, pseudomonads, *Bacillus cereus*, anaerobes. **Bacteraemic**

infection: *Candida* spp., *Staphylococcus aureus*, *Streptococcus pneumoniae*, Gp A β-haemolytic streptococci, coryneforms.
Microbiological investigations: Gram stain and culture of aspirated material. Blood cultures.
Antibiotic management: Systemic, topical and intravitreal antibiotics, guided by the results of microscopy and culture. Specialist referral is obviously very urgent; vitrectomy may be a vital component of therapy ☏.

Orbital infections

Infection confined to the eyelid and superficial tissues anterior to the orbital septum is referred to as **preseptal cellulitis**. Deeper infection is referred to as **periorbital** or **orbital cellulitis**.

Preseptal cellulitis
Risk factors: Usually secondary to laceration or minor trauma. Occasionally secondary to facial cellulitis or an infected Meibomian cyst (➤81).
Clinical features: Pain, swelling and erythema of the eyelid. Low-grade fever. Proptosis and impairment of ocular mobility are **not** seen; if present they suggest orbital cellulitis.
Organisms: *Staphylococcus aureus*, Gp A β-haemolytic streptococci, *Haemophilus influenzae* type B (particularly in children prior to introduction of Hib vaccination). Anaerobic infection may follow trauma, especially bite injuries, and is suggested by foul-smelling discharge and tissue necrosis.
Microbiological investigations: Gram stain and culture of pus. Blood cultures.
Other investigations: CT/MRI if there is suspicion of orbital spread.
Antibiotic management: Flucloxacillin. If *Haemophilus influenzae* is suspected, give cefotaxime **or** co-amoxiclav. See also bites (➤90).

Orbital cellulitis
Infection within the tissues of the orbit.
Risk factors: Usually by direct spread from ethmoid or frontal sinusitis (➤15). Less often following surgery or trauma, otitis media, dental infection or facial cellulitis.
Clinical features: Fever, headache, toxaemia,

eyelid oedema, rhinorrhoea, pain and tenderness over the eye. Limited, painful eye movement. Progressive untreated infection causes displacement of the globe by subperiosteal collection of pus extending directly from the infected adjacent sinus, ophthalmoplegia and severely reduced visual acuity.

Cavernous sinus thrombosis may occur with headache, eye pain, neck stiffness, swelling over the forehead and eyelids. Ophthalmoplegia and papilloedema occur. The patient is extremely unwell, with altered level of consciousness. The condition is bilateral.

Organisms: *Streptococcus pneumoniae*, *Staphylococcus aureus* (especially post-surgery or trauma), Gp A β-haemolytic streptococci, *Streptococcus 'milleri'*, *Haemophilus influenzae* and other fastidious Gram-negative rods, anaerobes. In elderly diabetics or immunocompromised patients fungal sinusitis due to *Mucor* spp., *Aspergillus* spp., *Fusarium* spp. and *Rhizopus* spp. may involve the orbit.

Microbiological investigations: Gram stain and culture of aspirated material. Blood culture. LP is indicated if there is meningism. Biopsy is often needed to establish the diagnosis of fungal infection.

Other investigations: Sinus X-rays, CT/MRI scanning to examine sinuses and delineate extent of infection.

Differential diagnosis: Preseptal cellulitis — in this condition, limitation of eye movement and impaired visual acuity do not occur.

Antibiotic management: Initially cefotaxime + metronidazole, guided thereafter by microbiology results.

Supportive management: Surgical intervention to drain collections of pus.

Complications: Meningitis.

> **Practice point:** Always check visual acuity in any patient with suspected eye infection.

Dacryocystitis

Infection of the lacrimal sac, usually secondary to obstruction of the nasolacrimal duct.

Clinical features: Pain, swelling and tenderness in the nasal corner of the eye below the mediocanthal ligament.

Organisms: *Staphylococcus aureus*, *Streptococcus pneumoniae*, Gp A β-haemolytic streptococci; *Actinomyces israelii*.

Microbiological investigations: Gram stain and culture of pus.

Antibiotic management: Local antibiotic ointment/drops **and** systemic flucloxacillin are required. *Actinomyces israelii* infection responds to local debridement.

Supportive management: Ophthalmological referral for duct irrigation or drainage is usually required ☎.

9: Skin Infections

In normal skin infection is prevented by physical integrity, dryness and regular shedding of the stratum corneum, free fatty acids and low pH of sebum, and normal cellular and humoral immune function. The normal cutaneous flora consists of a restricted range of organisms, most of which are opportunist pathogens in certain circumstances (Table 26).

Impetigo

Superficial infection of the stratum corneum, usually confined to the face.

Risk factors: Minor trauma, underlying dermatitis (e.g. atopic eczema). Nasal carriage of *Staphylococcus aureus*. Commonest in children.

Clinical features: Vesicles and pustules on an erythematous base, which burst leaving yellow-brown scabs. It is non-scarring. Persistence of flaccid blisters ('bullous impetigo') suggests staphylococcal infection (usually due to phage type 71). **Ecthyma** is a variant of impetigo which is common in debilitated, malnourished or alcoholic patients causing scarring ulceration on the legs.

Organisms: *Staphylococcus aureus* or Gp A β-haemolytic streptococci, often mixed.

Microbiological investigations: Usually unnecessary.

Antibiotic management: Topical mupirocin **or** oral flucloxacillin.

Folliculitis

Inflammation of the hair follicles.

Risk factors: Commonest in children. Moist warm conditions and tight clothing.

Clinical features: Erythematous papules and pustules around hairs, usually occurring in crops.

Organisms: *Staphylococcus aureus*. *Pseudomonas aeruginosa* causes 'hot-tub folliculitis' associated with contaminated Jacuzzis and hot tubs.

Antibiotic management: Flucloxacillin is used in

Table 26 Normal cutaneous flora

Organism	Location	Disease associations
Staphylococcus aureus	Anterior nares, skin folds	See text
Staphylococcus epidermidis *Micrococcus* spp.	All skin	Prosthetic materials and line infections
Corynebacterium spp. 'diphtheroids' *Bacillus* spp. *Brevibacterium* spp.	Moist areas	Erythrasma (≻92), prosthetic materials and line infections
Gram-negative bacilli, commonly *Acinetobacter* spp.	Moist skin	UTI, prosthetic materials and line infections
Propionibacterium acnes	Sebaceous glands	Acne vulgaris (≻92)
Pityrosporum orbiculare	Back and chest	Pityriasis versicolor, seborrhoeic dermatitis (≻92)
Candida albicans	Mucous membranes and moist skin	Candidiasis

extensive or prolonged folliculitis. Hot-tub folliculitis is usually self-limited.

Cutaneous abscesses (boils, furuncles and carbuncles)

Localised pyogenic skin infection, usually arising in an infected hair follicle.

Risk factors: Boils and carbuncles are common infections in normal hosts. Recurrent infection suggests diabetes mellitus, poor hygiene or nasal carriage of virulent *Staphylococcus aureus* strains.

Clinical features: A tender nodule, usually surmounted by a pustule through which a hair merges. A **furuncle** is an isolated cutaneous abscess or boil. Systemic features of infection are unusual. When several adjacent furuncles coalesce and drain through multiple orifices, this is termed a **carbuncle** and fever and toxaemia are more likely.

Organisms: *Staphylococcus aureus*, but often culture-negative. Mixed infection by coliforms, anaerobes and other Gram-positive cocci is more likely in perineal abscesses.

Microbiological investigations: Gram stain and culture of pus. Blood cultures in severe infection.

Antibiotic management: Flucloxacillin if there is significant surrounding cellulitis or failure to resolve. Co-amoxiclav is suitable for initial treatment of perineal abscesses, until results of microbiology are available.

Supportive management: Incision and drainage is usually required. Patients at risk of endocarditis should receive antibiotic prophylaxis for this procedure: For patients with prosthetic valves, flucloxacillin 1 g iv before and 6 hours after, **plus** gentamicin 120 mg with first dose. For non-prosthetic valves, flucloxacillin, 500 mg po at the same timings.

Complications: Systemic infection with metastatic abscess.

Special forms of cutaneous abscess
BOILS ON THE UPPER LIP AND NOSE
Boils in the 'dangerous triangle' carry the special risk of cavernous sinus thrombosis (➤86). They should not be incised or manipulated. Warm soaks may encourage pointing and flucloxacillin should be given.

PERIANAL ABSCESS
If infected with gut flora, often associated with fistula in ano.

HYDRADENITIS SUPPURATIVA
A chronic suppurative disease of apocrine glands in genital, axillary and perianal areas. Plugging of glands leads to proximal dilatation, rupture and infection with local normal flora. Sinus track formation and scarring follow.

Organisms: Mixed flora, including non-sporing anaerobes, *Streptococcus 'milleri'*, staphylococci, diphtheroids and coliforms.

Management: Incision and drainage of abscesses, antibiotics if inflamed and systemically unwell: flucloxacillin **plus** metronidazole, or co-amoxiclav.

BREAST ABSCESS
During lactation, *Staphylococcus aureus*, β-haemolytic streptococci and normal skin flora are usually involved. Incision and drainage may be required. Flucloxacillin or co-amoxiclav is given. Recurrent abscesses, often associated with diabetes mellitus or nipple inversion, may involve mixed anaerobic flora and may require excision of nipple ducts.

Cellulitis

Acute spreading infection of the subcutaneous tissues.

Risk factors: Minor trauma, dermatitis. Peripheral vascular disease. Impaired lymphatic drainage, often following previous attacks of cellulitis. Site of saphenous vein harvest for coronary artery bypass surgery.

Clinical features: Erythema, tenderness, swelling and warmth sometimes with bullae and desquamation. Fever, rigors. Lymphadenitis.

Organisms: Gp A β-haemolytic streptococci, *Staphylococcus aureus*. *Haemophilus influenzae* type B (previously predominantly in children, but a disease of adults since the advent of Hib vaccination). See also wound infections. Rarely *Streptococcus pneumoniae*, *Pasteurella multocida* (bite wounds ➤90).

Microbiological investigations: Local cultures are often negative. Swab any visible lesions (e.g. cracked skin between toes). Blood cultures.

Differential diagnosis: Venous thrombosis.

Antibiotic management: Flucloxacillin, iv in severe infections. If streptococcal infection alone is confirmed, benzylpenicillin. In children with facial cellulitis, initial therapy includes cover for *Haemophilus influenzae*: co-amoxiclav or parenteral or broad-spectrum cephalosporin.

Complications: Permanent scarring, lymphatic damage and lymphoedema, recurrence.

Particular forms of cellulitis

ERYSIPELAS

A clinically distinct form of cellulitis with a sharply demarcated raised edge, usually on the face or limbs, which may advance rapidly. It is usually due to Gp A β-haemolytic streptococci.

ERYSIPELOID

A rare infection due to *Erysipelothrix rhusiopathiae* (➤182). It presents as a tender purple well demarcated cellulitis of the fingers or hand, in those who handle raw fish and poultry. Give benzylpenicillin (erythromycin if penicillin-allergic).

HAEMOPHILUS INFLUENZAE
FACIAL CELLULITIS

(See comments above on age incidence.) Typically causes a purple cellulitis with indistinct margins over the face and arms.

BLISTERING DISTAL DACTYLITIS

Due to Gp A β-haemolytic streptococci with or without *Staphylococcus aureus*. It presents as a painful superficial bulla over the finger pulp in children. Incision and drainage and systemic flucloxacillin are required.

Wound infection

Risk factors: Damage to the physical integrity of the skin is the most important risk factor for infection. Wound infection can follow traumatic or surgical wounds. Predisposing factors include chronic illness and debility, diabetes, cirrhosis and alcoholism, trauma to

mucosae allowing inoculation of normal flora, foreign body, *Staphylococcus aureus* nasal carriage.

Clinical features: Erythema, warmth, tenderness, swelling and a purulent exudate. Postoperative fever. Failure to heal and dehiscence are important sequelae of surgical wound infection.

Organisms: *Staphylococcus aureus*, Gp A β-haemolytic streptococci. Contaminated accidental wounds and abdominal surgical wounds are infected by normal local mucosal flora including coliforms, *Clostridium* spp. and non-sporing anaerobes, and *Streptococcus 'milleri'*.

Microbiological investigations: Gram stain and culture of pus. Blood cultures if unwell.

Antibiotic management: Topical antibiotics are **not** indicated. Initial treatment depends on clinical situation and results of microbiology. Flucloxacillin is given initially, unless the wound is heavily contaminated or is an abdominal or mucosal surgical wound, in which case cover should be extended to coliforms and anaerobes, e.g. benzylpenicillin + gentamicin + metronidazole, **or** cefotaxime + metronidazole.

Supportive management: Drain pus, debride devitalised tissue and remove foreign bodies—this is more important than choice of antibiotic therapy. Establish tetanus vaccination status (➤218). See also Table 27 for special forms of wound infection.

Severe tissue infections

These may be classified by microbial aetiology, e.g. due to a single species such as Gp A β-haemolytic streptococci or *Clostridium perfringens*, or polymicrobial, often due to a mixture of Gram-negative aerobes and anaerobes. They may also be classified by anatomical site of infection, e.g. myositis, fasciitis. Certain clinical syndromes, such as clostridial myonecrosis or necrotising fasciitis due to Gp A β-haemolytic streptococci, are well defined, but very similar clinical features can result from polymicrobial infections, in which case the results of Gram stain and culture only identify a subset of the organisms responsible. **Early surg-**

Table 27 Special forms of wound infection

Risk factors	Organisms	Management	Comments
Freshwater contamination	*Aeromonas hydrophila* (➤196)	Cefotaxime	
Seawater contamination	*Vibrio vulnificus* (➤196) and other vibrios	Cefotaxime **or** doxycycline **plus** gentamicin	May range from mild cellulitis to severe bacterial myositis
Animal bites (monkey bites carry a special risk of monkey herpes B infection ☞)	*Pasteurella multocida* (➤209),*Capnocytophaga canimorsus* (DF-2) (➤208), non-sporing anaerobes, oral streptococci, staphylococci	Thorough cleansing. Give prophylactic antibiotics. Co-amoxiclav, **or** co-trimoxazole **plus** metronidazole	Establish need for tetanus treatment (➤218). Consider rabies if appropriate travel history (➤257)
Human bites	Non-sporing anaerobes, oral streptococci, staphylococci, *Eikenella corrodens* (➤212)	Thorough cleansing. Give prophylactic antibiotics. Co-amoxiclav, **or** erythromycin **plus** metronidazole	
Swimming-pool granuloma (fish-tank granuloma)	*Mycobacterium marinum*	Rifampicin and ethambutol	(➤231)

ical referral is essential as prompt debridement is necessary to avoid death in most severe tissue infections. **High-dose parenteral antibiotics**, including cover for Gram-negative aerobes and anaerobes, clostridia and Gp A β-haemolytic streptococci should be used in all cases initially (e.g. penicillin + gentamicin + metronidazole).

Gas gangrene (clostridial myonecrosis)
Necrotising gas-forming infection of muscle with systemic toxaemia. The presence of gas in the tissues is not pathognomonic of clostridial infection—it also occurs in infection with coliforms or non-sporing anaerobes.
Risk factors: This rare condition usually follows traumatic injury with wound contamination. Anaerobic devitalised tissue provides the environment for clostridial growth. Also occurs rarely following intestinal or biliary surgery and very rarely spontaneously, either by contiguous or metastatic spread from a colonic carcinoma or diverticular abscess, or in neutropenic patients.
Clinical features: Severe necrotising cellulitis and myositis with tissue gas and severe systemic toxaemia. Usually occurs 1–4 days after

trauma (range 8 h–3 weeks). Pain, fever, hypotension, oedema of affected skin with haemorrhagic bullae and unpleasant odour. At operation, muscles have a characteristic appearance, initially pale and oedematous, with tissue gas and a serous discharge, progressing to frank gangrene. Intravascular haemolysis, DIC and renal failure are also seen. Frequently fatal, even with optimum management.
Organisms: *Clostridium perfringens* (80%) (➤216), *Clostridium novyi (oedematiens)*, *Clostridium septicum*.
Microbiological investigations: Microscopy of tissue samples shows brick-shaped Gram-positive rods and scanty pus cells. Culture may be positive, but **the diagnosis is clinical** because of the urgent need for surgical debridement.
Other investigations: X-rays, CT and USS may help to localise and delineate infection.
Differential diagnosis: Necrotising fasciitis (see below).
Antibiotic management: Benzylpenicillin + gentamicin + metronidazole should be given to cover the possibility of mixed or secondary

infection with coliforms and non-sporing anaerobes.

Supportive management: Resection of all dead tissue is essential. Hyperbaric oxygen therapy is used although there has been no controlled clinical trial.

Comments: See also puerperal uterine infection by *Clostridium perfringens* (➤216).

Necrotising fasciitis (including synergistic gangrene, streptococcal gangrene, 'hospital gangrene')

Acute necrotising cellulitis involving the dermis, subcutaneous fat and superficial fascia.

Risk factors: Usually postsurgical, with exposure to bowel flora. May be spontaneous, following, e.g., urinary tract infection, urethral diverticulae or perianal suppuration. Predisposing factors include diabetes, age, gross obesity and intercurrent illness. It complicates minor skin wounds, particularly if due to Gp A β-haemolytic streptococci. Necrotising fasciitis due to Gp A β-haemolytic streptococci has been referred to in the past as 'hospital gangrene'.

Clinical features: Rapidly spreading painful cellulitis, often with tissue gas and foul odour. Physical signs such as erythema and induration may be less than expected, given the degree of tissue destruction subsequently found at operation. Diagnosis is often suggested by failure to improve on antibiotics, very rapid progression, systemic toxicity or development of cutaneous anaesthesia and gangrene. At surgical exploration, there is disintegration of the superficial fascial plane with extensive undermining.

Fournier's gangrene is a particular form of necrotising fasciitis affecting the male genitalia. Patients are usually >50 years and often diabetic. Infection follows surgery, minor trauma, local sepsis or UTI. Onset is rapid with systemic toxicity, genital swelling and gangrene which may extend up the abdominal wall and down the thighs. The penile and scrotal skin may slough.

Organisms: Mixed infection with coliforms and anaerobes, or Gp A β-haemolytic streptococci (~30%).

Microbiological investigations: Gram stain and culture of exudate, biopsy material or tissue fluid aspirated from the advancing edge. Blood cultures.

Other investigations: X-rays, CT and USS may demonstrate tissue gas and help to delineate infection.

Differential diagnosis: Streptococcal cellulitis (➤88). Clostridial myonecrosis (➤90).

Antibiotic management: Penicillin + gentamicin + metronidazole initially, guided thereafter by the results of microbiology.

Supportive management: Immediate surgical intervention is required to deroof undermined areas and remove all necrotic tissue. Radical debridement is essential.

MELENEY'S SYNERGISTIC GANGRENE
A rare, slowly progressive synergistic wound infection that occurs following surgery and is usually caused by *Streptococcus 'milleri'* and *Staphylococcus aureus* and often involving non-sporing anaerobes. It is not associated with systemic toxicity. Surgical debridement, flucloxacillin + metronidazole are indicated.

Bacterial myositis (pyomyositis)

Bacterial infection of muscle. Rare in the developed world, commoner in the tropics ('tropical pyomyositis').

Risk factors: There is antecedent trauma in 25%. Other cases occur in apparently healthy individuals and are presumed secondary to bacteraemia.

Clinical features: Induration and tenderness of muscles, usually quadriceps, progressing to fluctuance and abscess formation. Multiple abscesses occur in 40%.

Organisms: *Staphylococcus aureus*, Gp A β-haemolytic streptococci, *Aeromonas* spp., as well as many other less common organisms.

Microbiological investigations: Gram stain and culture of aspirated material. Blood cultures.

Other investigations: Leucocytosis. Creatine kinase is usually normal. USS, CT and MRI will delineate abscesses and guide aspiration for diagnosis and treatment.

Differential diagnosis: Cysticercosis (➤280), trichinosis (➤284).
Antibiotic management: Flucloxacillin initially, guided thereafter by microbiology.
Supportive management: Aspiration or incision and drainage.

Acne vulgaris

Inflammation of the seborrhoeic follicles. Acne is multifactorial in origin, due to increased, androgen-driven sebum production, hyperkeratosis of the follicular epithelium with plug formation and growth within the follicle of *Propionibacterium acnes*.
Management:
Mild cases: Regular, thorough cleansing using a detergent preparation followed by application of a keratolytic/microbicidal agent such as benzoyl peroxide.
Moderate cases: Long-term topical or oral tetracycline (250 mg 12-hly po) or erythromycin (250 mg 12-hly po). Topical clindamycin is also very effective.
Severe cases: These merit dermatological referral for consideration of topical retinoin or systemic isotretinoin. Because of the real risk of teratogenicity, the latter is only available for use under consultant dermatologist supervision.

Seborrhoeic dermatitis

Scaling and greasiness of the scalp, forehead, interscapular, sternal and intertriginous regions, caused by hypersensitivity to and overgrowth of commensal skin fungi, in particular *Pityrosporum orbiculare*. Ketoconazole shampoo and topical miconazole/hydrocortisone cream are effective. Topical hydrocortisone alone is often sufficient.

Cutaneous fungal infections ('dermatophytoses')

Ringworm (tinea) is particularly common in children, and in adults with poor personal hygiene or occupational exposure to animals.
Clinical features: Vary depending on the site of infection. **Tinea capitis** (scalp ringworm)

presents as an area of erythema and scaling on the scalp with hair loss and pustule formation. **Kerion** describes a large boggy inflammatory mass on the scalp with multiple pustules and overlying hair loss. Infection is acquired by person-to-person spread or via fomites such as infected hairbrushes or bedding. **Tinea barbae** affects the beard area, usually in men with rural occupations or animal contact. **Tinea corporis** presents as a pruritic scaly erythematous papule with a raised edge and central healing. **Tinea cruris** describes infection of the groin. It is common in men, and humidity and tight-fitting clothing are predisposing factors. **Majocchi's granuloma** occurs on the legs and arms, particularly in women after shaving. It presents as multiple red pustules that coalesce to form an inflamed plaque. **Tinea pedis** (athlete's foot) causes itching, soreness and maceration between the toes. Warmth, humidity and occlusion predispose. Fungal infection of the **nails** causes subungual hyperkeratosis with lifting of the free edge of the nail.
Organisms: *Microsporum* spp., *Trichophyton* spp., *Epidermophyton* spp. (➤289).
Microbiological investigations: Microscopy of KOH preparation of scrapings or hair. Culture.
Differential diagnosis: Seborrhoeic dermatitis, psoriasis, eczema.
Antibiotic management: Topical miconazole **or** clotrimazole. For scalp infection, griseofulvin 500 mg 24-hly for 4 weeks, or 2 weeks after clinical resolution. Terbinafine is a newer alternative which is effective with shorter courses of treatment. Fungal nail infections require systemic treatment for 3–6 months.
Supportive management: Attention to risk factors, such as close-fitting clothes or shoes.

Erythrasma

Superficial cutaneous infection by *Corynebacterium minutissimum*, commonest in tropical climates.
Clinical features: Maceration, scaling erythema in toe webs. Red-brown well-demarcated irregular patches over dry skin. Skin fluoresces red/pink in UV light (Wood's lamp).

Table 28 Causes of erythema nodosum

Streptococcal infection	(➤170)	Leprosy	(➤230)
Tuberculosis	(➤29)	Blastomycosis	(➤293)
Sarcoidosis		Coccidioidomycosis	(➤293)
Lymphogranuloma venereum	(➤72)	Ulcerative colitis	
Cat-scratch disease	(➤237)	Crohn's disease	
Psittacosis	(➤22)	Leukaemia	
Infectious mononucleosis	(➤105)	Lymphoma	
Tularaemia	(➤212)	Sulphonamides	(➤302)
Histoplasmosis	(➤293)	Pregnancy	
Yersinia spp.	(➤194)	Oral contraceptive pill	

Management: Topical miconazole. Vigorous washing. Whitfield's ointment.

Erythema nodosum (EN)

Tender red swellings on the front of the shins, and sometimes also on the thighs and forearms. Pathologically there is small-vessel vasculitis in the deep dermis and subcutaneous tissue. A number of infectious and non-infectious diseases are associated with EN (Table 28).

Herpes simplex skin infections

Herpes simplex virus (HSV) rarely infects intact skin; primary cutaneous infection is associated with trauma or pre-existing skin disease. Primary infection is often asymptomatic. Both primary and recurrent disease are associated with the development of painful vesicles that progress to pustules and then scabs, healing without scarring.

Primary cutaneous HSV infection
Clinical features: Traumatic herpes ('herpes gladiatorum', 'scrumpox') results from contamination of broken skin by infectious saliva or vesicle fluid. There is a localised vesicular rash with lymphadenopathy, fever and constitutional symptoms. Recurrences are common. There may be a prodrome of itching, pain or paraesthesia, and lymphadenopathy is common. Severe HSV infection occurs in patients with eczema or other skin disease (e.g. pemphigus or burns) which allows extensive viral replication and easy spread. Severe

infection in patients with atopic eczema **(Kaposi's varicelliform eruption, 'eczema herpeticum')** causes widespread vesicular rash and severe constitutional symptoms. In young children the infection may be fatal due to disseminated visceral involvement. HSV causes **paronychia** ('whitlow'), particularly in health professionals exposed to HSV-1-infected saliva, in children with herpes stomatitis (➤102) and in adults with genital herpes. Itching, pain and erythema of the terminal phalanx develop 2–7 days after exposure, followed by a vesicular eruption which resolves after ~10 days. Pain can be severe; recurrence and local lymphadenopathy are common.

Organisms: Most cutaneous HSV infections are due to HSV-1.

Microbiological investigations: Viral culture from vesicle fluid. Serology.

Recurrent cutaneous HSV infection
Recurrent infection occurs after the unusual cutaneous primary infections described above, but the most common manifestation is **herpes labialis** ('cold sores'), which are due to reactivation of HSV-1 infection in the trigeminal ganglion. Genital herpes, due to reactivation usually of HSV-2, in the sacral ganglia, is discussed elsewhere (➤66).

Clinical features: After a prodrome of pain and itching lasting from 6 to 48 hours, a small cluster of erythematous papules develops on the lip, usually at the vermilion border, and most commonly on the outer third of the lower lip. The papules rapidly develop into vesicles, which crust over and heal within 2–3 days. Herpes labialis is frequently precipitated by external stimuli, such as bright sunlight, or by intercurrent illness or fever. Classically, the sores appear during the course of bacterial pneumonia (hence 'fever sores').

Management: Oral acyclovir may shorten the duration of the primary attack, but it is less effective for recurrent attacks. Topical acyclovir is not very effective and is not recommended.

Molluscum contagiosum

A wart-like skin condition caused by poxvirus infection.

Risk factors: Infection occurs worldwide, most commonly in young adults. Transmission occurs by direct, including sexual, contact.

Clinical features: Firm raised umbilicated flesh-coloured nodules develop on the skin anywhere on the body except the palms and soles. Typically occur on the face and genitalia. Lesions persist for months or years.

Organisms: Poxvirus: molluscipoxvirus (➤245).

Microbiological investigations: Diagnosis is clinical. Routine culture of virus is not possible.

Supportive management: There is no specific antiviral therapy. Treatment depends on ablation of lesions by curettage, cryotherapy or topical agents such as trichloracetic acid.

Comments: In immunocompromised patients, particularly those with AIDS, molluscum contagiosum causes bigger and more numerous lesions, which can be very disfiguring. Regular cryotherapy is required.

Orf (syn. contagious pustular dermatosis)

This occupational disease of sheep workers is caused by a parapoxvirus (➤245) and is acquired by direct contact with infected animals. It produces a raised fleshy purple plaque 1–2 cm in diameter on the hands or fingers of infected farmers and veterinary surgeons. A central vesicle develops, often with haemorrhage into the base. Spontaneous resolution occurs over a few weeks. Recovery is sometimes complicated by the development of a widespread itchy vesicular eruption, which has been described as a form of erythema multiforme and which is thought to be a manifestation of hypersensitivity.

10: Bone and Joint Infections

Septic arthritis

Bacterial joint infection.

Risk factors: Usually secondary to haematogenous seeding of the highly vascular synovial membrane during bacteraemia; occasionally due to direct spread from bone or adjacent tissues. Pre-existing joint disease, (e.g. rheumatoid arthritis (RA), crystal synovitis, severe osteoarthritis, haemarthrosis) and chronic systemic disease (e.g. malignancy) or IVDU predisposes. Direct intra-articular inoculation, iatrogenic or traumatic, is a rare cause of infection, except in the case of prosthetic joint infection. In young adults consider disseminated gonococcal infection (➤66).

Clinical features: Rapid onset, over days, of monoarthritis affecting (in descending order of frequency) knee, hip, ankle, wrist, shoulder, elbow or other synovial joint. There is more than one affected joint in 15–20% Joint is swollen, tender, red, warm and has very limited range of movement due to pain. Fever and leucocytosis are common, but not always present. Signs can be minimal with infected prosthetic joint or at certain locations, e.g. sacroiliac joints.

Gonococcal arthritis is a feature of disseminated gonococcal infection (➤66). It is three times commoner in women. Only 25%, mostly men, report concurrent symptoms of genital gonorrhoea. The incubation time ranges from 1 day to 2 months after sexual exposure. Usual presentation is migratory polyarthralgia followed by synovitis and tenosynovitis at more than one site (knees, wrists, ankles, hand and foot tendon sheaths). Most have skin lesions (macules, papules and pustules), although these may be scanty. Septic arthritis also occurs during **meningococcaemia** (➤74), although *Neisseria meningitidis* infection is more often associated with a sterile immune-mediated oligoarthritis.

Organisms: Adults: *Staphylococcus aureus* (90% of cases complicating RA), streptococci, coliforms (particularly with malignancy, immunosuppression or IVDU), rarely *Streptococcus pneumoniae. Neisseria gonorrhoeae* and *meningitidis*. In children under 2 years: *Haemophilus influenzae, Staphylococcus aureus*. In neonates, *Staphylococcus aureus*, coliforms and Gp B β-haemolytic streptococci. Arthritis is also associated with *Brucella* spp. (➤209), *Salmonella* spp. (➤190). *Mycobacterium tuberculosis* (➤30).

Microbiological investigations: Immediate joint aspiration is mandatory. Fluid may be inoculated directly into blood culture bottles, but also send some in a sterile universal for Gram stain and conventional culture. Neutrophil counts on synovial fluid are usually high but do not differentiate from non-infectious causes. Fluid should always be examined for crystals, but their presence does not exclude sepsis, particularly as crystal arthropathy predisposes to septic arthritis. Synovial fluid culture is positive in >90% of cases due to *Staphylococcus aureus*, and blood cultures are positive in ~50%. Mycobacterial and fungal cultures should be requested in more chronic cases in groups at risk. USS, CT and MRI are used to assess the presence of and assist drainage of effusions from difficult joints such as hip and sacroiliacs. Synovial biopsy may be necessary to diagnose TB. In gonococcal arthritis, blood cultures are positive in <10% and synovial fluid culture in ~25%; genital cultures (➤65) are positive in the majority.

Other investigations: X-rays are often normal early in disease. Earliest finding is joint effusion with displacement of the fat pads, followed by periarticular osteoporosis, joint space narrowing and erosions. Bone scan can be helpful in localising infection and in differentiating between septic arthritis and overlying cellulitis.

Differential diagnosis: RA, crystal synovitis, seronegative spondarthritides, Reiter's syndrome, viral arthritis (e.g. due to rubella (➤101), rubella vaccination, parvovirus (➤107) or hepatitis B (➤49)), reactive arthritis (➤97), Lyme disease (➤224).

Antibiotic management: Depends on clinical situation and results of initial Gram stain and culture. **Gram-positive cocci seen:** flucloxacillin, unless there is reason to suspect MRSA (➤167) when vancomycin is used. **Gram-negative cocci seen:** cefotaxime. If *Neisseria gonorrhoeae* subsequently grown and shown to be penicillin-sensitive, change to benzylpenicillin. **Gram-negative bacilli seen:** cefotaxime + gentamicin. **Negative Gram stain:** adult with risk factors listed above: flucloxacillin + gentamicin; children and healthy young adults: cefotaxime. Therapy can be modified when culture results are available. Disseminated gonococcal infection characteristically responds rapidly (within 1–3 days) to appropriate antibiotics. Duration of therapy: 7–10 days for *Neisseria gonorrhoeae*. Other organisms 3–4 weeks, depending on response.

Supportive management: Joint drainage is required and is achieved by needle aspiration of peripheral joints. Axial joints usually need open surgical drainage. Rheumatological and/ or orthopaedic referral is essential ☎.

Complications: During recovery, a sterile 'postinfectious' arthritis may affect the joint. Differentiation from relapse depends on Gram stain and culture of synovial fluid.

> **Practice point:** Acute monoarthritis is septic until proven otherwise, and should be aspirated.

Prosthetic joint infection

Approximately 1% of joint prostheses will become infected. The majority are acquired during the original operation; occasionally infected later by bacteraemia.

Clinical features: Loosening of the prosthesis is more common and does not necessarily indicate infection, but predisposes towards it. Fever and local signs are not always present. Progressive pain made worse by activity is characteristic, although a good range of passive movement may be preserved.

Organisms: *Staphylococcus aureus* and *epidermidis*, coliforms, enterococci; many other species reported less often.

Investigations: ESR and CRP are usually raised and this is useful evidence of infection. Indium white cell scan may also be helpful. Aspiration around the prosthesis may yield the causative organism.

Management: Removal of the prosthesis, and antibiotics guided by culture.

Reiter's syndrome (RS)

Immune-mediated arthritis, conjunctivitis and mucocutaneous lesions associated with urethritis due to *Chlamydia trachomatis* (➤66) or bacillary dysentery.

Risk factors: Strongly associated with possession of HLA B27, 80% of cases being B27-positive. Commoner in males.

Clinical features: Onset occurs between a few days and 4 weeks after infectious illness. Acute-onset asymmetrical oligoarthritis affecting (in decreasing order of frequency), ankles, knees, metatarsophalangeal joints, proximal interphalangeal toe joints, wrists, sternocostal and sacroiliac joints. Most patients have two or more affected joints. Inflammation occurs at the points of insertion of tendons ('enthesopathy') causing Achilles tendinitis and 'sausage' swelling of digits. Conjunctivitis is usually bilateral and mild. Rarely anterior uveitis develops. Urethritis presents as mucopurulent urethral discharge with dysuria. The meatus may be swollen and red. In postdysenteric RS, sterile urethritis may develop 1–2 weeks after diarrhoea. Skin lesions include superficial painless ulceration of the glans penis, which is either localised or encircles the glans (circinate balanitis), and crusted scaling papules usually on the soles, palms, trunk and genitals (keratoderma blenorrhagica). Oral ulceration also occurs. Eye and skin involvement is unusual post-dysentery. Arthritis resolves slowly over months, and does not usually cause permanent joint damage, although this may occur. Recurrences occur, often triggered by sexual exposure. Heart block and aortic regurgitation occur rarely in patients with severe long-standing disease.

Organisms: *Chlamydia trachomatis* (➤233), *Salmonella* spp. (➤190), *Shigella* spp. (➤192), *Yersinia enterocolitica* (➤194).
Microbiological investigations: Urethral smear and culture for *Chlamydia trachomatis* and *Neisseria gonorrhoeae* (➤65). Aspiration and culture of synovial fluid to exclude septic arthritis (➤95). Synovial fluid usually contains 5000–20000 WBC/μl (usually >50000 WBC/μl in septic arthritis) and culture is negative. Stool culture. Yersinia serology (➤194).
Other investigations: Leucocytosis and raised ESR are common.
Differential diagnosis: Gonococcal arthritis (➤95). Rheumatoid arthritis, psoriatic arthritis, ankylosing spondylitis, inflammatory bowel disease.
Antibiotic management: Tetracycline is given for chlamydial urethritis. Prolonged tetracycline treatment for 3 months speeds resolution of arthritis in postvenereal but not dysenteric cases.
Supportive management: Non-steroidal anti-inflammatory drugs. Intraarticular steroid injections and immunosuppression in severe cases. Rheumatological referral is recommended.
Comments: The term **reactive arthritis** is used to describe post-dysentery arthritis without the eye or cutaneous features of Reiter's disease.

Viral arthritis

A symmetrical peripheral arthritis, superficially resembling rheumatoid arthritis, complicates a number of infections, particularly parvovirus (➤107), rubella and rubella immunisation (➤101) and hepatitis B (➤49), but also mumps (➤102), enteroviruses (➤251), herpesviruses (➤241) and adenoviruses (➤240). Joint symptoms are usually mild, of sudden onset and brief duration, and often occur early in the illness at the same time as skin rash. Joint damage can be more severe and persistent, particularly after parvovirus and rubella infections. Serological confirmation of infection should be sought as a firm diagnosis helps to differentiate from rheumatoid arthritis. Arthritis is a prominent feature of some arthropod-borne alphavirus infections

such as chikungunya, O'nyong-nyong, Ross River virus and Sindbis (➤253).

Osteomyelitis

Infection of bone, including periosteum, cortical bone and medullary cavity, leading to progressive destruction of bone and deposition of new bone. May be acute (over weeks) or chronic (months to years). **Sequestrum** is dead bone that is devoid of blood supply. It acts as a foreign body and must be removed before antibiotics will be effective. Periosteal new bone formation is referred to as **involucrum**. Osteomyelitis arises by two main mechanisms: **haematogenous** spread during bacteraemia and by spread from a **contiguous focus** of infection.
Risk factors: Bacteraemia. Contiguous soft-tissue infection, such as frontal sinusitis, leading to local osteomyelitis with oedema of the forehead ('Pott's puffy tumour'). Local predisposing factors include previous trauma, particularly open fractures, foreign bodies, including prosthetic implants, vascular insufficiency. Rarely cranial radiotherapy causes osteoradionecrosis, which predisposes to subsequent osteomyelitis. Sickle-cell disease, diabetes mellitus, IVDU are also risk factors.
Clinical features: Fever, rigors, bone pain, local swelling, tenderness and erythema. These classic features are seen in acute haematogenous osteomyelitis, and are often mild or absent in disease due to contiguous infection. **Haematogenous** infection classically affects the metaphyses of long bones (esp. tibia and femur) in children and the vertebrae of adults. **Contiguous** osteomyelitis is commonly secondary to open fractures, hip replacements and in the sacrum secondary to decubitus ulcers. **Brodie's tumour** (primary subacute pyogenic osteomyelitis) presents subacutely with pain and low-grade fever. It affects the lower limb in patients under 20 years. **Chronic osteomyelitis** usually presents with sinus formation and discharge. Systemic features are uncommon and local signs tend to be less prevalent. It is difficult to eradicate without extensive surgical debridement.
Organisms: Neonates: *Staphylococcus aureus*, Gp B β-haemolytic streptococci, coliforms (especially *Salmonella* spp. worldwide). **Chil-**

dren < 6 years: *Staphylococcus aureus*, *Staphylococcus epidermidis*, streptococci, *Haemophilus influenzae*. **Adults:** *Staphylococcus aureus*. **Elderly/immunocompromised patients:** *Staphylococcus aureus*, coliforms, pseudomonads. **Children with sickle-cell disease:** *Salmonella* spp. Mixed infection is common in disease due to vascular insufficiency. Anaerobic infection occurs particularly in the diabetic foot (➤221), dental sepsis, in lower-limb fractures, in osteomyelitis underlying venous ulceration and in deep human bite wounds. Brodie's tumour is always due to *Staphylococcus aureus*.

Microbiological investigations: Accurate microbiological diagnosis is very important. Send blood cultures if systemically unwell. Culture of sinus pus should be performed, but may not accurately reflect organisms present in bone, unless *Staphylococcus aureus* is isolated. Needle aspiration under radiological guidance should be performed early; open biopsy is more sensitive.

Other investigations: Leucocytosis and raised ESR are likely. **Plain X-rays are usually normal early in disease**. Soft-tissue swelling and periosteal elevation are seen after 1–2 weeks and lytic changes and sclerosis even later. Technetium bone scan is sensitive and is usually positive at presentation. It may be difficult to interpret if there is contiguous soft-tissue infection. CT and MRI scanning are particularly helpful for vertebral disease. Alkaline phosphatase is usually normal.

Differential diagnosis: Includes sickle-cell crisis. Primary and metastatic tumour. Tuberculous osteomyelitis (➤30).

Antibiotic management: Antibiotics penetrate chronically infected bone poorly, so prolonged treatment is required, initially parenteral. **Empirical therapy** before organism is isolated as follows. **Neonates:** flucloxacillin + gentamicin. **Children <6 years:** flucloxacillin + ampicillin **or** co-amoxiclav **or** cefotaxime. **Adults:** flucloxacillin (+ gentamicin if elderly or immunocompromised). **Treatment of particular organisms** as follows. *Staphylococcus aureus*: flucloxacillin (+ oral fucidin if severe). MRSA: vancomycin. Streptococci: benzylpenicillin. *Haemophilus influenzae*:

ampicillin if sensitive, **or** cefotaxime. Coliforms: cefotaxime **or** ciprofloxacin. *Pseudomonas aeruginosa*: azlocillin **or** ceftazidime ± gentamicin. **Suppression of chronic osteomyelitis:** flucloxacillin (for Gram-positives); ciprofloxacin (for Gram-negatives). Oral treatment of Gram-negative osteomyelitis possible with ciprofloxacin, but only where the organism has been isolated and shown to be sensitive and compliance guaranteed.

Suppportive management: Drainage is indicated if there is a poor response to appropriate antibiotic therapy. Surgery may be required for diagnosis or for debridement and removal of sequestra. Osteomyelitis of the femoral head is usually drained to prevent the development of septic arthritis. Early orthopaedic consultation advised.

Complications: Recurrence. Chronic osteomyelitis causes amyloidosis. Rarely, carcinoma occurs in the sinus tract.

Comments: Septic arthritis is an unusual complication in adults because the epiphyseal plate provides a physical barrier to spread of infection. It is much more likely in infants, in whom the plate has yet to develop.

Vertebral osteomyelitis

Osteomyelitis of the vertebral body is usually haematogenous in origin, and retrograde venous spread from the genitourinary tract occurs rarely.

Risk factors: Patients are usually elderly. IVDU also predisposes.

Clinical features: Usually presents subacutely. Clinical signs may be minimal, and diagnosis is frequently delayed. Back pain and raised ESR in an elderly patient should alert. Spinal tenderness and referred root pain. Neurological complications such as paraplegia or meningitis are rare.

Organisms: *Staphylococcus aureus*, *Salmonella* spp., coliforms, *Pseudomonas aeruginosa* (esp. IVDU), streptococci, fastidious Gram-negative bacteria.

Microbiological investigations: Blood cultures. Biopsy is essential if blood cultures negative. Open biopsy is much more sensitive than needle aspiration.

Other investigations: Raised ESR. Plain X-rays may be normal in early disease. Radiological involvement of the disc favours infection (pyogenic or TB) rather than tumour.

Differential diagnosis: Tuberculous osteomyelitis. Metastatic carcinoma (especially prostatic).

Antibiotic management: As above for osteomyelitis.

> **Practice point:** Minimal tenderness on vertebral percussion may be the only sign of vertebral osteomyelitis.

Diabetic foot infections

A common cause of hospital admission and amputation. Diabetics are prone both to cellulitis, due to Gp A β-haemolytic streptococci, and to infections of deep tissues and bone with mixed bacteria.

Risk factors: Ischaemia due to peripheral vascular disease, neuropathy and defective immune function, particularly phagocytosis, contribute to pathogenesis. Poor diabetic control, smoking, hypertension and hyperlipidaemia.

Clinical features: Commoner in elderly type 2 diabetics. Many patients have long-standing ulceration. Warmth, redness, swelling and exudate suggest infection but tenderness is usually absent due to neuropathy. There may be crepitus and foul odour. Concomitant evidence of peripheral vascular disease (absent pulses, bruits, atrophic skin) and neuropathy. Unexplained poor diabetic control suggests underlying infection. Fever is unusual.

Organisms: Polymicrobial infection is common. *Staphylococcus aureus*, non-sporing anaerobes, *Staphylococcus epidermidis*, streptococci including β-haemolytic Gp A and B and *Streptococcus 'milleri'*, enterococci, coliforms and coryneforms.

Microbiological investigations: Local sinus cultures are misleading, unless *Staphylococcus aureus* is isolated. Isolation of coliforms and pseudomonads from ulcers and sinuses is particularly likely to represent superficial colonisation. Curettings from ulcer base or material removed at surgical debridement is more likely to represent organisms responsible. Blood culture if systemically unwell.

Other investigations: Plain X-ray for osteomyelitis and gas in tissues. Bone scan may be difficult to interpret because of overlying soft-tissue infection.

Antibiotic management: For mild cases, oral flucloxacillin + metronidazole or co-amoxiclav. In severe infection, iv flucloxacillin + gentamicin + metronidazole or cefotaxime + metronidazole.

Supportive management: Control hyperglycaemia. A full discussion of the indications for and timing of reconstructive surgery and amputation is beyond the scope of this manual. Early orthopaedic consultation is advised.

Comments: Prevention of diabetic foot ulcers depends on good glycaemic control, careful foot care with regular chiropody, correctly fitting shoes and patient education, and attention to other risk factors such as smoking, hypertension and hyperlipidaemia.

11: Paediatric Infections

This chapter considers infections which occur most often in childhood, and the important differences between bacterial infections in children and adults.

Common viral infections of childhood

Measles (syn. rubeola, morbilli) ✉ ①
Organism: Family paramyxovirus: morbillivirus (➤248).
Epidemiology: Prior to immunisation, infection was widespread in all communities (>90% infected by age 20). Since immunisation, measles is much less common, usually occurring in unimmunised adolescents. Measles-related deaths are now extremely rare in the developed world. In developing countries infection occurs in epidemics and is severe and an important cause of death.
Reservoir: Humans.
Transmission: Highly contagious. Droplet spread via respiratory route.
Incubation period: Seven to 18 days. Mean 10 days to prodrome, 14 days to rash.
Infectious period: Just before onset of symptoms to 4 days after appearance of rash.
Clinical features: Prodrome 2–4 days with malaise, fever, coryza, conjunctivitis and cough. Fever peaks after the onset of rash and resolves over the next 3 days. Fever persisting beyond the third day of rash suggests secondary bacterial infection. **Koplik's spots** are pathognomonic, 1–2 mm white spots on an erythematous base on the buccal mucosa appearing first opposite the lower molar teeth, 2 days before the rash. **Rash** appears 2–4 days after onset – a blanching erythematous maculopapular eruption starting behind the ears, rapidly involving the forehead and then spreading caudally so that the face, trunk, buttocks and legs are involved by the third day. May be confluent. As it fades, it leaves non-blanching 'staining' due to capillary haemorrhage. Rash lasts 1 week and ends with fine

desquamation. Soles and palms are spared and do not desquamate (in contrast to scarlet fever ➤108).

The majority have **pulmonary involvement**, which, although usually mild, accounts for 90% of deaths due to measles. Direct viral involvement causes bronchiolitis and giant-cell pneumonia, giving bilateral hyperinflation and diffuse fluffy infiltrates on CXR. It is difficult to distinguish from secondary bacterial pneumonia, usually due to *Staphylococcus aureus, Haemophilus influenzae* or group A β-haemolytic streptococci. Severe infection is particularly likely in immunocompromised patients and dramatic desquamating skin infection in malnourished children is a common cause of death in the developing world.

Diarrhoea, vomiting, abdominal pain, severe pharyngitis and cervical lymphadenopathy may occur. In severe cases, generalised lymphadenopathy and splenomegaly may be seen. Myocarditis, pericarditis and hepatitis occur rarely. Encephalitis, which may be severe and leave permanent neurological sequelae, occurs in ~1 in 1000 cases.

Modified measles describes a less severe form, often with a prolonged incubation period, seen in those with partial immunity (infants with maternal antibodies, recipients of immunoglobulin, previously immunised patients).

Atypical measles is a rare form occurring in previously immunised individuals. Early symptoms include high fever and headache. The rash appears peripherally and may be maculopapular, urticarial or vesicular. Pulmonary involvement with dyspnoea and nodular changes on CXR are common. Patients are often very unwell and the illness may last 2 weeks or more. Diagnosis is confirmed by demonstrating a large rise in specific antibodies.
Investigations: Diagnosis is clinical, but can be confirmed by serology.
Specific management: None.

Supportive management: Symptomatic relief. Treatment of complications including antibiotics for secondary bacterial infection.

Complications: Bacterial otitis media (➤15) and pneumonia (➤22). **Subacute sclerosing panencephalitis (SSPE)** is a very rare (~1 in 100 000 cases) complication due to persistent measles infection. Onset is insidious and occurs 6–8 years after measles, with behavioural and intellectual changes progressing to myoclonic spasms, focal neurological deficits, coma and death, usually within 3 years.

Immunisation: Single-dose live vaccine gives 90–95% protection (➤337).

Comments: Infection in pregnancy can cause abortion or stillbirth, but does not cause congenital malformation. Infants born to immune mothers are protected by maternal antibody for 6–9 months. These antibodies interfere with immunisation which is therefore not recommended in UK before age 12 months. In developing countries, where death due to measles is common before that age, it needs to be given earlier, and repeated.

Rubella (syn. German measles) ✉ ①
Organism: Family togaviridae: rubivirus (➤253).
Epidemiology: A worldwide disease of childhood. Its significance lies entirely in the ability of maternal infection during pregnancy to cause congenital malformation (➤102).
Reservoir: Humans.
Transmission: Droplet spread by the respiratory route.
Incubation period: Sixteen to 18 days (range 14–23).
Infectious period: One week before and 4 days after the onset of rash. Infants with congenital rubella syndrome (CRS) often continue to excrete virus in pharyngeal secretions and urine for many months after birth.
Clinical features: Frequently asymptomatic, especially in children. Adults present with 1–5-day prodrome with headache, fever and upper respiratory symptoms. Onset of disease in children occurs with rash; this consists of discrete maculopapular patches of erythema, starting on the face and spreading to the rest of the body. Typically there is generalised

and particularly postauricular lymphadenopathy, splenomegaly and conjunctivitis. Arthralgia occurs in the majority of adults. Some patients develop a symmetrical peripheral arthritis (➤97). This usually lasts 5–10 days and resolves, but is sometimes severe or persistent, resembling rheumatoid arthritis. Thrombocytopenia, Guillain–Barré syndrome and encephalitis (1 in 5000 cases) occur rarely.

Investigations: Clinical diagnosis is unreliable and serological confirmation must be sought whenever pregnancy is a possibility. Acute infection is diagnosed by demonstrating specific IgM or a greater than fourfold rise in IgG titres between acute and convalescent sera. Serum taken earlier than 1 week or later than 3 weeks after onset of rash can give a false negative IgM.

Exposure to rubella in pregnancy: Any pregnant woman with suspected rubella or exposure to rubella requires serological screening, irrespective of a history of immunisation, clinical rubella or a previous positive rubella antibody test. Serum should be taken as soon as possible. ✆ Close liaison with the virology lab is required, as further serum samples will be needed. If current rubella infection is confirmed, parents need counselling on the risk of CRS and termination (➤102).

Immunisation: Immunisation with measles/mumps/rubella (MMR) vaccine is currently recommended for all children between 12 and 15 months old. Females of 10–14 years old should be given single-antigen rubella vaccine unless there is documented evidence that they have received MMR. Non-pregnant seronegative women of childbearing age should be vaccinated and advised not to risk pregnancy for 1 month after vaccination. All women should be screened in every pregnancy for rubella antibodies, irrespective of a previous positive antibody report. Immunisation of seronegatives should not be performed during pregnancy, although there is no evidence that this is harmful. Immunisation must be given post-delivery.

Specific management: None. Human immunoglobulin should be given to pregnant women exposed to rubella who will not consider termination under any circumstances, although its benefits are controversial.

CONGENITAL RUBELLA SYNDROME (CRS)
The risks of CRS following maternal rubella depend on the stage of pregnancy at which infection occurs: <10 weeks, risk ~90%; 11–12 weeks, ~30%; 13–20 weeks, <10%; >20 weeks, risk very low.
Clinical features: Of neonates with CRS, 50% appear normal at birth. Affected children usually have low birth weight. Clinical features are transient, permanent or developmental. **Transient** features include hepatitis, hepatosplenomegaly and jaundice, thrombocytopenia, chronic rubelliform rash, haemolytic anaemia, hypogammaglobulinaemia, lymphadenopathy, encephalitis and diarrhoea. These features can be severe, but usually resolve over the first few weeks of life. **Permanent** features include the classical triad of patent ductus arteriosus, cataracts and nerve deafness. Deafness is the commonest manifestation of CRS affecting ~80% of cases. It is usually bilateral and reflects central or peripheral neurological damage. Other common defects include pulmonary artery stenosis and pulmonary valvular stenosis, retinopathy, cloudy cornea and glaucoma, microcephaly, mental retardation and spastic diplegia. **Developmental** defects present later in life. Children with CRS have a greatly increased risk of developing insulin-dependent diabetes mellitus (20% by age 35) and hypo- or hyperthyroidism. Hearing loss and ocular defects may also be progressive.
Diagnosis: The assessment of a child with congenital defects consistent with intrauterine infection includes consideration of other potential causes (TORCH screening ➤111). Congenital rubella infection is confirmed by identifying antirubella IgM in the neonate, isolating rubella virus or demonstrating the persistence of specific IgG after 12 months, when maternally derived IgG levels should have waned.

Mumps (syn. infectious parotitis) ✉ ①
Organism: Family paramyxovirus: paramyxovirus (➤248).

Epidemiology: In the absence of immunisation, infection is widespread and frequently asymptomatic.
Reservoir: Humans.
Transmission: Droplet spread by the respiratory route.
Incubation period: Twelve to 25 days.
Infectious period: One week before parotitis and up to 10 days thereafter.
Clinical features: There is a 2–3-day prodrome with malaise, headache, fever and anorexia. Progressive pain and swelling develop in one or both parotid glands, peaking at 2–3 days and resolving over the following week. There is often associated swelling of sublingual and submandibular glands. Meningoencephalitis is commoner in postpubertal patients (➤77). It is rarely complicated by permanent nerve deafness (1 in 20 000 cases of mumps) or facial palsy. Other rare neurological complications include acute cerebellar ataxia and transverse myelitis. Orchitis occurs in ~20% of postpubertal males. It is usually unilateral, so sterility is rare. Oophoritis also occurs, causing pelvic pain and tenderness. Orchitis and meningitis can occur before or without parotitis. Pancreatitis occurs in <10% of cases and presents with abdominal pain and tenderness, nausea and vomiting days to weeks after parotitis. Resolution usually occurs in 7–10 days. Thyroiditis, myocarditis and arthritis are very rare.
Investigations: Diagnosis is confirmed by specific serology.
Differential diagnosis: Bacterial parotitis. Viral and bacterial meningitis (➤74). Bacterial epididymo-orchitis (➤60).
Immunisation: Immunisation is recommended at age 12–15 months as part of the MMR vaccine (➤337). Vaccine may also be given to susceptible adults, but antibody responses develop too slowly for this to be useful as protection after exposure to mumps.

Practice point: Serum amylase is raised in uncomplicated mumps parotitis.

Primary herpes simplex virus (HSV) infection (herpetic stomatitis)
Organism: Family herpesviridae: HSV1 (➤241).

Epidemiology: More than 80% of primary HSV infections are asymptomatic. In children > 6 months and <5 years old, acute gingivostomatitis may occur. May also occur in adults, in whom it is usually less severe.

Reservoir: Humans.

Transmission: Usually from an adult with herpes labialis or from another infected child.

Incubation period: Three to 6 days (range 2–14 days).

Infectious period: Virus is secreted in saliva for many weeks following acute infection. Periods of asymptomatic viral shedding also occur. Isolation, ①, is recommended for children with disseminated infection.

Clinical features: Abrupt onset of fever, anorexia, listlessness and sore mouth, followed by severe ulcerative gingivostomatitis with local lymphadenopathy. Vesicles (1–3 mm) form on buccal mucosa, rupture and coalesce, leaving painful ulceration. Salivation and drooling are prominent. Herpetic vesicles develop in areas contaminated by highly infectious saliva, including perioral skin, eye (➤84), fingers and vulva.

Investigations: Diagnosis is confirmed by culture of HSV from saliva, and by a rise in specific antibody titres.

Differential diagnosis: *Candida albicans* (➤291). *Capnocytophaga ochracea* (➤208). Other viral causes of oropharyngeal ulceration include Coxsackieviruses (hand, foot and mouth disease or herpangina ➤108) and echoviruses (➤251).

Specific management: Topical acyclovir is of **no** benefit. Systemic or intravenous acyclovir speeds healing and is particularly useful in the immunocompromised host.

Supportive management: Maintenance of adequate fluid input may require parenteral therapy.

Varicella (syn. chickenpox) ⊠ (Scotland only) ①

Organism: Family herpesviridae: varicella zoster virus (VZV, syn. herpes zoster) (➤243).

Epidemiology: VZV infection occurs worldwide. Seroprevalence at age 20 is typically ~95%. Primary infection with VZV causes chickenpox, which is primarily a disease of childhood, although it occurs at any age and is more severe in adults, with a higher incidence of serious complications such as pneumonitis. Reactivation of latent VZV in sensory ganglia causes herpes zoster (syn. shingles).

Reservoir: Humans.

Transmission: Person to person by direct contact or droplet spread from cases of chickenpox or herpes zoster.

Incubation period: Thirteen to 21 days.

Infectious period: From 2 days before the onset of rash until the lesions are crusted. Scabs are non-infectious.

Clinical features: There is a mild prodrome of malaise, fever, headache and rhinitis. The rash develops as crops of vesicles, each appearing on an erythematous base ('dewdrop on a rose petal'). Vesicles rapidly progress to umbilicated papules, pustules and scabs. Distribution is typically central on head, trunk and arms, and also the palate or gums. New crops continue to appear for up to 7 days. Fever remains elevated for 4–5 days after onset of rash. Bacterial superinfection of the rash is common (esp Gp A β-haemolytic streptococci). Many patients have mild viral hepatitis. Mucositis may cause dysuria.

Varicella **pneumonitis** is commoner in immunocompromised patients and adults especially if they smoke or are pregnant. It can progress rapidly, with hypoxia and tachypnoea. CXR shows widespread patchy shadowing. If severe, intubation and ventilation are required, and there is significant mortality. Residual pulmonary fibrosis and CXR calcifications may occur in survivors. Pulmonary disease during varicella is often due to secondary bacterial pneumonia, usually with *Streptococcus pneumoniae*, *Haemophilus influenzae* or *Staphylococcus aureus*. Staphylococcal septicaemia may occur. **Encephalitis** presenting with cerebellar ataxia occurs very rarely. It may be fatal, but usually resolves in the immunocompetent host. **Thrombocytopenia** and **disseminated intravascular coagulopathy** occur very rarely and may cause haemorrhagic varicella, with bleeding into vesicles.

Investigations: Usually diagnosed clinically. Light microscopy of vesicle contents reveals multinucleate giant cells (Tzanck preparation); electron microscopy shows large numbers of herpesvirus particles. Commercial kits are available for the detection of VZV antigens in vesicle fluid. Retrospectively diagnosis is confirmed by serology.

Differential diagnosis: In atypical cases, vesicular impetigo due to *Staphylococcus aureus* or Gp A β-haemolytic streptococci can be confused (➤87). Other infectious vesicular rashes include herpes simplex infection (➤93), hand, foot and mouth disease (➤107) and disseminated gonococcal infection (➤65). Noninfectious causes include Stevens–Johnson syndrome, pemphigus and pemphigoid.

Specific management: Acyclovir is indicated in the following circumstances: immunocompromised patients (including those with AIDS), adults with varicella, neonates, and if there is evidence of severe or disseminated disease, in particular, ophthalmic disease, pneumonitis or encephalitis. Acyclovir is given intravenously 10 mg/kg 8-hly for 7–10 days. Dose is reduced in renal failure and a good throughput of fluid should be maintained to avoid crystalluria. Antibiotics are required for secondary bacterial infection of rash or lower respiratory tract. Some physicians give parenteral flucloxacillin to all adult cases because of the small risk of staphylococcal septicaemia.

Supportive management: Symptomatic relief with calamine lotion and analgesia/antipyretics.

Complications: Chickenpox is typically a mild infection; morbidity and mortality are related to particular clinical circumstances:

Infection in pregnancy: Pregnant women with varicella have an increased risk of severe pneumonitis (~10%). Acyclovir should be given at the first sign of respiratory distress. If infection occurs at less than 26 weeks' gestation there is a small risk of foetal malformation (microcephaly, hydrocephalus, limb hypoplasia, cutaneous scarring and ophthalmic defects). The risk is highest during the first trimester (~3%). Infection around delivery may be followed by neonatal infection, which can be severe.

Infection in neonates: Neonates of mothers who develop varicella <5 days before or shortly after delivery will not be protected by maternal IgG and are at risk of developing severe disseminated infection. They should receive acyclovir and VZIG (see below). Herpes zoster during pregnancy poses no threat to mother or child since, by definition, the mother will have anti-VZV IgG which will protect the neonate.

Infection in the immunocompromised: Severe skin eruption with haemorrhage is more common, and dissemination to internal organs, with hepatitis, pneumonitis, pancreatitis and encephalitis occurs more frequently and can be fatal.

Reye syndrome was in the past most often associated with varicella and aspirin use in children. Now that the use of aspirin in childhood is discouraged, Reye syndrome has become much less common.

Immunisation: A live attenuated vaccine is used in some countries (e.g. Japan) but is not licensed in the UK. It is available on a named-patient basis for immunocompromised patients such as children with leukaemia.

Varicella zoster immune globulin (VZIG) is prepared from donors with high-titre antibodies against VZV and is only available in small quantities. It does not prevent infection but modifies its severity and is given to the following groups **after exposure to chickenpox or herpes zoster**:
• VZV-seronegative immunosuppressed patients on high-dose steroids (⩾ 2 mg/kg/day of prednisolone for >1 week within 3 months of exposure).
• Bone marrow transplant recipients and patients with debilitating disease, irrespective of a history of chickenpox.
• Infants less than 4 weeks old whose mothers develop chickenpox 1 week before to 4 weeks after delivery, or who are exposed to VZV from another source and whose mothers have no history of chickenpox or are seronegative.
• Infants less than 4 weeks old in contact with VZV who are born at less than 30 weeks' gestation or with birth weight less than 1 kg. These may not have maternal antibody despite a positive maternal history.
• Pregnant women who are VZV-seronegative.

- VZV-seronegative patients with symptomatic HIV infection.

Herpes zoster (syn. shingles) ①
Reactivation of VZV in sensory nerve ganglia causes herpes zoster.
Epidemiology: Occurs at any age but is commoner in the elderly. Also frequent in the immunocompromised, in whom disseminated disease is more likely. Second and third attacks occur but are unusual.
Clinical features: Pain, often severe or burning, localised to a single dermatome followed after 1–4 days by a vesicular eruption which progresses through the same stages as varicella (papules, vesicles, pustules and scabs) and is confined to the same dermatome with sharp demarcation in the midline. Commonly involved areas are the thoracic dermatomes and the ophthalmic division of the trigeminal nerve (➤84). Patients are often systemically unwell with fever, headache, mild confusion. Rarely viral meningitis or encephalitis may ensue. A few disseminated lesions outside the dermatome are commonly seen in normal hosts. In the immunocompromised, widespread progressive dissemination can occur. Very severe zoster is rarely accompanied by weakness of the muscles supplied by the same spinal root. Involvement of particular nerve roots causes a number of specific syndromes (Table 29).

Healing occurs with scarring after 1–4 weeks. Postherpetic neuralgia persisting beyond 1 month after healing is an infrequent occurrence. It is more likely in elderly female patients, may be severe, and usually resolves over 6–24 months.
Management: **Parenteral** acyclovir speeds resolution of zoster and is given to immunocompromised patients or those with specific syndromes mentioned above. Topical and oral acyclovir may speed resolution if treatment is started early.

Infectious mononucleosis (IM)
(syn. glandular fever)
Organism: Family herpesviridae: Epstein–Barr virus (EBV) (➤243).
Epidemiology: Common in all populations. In developed countries adult seroprevalence is >90%. Infection under 5 years is common (seroprevalence ~50%) but usually asymptomatic. Further peak of seroconversion occurs during adolescence. Of these cases, 50% result in infectious mononucleosis, the rest being asymptomatic.
Reservoir: Humans.
Transmission: Person to person via saliva.
Incubation period: Thirty to 45 days.
Infectious period: EBV can be recovered from oral secretions for up to 18 months after infection; ~25% of asymptomatic seropositives shed virus in saliva. Transmission by blood transfusion has occurred.
Clinical features: Onset varies from acute to insidious. In young children, fever, sore throat, lymphadenopathy, malaise and anorexia are common. In adolescents and adults, non-specific features predominate and ton-

Table 29 Specific syndromes due to reactivation of Herpes zoster

Syndrome	Root	Clinical features
Ophthalmic (➤84)	V1. Rarely associated with ipsilateral III, IV and VI palsies	Pain in scalp. Corneal lesions and iridocyclitis. Rash over forehead, eyelid and nose
Geniculate (Ramsay-Hunt)	VII. Variable involvement of V, IX and X	Pain in ear canal, pinna and scalp. Facial nerve palsy. Tinnitus, vertigo, deafness, dysphagia. Vesicles on external auditory meatus, scalp, pinna and hemitongue
Vagal and glossopharyngeal	X, XI	Mucous membrane involvement only–soft palate and posterior pharynx. Pain in throat, dysphagia
Sacral	S1–4	Disturbance of micturition, haematuria

sillitis is often absent. Physical findings include generalised, particularly cervical, lymphadenopathy (95%), tonsillitis with tonsillar enlargement and exudate (85%), splenomegaly (50–75%), hepatomegaly (10–50%), petechial palatal haemorrhages (10%) and periorbital oedema (30%). Widespread maculopapular rash develops in a few patients; administration of ampicillin induces a florid pruritic rash in nearly all patients with IM. Most attacks resolve fully within 2–3 weeks.

Investigations: Peripheral WBC is increased to 10–50 × 10^9/l, with an absolute (>4 × 10^9/l) and relative (>50% of total WBC) increase in mononuclear cells, of which ≤20% are atypical lymphocytes. These are activated T lymphocytes, produced in response to virus-induced proliferation of B cells, and have a characteristic morphology with large nuclei, fine reticular chromatin pattern and abundant basophilic, often vacuolated, cytoplasm. Mild thrombocytopenia is common.

Heterophile antibodies: Patients with IM produce IgM antibodies that bind erythrocytes from other species (sheep and horses, but not guinea-pig kidney cells). Heterophile antibodies are also found in normal sera, and in some patients with lymphoma, but these usually bind to guinea-pig kidney cells. Several tests are available: The Paul–Bunnell test measures agglutination of sheep RBCs by patient's serum. In the Paul–Bunnell–Davidsohn test, the serum is first preabsorbed with guinea-pig kidney cells. In the monospot test, formalinized horse RBCs are agglutinated after preabsorption of serum on guinea-pig kidney cells. These tests are positive in 40% of patients during the first week of illness, 60% by week 2 and 80% by week 3. They are usually negative in children under 5 years. A positive test usually persists for 3–6 months after IM, and occasionally up to 1 year. Patients also make **specific antibodies** against viral antigens including viral capsid antigen (VCA) and nuclear antigens (EBNA). Anti-VCA IgM is a sensitive and specific indicator of recent infection. It is not available routinely but is useful in difficult cases.

Patients usually have mildly abnormal liver function and, occasionally, jaundice.

Differential diagnosis: Bacterial pharyngitis due to Gp A β-haemolytic streptococci (➤17). Other causes of mononucleosis, including CMV (➤243) and *Toxoplasma gondii* (➤264), are rare. In these conditions, heterophile antibodies do not occur. Diphtheria (➤181).

Specific management: None. Acyclovir is **not** indicated. Steroids are used for thrombocytopenia, haemolytic anaemia, neurological complications and myocarditis. If tonsillar enlargement threatens to cause airway obstruction, prednisolone should be given (60 mg/day for 5–10 days). Tracheotomy may be required. Avoid ampicillin/amoxycillin in patients who may have IM (➤17).

Complications: Tonsillar enlargement may be so severe as to threaten airway obstruction. Splenic rupture occurs in ~0.2% of patients. Abdominal pain is rare in IM and if it occurs splenic rupture should be excluded. Rarely, profound thrombocytopenia, with purpura and haemorrhage, occurs. Autoimmune haemolytic anaemia also occurs rarely. Neurological complications include encephalitis, presenting with cerebellar ataxia, viral meningitis, Guillain–Barré syndrome, Bell's palsy and transverse myelitis. These affect less than 1% of patients and usually resolve completely, but they account for most of the mortality and long-term morbidity associated with IM. Very rare complications include myocarditis, pericarditis and pneumonitis.

Boys who carry the very rare X-linked immunoproliferative syndrome (XLP) gene have a specific defect of the immune system that renders them susceptible to fatal acute IM, which occurs in >75% of XLP gene carriers. Features include massive hepatic necrosis, pancytopenia and lymphoma. The mean reported age of presentation is 6.5 years.

Comments: Postinfectious fatigue has been said to be a particular feature of IM, but in practice this is rare. There is no firm evidence to implicate EBV in the aetiology of the chronic fatigue syndrome (CFS, ➤243), and EBV serology has no part in the work-up of patients with CFS. Genuinely persistent active EBV infection has been reported very rarely. Patients have very high-titre specific anti-EBV antibodies and a variety of clinical features including pancytopenia, lymphadenopathy, hepatosplenomegaly, interstitial pneumonitis and hepatitis. They may respond to acyclovir.

EBV is associated with the development of African Burkitt's lymphoma and nasopharyngeal carcinoma, and polyclonal B-cell lymphomas in immunosuppressed patients, particularly those with AIDS (➤130). It is also responsible for oral hairy leucoplakia, which is a proliferation of the buccal mucosa on the lateral margins of the tongue seen in patients with HIV infection. It responds to acyclovir, but is associated with a poor prognosis and impending progression to AIDS (➤122).

Exanthem subitum ① (syn. roseola infantum, sixth disease)
Organism: Family herpesviridae: human herpesvirus type 6 (HHV-6) (➤244).
Epidemiology: Infection is worldwide and very common in children >4 months and <3 years.
Reservoir: Humans.
Incubation period: Ten days (range 5–15 days).
Infectious period: As with other herpesviruses, asymptomatic carriers may continue to excrete virus for many months.
Clinical features: Abrupt onset of fever lasting 3–5 days, followed by a rash, which develops on the back and neck and spreads to the chest and limbs. The feet and face are spared, and the rash typically lasts 2 days. There is mild malaise, vomiting, diarrhoea, cough, coryza, pharyngitis and lymphadenopathy.
Specific management: None.

Erythema infectiosum ① (syn. fifth disease, slapped-cheek disease)
Organism: Family parvovirus: parvovirus B19 (➤245).
Epidemiology: Worldwide distribution. Typically occurring in sporadic epidemics. Infection is commonest between 5 and 14 years. Seroprevalence typically 20% at 10 years, 50% at 50 years.

Reservoir: Humans.
Transmission: Person to person by respiratory droplet spread.
Incubation period: Four to 20 days.
Infectious period: Probably from before the onset of rash, but not thereafter.
Clinical features: After a short prodrome of myalgia, arthralgia, malaise and fever, the typical rash develops on the face. It is sharply demarcated, occasionally with a raised edge ('slapped cheek' appearance). After 1–2 days a maculopapular rash develops on the trunk, legs, arms and buttocks. After a few days, areas of clearing develop, giving the rash a characteristic lacy or reticulate appearance. The rash may fade and reappear over the following 3 weeks.
Investigations: Diagnosis can be confirmed by serology.
Specific management: None.
Complications: Infection in patients with haemolytic anaemias, such as sickle-cell disease, causes severe aplastic crises. Intrauterine infection infrequently causes fetal anaemia, hydrops fetalis and fetal death.

Arthritis is a common complication in adults. Arthralgia occurs in ~75% of cases in patients over 20 years. In 60% there is joint swelling, which superficially resembles the acute onset of rheumatoid disease. The vast majority recover with no residual joint damage. In children arthritis is much less common; under 9 years of age, only 5% have arthralgia and 3% have joint swelling.

Enteroviral infections
Enteroviral infections account for the majority of childhood febrile exanthemata, but only two —hand, foot and mouth disease and herpangina—produce a significantly characteristic clinical picture to allow easy identification. Transmission is typically by faeco-oral or respiratory route and incubation times are short (3–5 days). Viral excretion persists in stool for several weeks.

HAND, FOOT AND MOUTH DISEASE (syn. enteroviral vesicular stomatitis with exanthem)
Organisms: Coxsackievirus A16 (plus other serotypes) (➤251).

Clinical features: Pharyngitis with vesicles that burst, leaving 5–10 painful oral ulcers. Simultaneous vesicular rash on hands and feet. Resolves within 7–10 days. A very rare severe relapsing form is described.

HERPANGINA
(syn. enteroviral vesicular pharyngitis)
Organisms: Coxsackie A viruses (A1–10, A22) (➤251).
Clinical features: Vesicles and ulcers confined to the posterior pharynx, i.e. on the tonsillar pillars, soft palate and uvula. Constitutional symptoms include fever, headache, vomiting and myalgia.

Specific bacterial infections of childhood

Scarlet fever (syn. scarlatina) ✉ ①
Scarlet fever is caused by infection with streptococci that produce erythrogenic toxin. It usually accompanies streptococcal pharyngitis (➤17), but can also follow cutaneous infection. Streptococcal erythrogenic toxin is similar to the toxic shock syndrome toxin of *Staphylococcus aureus*.
Organisms: Group A β-haemolytic streptococci (➤170).
Epidemiology: Scarlet fever was common and frequently fatal in the nineteenth century, but its severity and frequency have waned since the 1920s. It is now rarely serious.
Clinical features: One or two days after onset of sore throat, rash appears on face, sparing the area around the lips ('circumoral pallor') and spreading to the neck, chest, back, trunk and limbs. Rash is a diffuse blanching erythema with punctate elevations around hair follicles that give a characteristic 'sandpaper' feel to the touch. It is accentuated in skin folds by capillary haemorrhage (Pastia's lines). Palms and soles are usually spared. Rash is followed by desquamation, which starts on the hands. The tongue is red with prominent papillae ('strawberry tongue').
Investigations: Throat swab. ASOT (➤170).
Differential diagnosis: Measles (➤100) and other viral exanthemata. Kawasaki's disease (➤154).

Specific management: Oral penicillin V or parenteral benzylpenicillin should be given.
Complications: Rheumatic fever (➤171), poststreptococcal glomerulonephritis (➤171), erythema nodosum (➤93).

Toxic epidermal necrolysis
(syn. scalded-skin syndrome, Ritter's disease, staphylococcal scarlet fever)
Staphylococcus aureus may produce an exotoxin that causes exfoliation of the upper layers of the epidermis ('exfoliatin'). The initial site of staphylococcal infection is usually minor and localised, but general skin colonisation may follow rapidly.
Organism: *Staphylococcus aureus* (➤165).
Clinical features: Abrupt onset of generalised skin erythema, followed after 1–2 days by wrinkling and separation of upper layers with even slight trauma, such as light stroking (Nikolsky's sign). Large sheets of skin peel off, leaving a raw tender surface. The rash fades over the next few days. There may be associated conjunctivitis, stomatitis and urethritis.
Investigations: *Staphylococcus aureus* is usually cultured from the skin.
Specific management: Flucloxacillin is the drug of choice. For penicillin-allergic patients, erythromycin or cefotaxime is given.

Pertussis (syn. whooping cough) ✉ ①
Organisms: *Bordetella pertussis* (➤208). *Bordetella parapertussis* and *Bordetella bronchiseptica* are unusual causes of a milder illness.
Epidemiology: Infection is seen worldwide, but is unusual in the UK since the advent of vaccination. Rarely proven in adults. Fears about vaccine side-effects in the past led to a decline in vaccine uptake, and a rise in reported cases and deaths. Vaccine uptake in UK is now ~90%. Σ ~400. Case fatality rate ~1:200 under 2 months of age, ~1:15000 in 1–4-year age-group.
Reservoir: *Bordetella pertussis* and *Bordetella parapertussis* have no animal reservoir, but *Bordetella bronchiseptica* causes illness in a wide range of mammals, including farm animals.

Transmission: Highly contagious. Person to person via the respiratory droplet route.
Incubation period: Seven days (range 6–20).
Infectious period: From the onset of illness to 2–3 weeks into the paroxysmal stage.
Clinical features: Clinical course is considered in three stages. **Catarrhal stage:** illness commences with symptoms of mild URTI, such as non-paroxysmal cough, coryza, conjunctivitis and sneezing. After 7–10 days the cough becomes more frequent and intense. Fever is low-grade or absent. **Paroxysmal stage:** the cough becomes very severe and frequent. Paroxysms, precipitated by many stimuli including eating, drinking, emotion or exercise, are characterised by repeated staccato coughing during a single prolonged expiration, followed by forceful inspiration giving rise to the 'whoop'. Whoop is often absent in infants and older patients. Paroxysms are associated with vomiting and exhaustion, and may cause facial/eyelid oedema, subconjunctival haemorrhage and erosion of the lingual frenulum. The paroxysmal stage lasts from 2 to 4 weeks. **Convalescent stage.** this lasts 2 weeks to 2 months, during which paroxysms become less severe and less frequent, although still triggered by intercurrent viral respiratory infections. Morbidity and mortality in pertussis occur in infants and are associated with the paroxysms of coughing, which cause feeding difficulties, choking, anoxia and apnoea.
Investigations: During the catarrhal stage there is a lymphocytosis. CXR may be normal or show dense markings radiating from the heart borders ('shaggy heart sign') due to peribronchial thickening. Culture of the organism requires special media. Clinical disease is very variable, therefore bacteriological confirmation essential. Pernasal swab is the sample of choice. Serology will confirm the diagnosis in retrospect.
Differential diagnosis: Other causes of respiratory tract infection (➤17). Inhaled foreign body.
Specific management: Erythromycin, given during the first 5 days of illness, shortens the duration of the paroxysmal stage. It should still be given after this time, but in this situation the main benefit is to render the patient non-

infectious to others. Treatment is given for 14 days. Isolation is necessary until 5 days' treatment have been completed. Co-trimoxazole is an alternative for patients allergic to erythromycin. Close contacts are given a 14-day course of erythromycin.
Complications: Atelectasis, particularly of the right upper lobe, is common during the paroxysmal stage. Other pulmonary complications include secondary bacterial infection (due to *Haemophilus influenzae, Streptococcus pneumoniae*, Gp A β-haemolytic streptococci, *Staphylococcus aureus*), suggested by fever and CXR changes. Pneumothorax, mediastinal and subcutaneous surgical emphysema and diaphragmatic rupture have been reported. There is no evidence of long-term pulmonary damage in survivors.

Neurological damage, including encephalopathy progressing to coma, and focal deficits, including hemiplegia, account for significant morbidity and mortality and are probably caused by anoxia during paroxysms or cerebral haemorrhage.
Immunisation: Recommended for all babies at 2 months as part of DTP vaccination (➤337). There is no transfer of protective maternal antibodies even in infants of mothers with documented history of pertussis or pertussis vaccination.

Bacterial infection in childhood

Children are susceptible to most of the bacterial infections described in the system-based chapters of this manual, but, in many cases, the expected range of infecting organisms varies with age. For example, prior to the introduction of Hib vaccine (➤337), children were particularly at risk from invasive infection by *Haemophilus influenzae* type B, which causes pneumonia, epiglottitis and meningitis in children but only rarely invasive infections in adults.
See:
- Pneumonia in children (➤27).
- Bacterial meningitis (➤74).
- Infectious diarrhoea (➤44).
- Haemolytic uraemic syndrome (➤188).

Antibiotic prescribing in children

Consult the British National Formulary for details of paediatric doses. Some antibiotics are relatively contraindicated in childhood (Table 30).

For some drugs there is insufficient data upon which to base recommendations for use/dosage below a certain age. For specified ages see Section 3 and consult manufacturer's data sheet.

CLINICAL SYNDROME
Henoch-Schönlein purpura (HSP)
An acute febrile illness of childhood and adolescence commonly affecting boys under 6 years old. Non-thrombocytopenic purpura, typically on the legs and buttocks, abdominal pain and diarrhoea (with or without blood), arthritis and glomerulonephritis. Preceding respiratory infection is common but no single pathogen has been implicated. Histology shows necrotising vasculitis. Suspect HSP in children with diarrhoea who develop arthritis or skin rash or who fail to recover promptly. Paediatric referral is recommended.

Neonatal infections

Infection in the neonate is common and requires a high level of awareness since neonates rarely manifest classical symptoms of infection seen in older patients (Table 31). Neonatal sepsis presenting early, within 5 days of birth, is usually due to infection acquired before or during birth (early neonatal infection—ENI). After 7 days or more after birth, it is due to infection acquired after birth (late neonatal infection—LNI).

Clinical features: Presenting signs are similar for both categories. Signs of infection are often subtle, and up to 10% of babies with positive blood cultures are asymptomatic. Even with proven meningitis neonates rarely have neck stiffness or bulging fontanelle. Fever (50%) or hypothermia (15%), dyspnoea (20%), apnoea (20%), cyanosis (25%), tachycardia or hypotension (25%), anorexia (30%), vomiting (20%), abdominal distension (20%) and diarrhoea (10%), hepatomegaly (30%) and jaundice (30%), bleeding diathesis (2–10%), lethargy (35%), irritability (15%) or fits (15%). Rarely disseminated enteroviral infection produces a clinical illness similar to bacterial sepsis.

Table 30 Common antibiotics to avoid in children

Drug	Adverse effect	Comments
Ceftriaxone	Displaces plasma bilirubin causing jaundice	Contraindicated under 6 weeks
Tetracyclines	Staining of teeth. Occasional dental hypoplasia	Avoid in pregnancy and children under 12 years
Chloramphenicol	Grey-baby syndrome. Agranulocytosis	Avoid in neonates if possible. Use only if specifically indicated
Sulphonamides	Displace plasma bilirubin, causing jaundice. Hypersensitivity reactions	Avoid in children, unless specifically indicated, e.g. for pneumocystosis
Quinolones	Cartilage damage and arthritis in young *animals*	Not licensed for use in children
Trimethoprim	Antifolate activity may interfere with haemopoiesis	Avoid in neonates. Contraindicated in pregnancy.
Ethambutol	Children may be unable to report visual symptoms if they develop optic neuritis	Avoid in children under 6 years
Nitrofurantoin	Haemolytic anaemia	Avoid in children under 3 months

Table 31 Features of early and late neonatal infection

	ENI	LNI
Acquisition	Usually from mother	Often by cross-infection (via staff hands) from other babies
Risk factors	Maternal perinatal infection, including infections causing disseminated intrauterine infection and congenital abnormalities (➤112), genital infections (e.g. HSV ➤66, or *Chlamydia trachomatis* ➤66) and infections acquired close to birth such as intra-amniotic infection (➤63). Prolonged rupture of membranes (PRM). Prolonged/difficult labour. Prematurity/low birth weight. Low APGAR score/need for resuscitation. Scalp electrodes	Congenital abnormalities. Prolonged admission to special care baby unit. Procedures and medical interventions, especially iv lines and umbilical artery catheters Less strongly associated with risk factors for ENI
Organisms	Gp B βHS (➤173), *Escherichia coli* (KI) (➤189), *Listeria monocytogenes*. Less often *Streptococcus pneumoniae* (associated with severe endometritis), other coliforms. Rarely anaerobes (particularly with PRM and intra-amniotic infection ➤63), Gp A βHS, *Haemophilus influenzae*	Gp B βHS (➤173), *Listeria monocytogenes*, *Staphylococcus aureus, Staphylococcus epidermidis*, *Serratia* spp., *Citrobacter* spp. and other coliforms, *Salmonella* spp. (tropics), *Candida albicans*, *Malassezia furfur*
Clinical features	Overwhelming generalised sepsis. ~30% have meningitis and mortality is high (~50%)	Meningitis ± bacteraemia. Skin sepsis

Practice point: Of healthy women, 25% carry Gp B βHS as a vaginal commensal. Treatment often does not eradicate the carrier state, but may reduce incidence of premature rupture of membranes (➤173).

Microbiological investigations: Culture of blood, urine and CSF. CXR. Leucocytosis is common; the normal ranges for infants differ with age (Table 32).

Antibiotic management: Early presumptive treatment with benzylpenicillin and gentamicin is commenced after cultures have been obtained. If Gp B βHS infection is confirmed, benzylpenicillin (+ initial gentamicin) is the agent of choice. Parenteral or broad-spectrum cephalosporins are alternatives (➤299).

Supportive management: A detailed discussion of the management of severely ill neonates is beyond the scope of this manual. Careful attention to airway, fluid balance and control of cross-infection are all vital. Urgent referral to neonatology/paediatric intensive care is essential.

Table 32 Normal ranges for neutrophils in neonates

Age	Total neutrophils × 10⁹/l
Birth	1.8–6.0
12 hours	7.8–14.5
1 day	7.2–12.6
2 days	3.6–8.1
≥5 days	1.8–5.4

Congenital infection– 'TORCH' screening

Disseminated intrauterine infection by a number of organisms causes fetal abnormalities. The acronym TORCH (**T**oxoplasma **O**ther **R**ubella **C**MV **H**SV) is used to describe these infections, which have the following in common: (i) mild or inapparent infection in the mother; (ii) wide range of severity in the infant; (iii) similarity of presentation with growth retardation and congenital defects; (iv) diagnosis by serology; and (v) long-term sequelae with progressive disease in childhood and adolescence if untreated.

Major congenital syndromes
For more detailed discussion of these conditions
see cross-references.

Toxoplasma gondii (➤264): After 1° maternal
infection during pregnancy, 33–50% of
fetuses will be infected. Infection may cause
abortion. Of infected fetuses, 10–20% show
evidence of congenital disease, including
petechiae, hepatosplenomegaly, maculopapular rash and interstitial pneumonitis.
Choroidoretinitis, microcephaly and intracerebral calcification are seen. The risk of
fetal infection is lowest during the first
trimester, but the consequences are more severe then. Conversely, infection later in pregnancy is more likely to result in fetal infection,
but the degree of congenital abnormality is
less. Maternal infection > 6 months before
conception does not result in fetal infection,
but rare cases have been reported of fetal
infection and abnormality occurring when the
mother has definitely acquired infection during the 6-month period prior to conception.
Diagnosis is by serology, and treatment of the
neonate is essential.

Rubella (➤101): Fetal infection rate depends on
stage of pregnancy at which maternal infection occurs (➤102). Classic triad comprises
cataracts, deafness, patent ductus arteriosus.
Other cardiac lesions, microcephaly, mental
retardation are also seen. Diagnosis is by
serology or culture of virus from the
infant.

CMV (➤243): Infection occurs in 50% of fetuses
after 1° maternal infection during pregnancy,
but <5% after reactivation. Of infected
fetuses, 10% have disease after 1° infection,
but it is rare after reactivation. Hepatosplenomegaly, petechiae, thrombocytopenia,
intrauterine growth retardation. Microcephaly, encephalitis, intracerebral calcification, mental retardation. Diagnosis is by
serology.

HSV (➤66): Infection is acquired peripartum. Of
HSV-infected mothers, 40% have no history
of current infection or genital lesions. Of babies delivered via an actively infected birth
canal, 50% will become infected and nearly all
of these will manifest disease. Infection may
be localised to the eye or CNS, but usually

becomes disseminated with a vesicular rash,
hepatomegaly and jaundice, pneumonitis and
encephalitis. Diagnosis is by viral culture
and serology. Treatment with acyclovir is
essential.

Syphilis (➤67): The risk of infection is highest
during early syphilis (1° or 2°). Treatment of
the mother before 16 weeks' gestation will
prevent congenital disease. Neonates may
present with fulminant disease; hepatitis, pulmonary haemorrhage and intercurrent bacterial infection are common and mortality is
high. In less severe early congenital syphilis,
signs develop over the first 2–10 weeks of life,
including vesicular or bullous rash involving
the sole and palms, rhinitis (snuffles) and evidence of widespread visceral involvement.
Features of late congenital syphilis develop
throughout childhood and include interstitial
keratitis, Clutton's joints, Hutchinson's teeth,
meningoencephalitis and skeletal changes.
Diagnosis is by serology or dark-ground
examination of material from mucosal
lesions.

Parvovirus (➤107): Infection causes abortion
and stillbirth, or fetal anaemia and hydrops
fetalis.

Other agents transmitted vertically include HIV
(➤114), hepatitis B (➤49), EBV (➤243),
leptospirosis (➤226), VZV (➤103), enteroviruses (➤251), *Ureaplasma urealyticum* and
Mycoplasma hominis (➤233).

Specific neonatal infections

Ophthalmia neonatorum ⊠
Conjunctivitis affecting the newborn (➤83).
Organisms: *Chlamydia trachomatis*, *Neisseria
gonorrhoeae*, *Staphylococcus aureus*.

Otitis media
Not rare in the neonatal period (➤15).
Organisms: Coliforms, *Staphylococcus aureus*,
Haemophilus influenzae, streptococci.
Microbiological investigations: Tympanocentesis
may be indicated, particularly if otitis fails to
respond promptly to antibiotics, because progression to meningitis or generalised sepsis
may occur.

Antibiotic management: Ampicillin + gentamicin initially.

Pneumonia

Risk factors: Intrapartum aspiration of maternal cervicovaginal flora, or infected amniotic fluid. Congenital infections (➤112).

Clinical features: Physical signs of pneumonia are usually absent. Signs of generalised sepsis (➤110), respiratory distress and CXR changes are more often seen.

Organisms: Gp B β-haemolytic streptococci, *Staphylococcus aureus*, coliforms, viral infections including RSV (➤249), influenza (➤247).

Chlamydia trachomatis causes lower respiratory tract infection that develops between 4 and 12 weeks. There is a history of conjunctivitis in 50%. Signs include gradual onset of cough and inspiratory crepitations. CXR shows patchy infiltrates. Many affected children have eosinophilia.

Necrotising enterocolitis

A severe infection of unknown cause. Pathogenesis may be related to temporary anoxia or other trauma to the bowel allowing invasion of the epithelium by gut organisms.

Risk factors: Occurs sporadically and as nursery epidemics. Associated with prematurity and umbilical artery catheter use. Usually occurs during the first 3 weeks, peaking at 3–10 days.

Clinical features: Fever, apnoea, lethargy. Abdominal distension, vomiting, blood in stools. In severe cases, there are signs of peritonitis, crepitus and cellulitis of the anterior abdominal wall. Perforation can occur and healing may be complicated by stricture.

Organisms: No single causative pathogen has been identified. Blood cultures are often positive with intestinal flora.

Investigations: AXR shows ileus, bowel distension, pneumatosis intestinalis, portal vein gas or free peritoneal gas.

Antibiotic management: Benzylpenicillin + gentamicin + metronidazole.

Supportive management: It is necessary to stop oral feeding and institute parenteral nutrition. Full paediatric intensive care is required, and mortality is high.

Urinary tract infection

Risk factors: Structural abnormality of the urinary tract.

Clinical features: Non-specific features of infection with fever and vomiting.

Organisms: *Escherichia coli, Klebsiella* spp., enterococci.

Microbiological investigations: Clean-catch urine or suprapubic aspirate.

Other investigations: Imaging of urinary tract should be performed in all cases to exclude structural abnormality.

Neonatal skin infections

There include cellulitis, Ritter's disease (toxic epidermal necrolysis or 'scalded-skin' syndrome ➤108), and oomphalitis (infection of the umbilical stump). Oomphalitis may cause ascending phlebitis resulting in peritonitis or generalised sepsis. It is usually due to *Staphylococcus aureus*, streptococci and coliforms. Careful local toilet is required. If severe, flucloxacillin and gentamicin are required.

12: HIV Infection and AIDS

Epidemiology

Acquired immunodeficiency syndrome (AIDS) was first described in 1981 in 16 homosexual men in the USA. The causative agent, human immunodeficiency virus (HIV), was isolated in 1983. Since then HIV infection has been reported from almost all countries and in 1993 WHO estimated ~14 million infected people worldwide, over half of whom live in sub-Saharan Africa, and ~3 million cases of AIDS worldwide. In the UK there have been ~10 000 AIDS cases to 1994, and ~20 000 reported HIV infections. Patterns of transmission vary between countries. In UK, USA and Europe, infection has largely been confined to homosexual men and intravenous drug users, with comparatively small numbers of heterosexually acquired infections. In the developing world, heterosexual transmission is much more important, and this accounts in part for the greater prevalence of HIV infection there. The prevalence of genital ulcers, in particular chancroid (➤71), is thought to be an important factor.

Virology

Key biological features: HIV-1 and HIV-2 are members of the lentivirus family of human retroviruses. Virus attaches to host cells via specific binding of the viral envelope glycoprotein gp120 to the host membrane protein CD4. This accounts for its preference for infecting CD4+ helper T lymphocytes, macrophages and other antigen-presenting cells. The viral RNA genome is transcribed into DNA, which then integrates into the host genome. A very large number of **immunological defects** have been described in AIDS, affecting all the components of the immune system. The most important abnormalities are:

• a severe decline in the number of CD4+ helper T lymphocytes, associated clinically with impaired cell-mediated immunity and

the development of opportunist infections and malignancies;

• hypergammaglobulinaemia, which is associated clinically with the development of a wide range of autoantibodies, idiopathic thrombocytopenia and a high incidence of severe drug allergies.

HIV-2 is found mainly in W Africa. It shares only 45% sequence identity with HIV-1. Antibodies against one type do not always bind to the other type, so antibody assays now detect both viruses. HIV-2 differs from HIV-1 in the following ways:

• transmission rates appear to be lower;
• is less pathogenic *in vitro*;
• the time to development of AIDS is probably longer with HIV-2 than HIV-1.

In the following sections no further distinction will be made between HIV-1 and HIV-2.

Transmission

Well-defined routes of transmission exist:

• By **sexual contact**, both homo- and heterosexual, male to female and vice versa. Risk of transmission is highest with rectal intercourse. Other factors which promote infectivity are very early or advanced HIV infection, genital ulcer disease and other STDs. Factors which increase susceptibility to infection include rectal or traumatic intercourse, use of oral contraceptives, cervical ectopy and concurrent genital ulcer disease and other STDs.

• **Blood-borne**, in particular IVDU but also by transfusion of blood/blood products. In the UK blood for transfusion is now screened for anti-HIV antibodies and high-risk blood and tissue donors are excluded by questionnaire. In addition, blood products such as factor VIII are heat-treated.

• **Vertical transmission.** Approximately 20% of children born to HIV+ mothers are infected. This rate is reduced by zidovudine treatment. Some of these are infected postnatally by breast-feeding, which should be avoided where safe alternative methods of feeding are available. Diagnosis of infection in children is difficult, due to passively acquired maternal antibodies which may persist for up to 18 months. Viral culture, antigen detection and PCR may confirm infection.

Casual and household contact is not associated with transmission.

Natural history of infection

Incubation: Following infection there is an asymptomatic period of 2–4 weeks during which all tests for HIV antibodies and antigens are negative.

Seroconversion: This is accompanied by a febrile illness in ~50% of cases, although it may not be recognised as such. Clinical features are variable but include fever, malaise, headache, pharyngitis, generalised lymphadenopathy and a maculopapular rash. Features suggesting primary HIV infection rather than any other flu-like illness include the skin rash, mucocutaneous ulceration (mouth, oesophagus, anogenital area), neurological involvement (meningoencephalitis, peripheral neuropathy, retro-orbital pain and photophobia) and oral candidiasis. Initial lymphopenia followed by an atypical lymphocytosis may occur. Mild thrombocytopenia and abnormal liver function tests are common. Specific antibody tests for HIV become positive between 2 and 6 weeks after the onset of the seroconversion illness. Differential diagnosis includes rubella (➤101), infectious mononucleosis (➤105), secondary syphilis (➤67) and disseminated gonococcal infection (➤66). Resolution occurs over 2–4 weeks.

Latency: Following infection patients remain free from serious illness for a variable number of years. After an initial asymptomatic period, they may develop constitutional symptoms (e.g. fever, malaise and weight loss), manifestations of mild immunodeficiency (e.g. oral candidiasis, cutaneous herpes zoster or herpes simplex, or bacterial infections) or manifestations of immunodysregulation (e.g. immune thrombocytopenia, multiple drug allergies or

seborrhoeic dermatitis). This phase of HIV-related illness was previously referred to as AIDS-related complex (ARC). There may be persistent generalised lymphadenopathy but this is not a prognostic indicator for progression to AIDS.

Progression to AIDS: This is defined in the UK by development of one of the AIDS-defining illnesses listed in Table 33. Prior to the introduction of prophylaxis against *Pneumocystis carinii* pneumonia (PCP), patients often presented with this infection, usually after the CD4 count had fallen below 200 cells/μl. In the USA, a CD4 count below 200 cells/μl is considered diagnostic of AIDS, but this definition has not been adopted in the UK.

The median time from infection to the onset of AIDS in the developed world is about 10 years, although some patients progress rapidly within 2 years of infection, and there are also reports of 'long-term survivors' known to be infected for 12–15 years who have yet to develop clinical illness. Survival following the diagnosis of AIDS also varies widely depending on the nature of the AIDS-defining event, but is about 1–2 years in the developed world. Immunological abnormalities may be demonstrated in almost all HIV-seropositive individuals from early in the asymptomatic latent stage, and it is likely that all infected persons will eventually progress to AIDS. Many patients become extremely unwell or even die before they acquire a strict AIDS-defining diagnosis.

AIDS in children: The average age of onset of immunodeficiency in perinatally infected children in the USA is 5 to 10 months. Few infected infants remain well beyond 3 years of age, and their median survival after diagnosis of AIDS is ~9 months. Children with AIDS present in a number of ways, including failure to thrive and developmental delay, hepatosplenomegaly and lymphadenopathy, recurrent bacterial infection or with the opportunistic infections common in adults, particularly candidiasis and *Pneumocystis carinii* pneumonia. Some manifestations of AIDS are unique to children, such as salivary gland enlargement and lymphoid interstitial

Table 33 AIDS indicator diseases (UK definition)

AIDS indicator disease	Comments and qualifications
Bacterial infections, recurrent or multiple	In a child less than 13 years
Candidiasis	Affecting oesophagus, trachea, bronchus or lungs
Cervical carcinoma	Invasive
Coccidioidomycosis	Disseminated or extrapulmonary
Cryptococcosis	Extrapulmonary
Cryptosporidiosis	With diarrhoea for greater than 1 month
Cytomegalovirus disease	Onset after age 1 month, not confined to liver, spleen and lymph nodes
Cytomegalovirus retinitis	
Encephalopathy (dementia) due to HIV	HIV infection and disabling cognitive and/or motor dysfunction, or milestone loss in a child, with no other causes by CSF examination, brain imaging or post-mortem
Herpes simplex	Ulcers for longer than 1 month or bronchitis, pneumonitis or oesophagitis
Histoplasmosis	Disseminated or extrapulmonary
Isosporiasis	With diarrhoea for greater than 1 month
Kaposi's sarcoma	
Lymphoid interstitial pneumonia and/or pulmonary lymphoid hyperplasia	In a child less than 13 years
Lymphoma	Burkitt's or immunoblastic or primary in brain
Mycobacteriosis	Disseminated, extrapulmonary or pulmonary
Pneumocystis carinii pneumonia	
Progressive multifocal leukoencephalopathy	
Recurrent non-typhoidal salmonella bacteraemia	
Recurrent pneumonia	Two episodes within 12 months
Toxoplasmosis of brain	Onset after age 1 month
Wasting syndrome due to HIV	Weight loss (over 10% of baseline) with no other cause, and 30 days or more of either diarrhoea or weakness with fever

pneumonia (LIP). LIP occurs in 40% of children, with nodular peribronchial infiltrates and hilar lymphadenopathy. LIP causes clubbing and progressive shortness of breath, which may respond to steroids; acute deterioration of ventilation is usually due to intercurrent infection. Neurological disease, in particular encephalopathy, is common and often severe.

Tests for HIV infection

A large number of commercial test kits for the detection of anti-HIV antibodies are available. Serum is initially screened by an ELISA-based method, and positive results are confirmed by Western blot or by immunoblotting using recombinant antigens. In almost all cases these tests are positive within 2–4 months of acquiring infection. Infection can also be demonstrated by viral culture, antigen detection or PCR for viral RNA. Test results should be interpreted in the clinical context. In particular, a positive result in a patient with no clinical features to suggest HIV infection and no risk factors should be treated with caution. Close liaison with the laboratory is essential.

CD4 counts

T lymphocytes may be divided on the basis of surface protein expression into two main categories: CD4+ (helper) T cells and CD8+ (cytotoxic/suppressor) T cells. HIV specifically infects and depletes the CD4+ subset, and the CD4 count falls as immunodeficiency develops. CD4 counts are subject to wide diurnal variation and the counting procedure itself is inaccurate, so at least two counts should be performed before management decisions are made. Some patients with very low counts may remain relatively well. Nevertheless, the CD4 count is the only widely used marker of immunological status and does allow approximate staging of infection.

Normal ranges for CD4 count are: absolute count >500 cells/μl, or 40–70% of total lymphocytes. The CD4/CD8 ratio should be >0.5. There is a small reversible decrease in CD4 count during the seroconversion illness. During the latent period there is a gradual decline in CD4 count. Opportunist infections are unusual before the count falls below 200 cells/μl. Below 100 cells/μl, infections, particularly PCP and disseminated *Mycobacterium avium-intracellulare* (MAI), are usual. Patients with end-stage disease typically have counts <50 cells/μl.

Management

General care of patients during latency and AIDS

Initial assessment includes estimation of the likely duration and route of infection and careful history and examination to exclude ongoing opportunistic infection and malignancy. Previous illnesses, especially STDs, should be reviewed. Baseline investigations should include: CD4 count, FBC, serology for CMV, toxoplasmosis, hepatitis C, hepatitis B and syphilis. A cervical smear should be performed and repeated at least annually in all HIV+ women. Information, education and social and psychological support are very important, and an integrated approach involving doctors, nurses, health advisers and other professionals is essential.

Follow-up visits should include examination for conditions that present insidiously, including skin (seborrhoeic dermatitis, superficial infections, Kaposi's sarcoma), mouth (candidiasis, oral hairy leucoplakia), lymph nodes (*localised* enlargement suggests infection or malignancy), fundi (chorioretinitis) and neurological system (AIDS dementia complex, peripheral neuropathy). CD4 count and FBC should be monitored every 3–6 months until the count is <50 cells/μl.

Antiretroviral therapy

Zidovudine (AZT, Retrovir®) inhibits viral reverse transcriptase and prevents viral replication *in vitro*. It prolongs survival in patients with AIDS and reduces vertical transmission. Early studies suggested that treatment started during the asymptomatic latent stage would delay progression to AIDS, but recent large controlled studies have failed to demonstrate any benefit from early treatment. At present, indications for zidovudine remain unclear. Some continue to advocate its routine use in all patients with CD4 counts <500 cells/μl.

We currently do not advise treatment until patients are symptomatic, and then prescribe 250 mg 12-hly. Zidovudine is of particular benefit in patients with AIDS dementia complex or thrombocytopenia. Main side-effects are haematological (anaemia, neutropenia) but these occur in a minority of patients. Nausea, headache and myalgia also occur. Most patients develop macrocytosis.

Didanosine (ddI) is used for patients who are unable to tolerate zidovudine, and is of similar efficacy. Adverse effects include peripheral neuropathy and pancreatitis.

Zalcitabine (ddC) causes peripheral neuropathy in many patients and is unsuitable for use as single-agent therapy. It may play a part in future combination therapies.

It is likely that future therapies for AIDS will consist of combinations of antiretroviral drugs, and clinical trials of zidovudine and didanosine, and other combinations, are in progress.

Prophylaxis

In contrast to antiretroviral therapy, the value of prophylactic antimicrobials against specific infections is firmly established (Table 34).

HIV patients often require simultaneous treatment with numerous agents, increasing the potential for interactions and additive side-effects of agents with similar toxicity (Table 35).

Table 34 Prophylaxis against opportunist infections in HIV+ patients

Organism	Indications for prophylaxis	Regimen	Comments
Pneumocystis carinii (➤119)	CD4 count <200 cells/µl or AIDS	Co-trimoxazole 960 mg daily, 3 days/week **or** inhaled pentamidine* (300 mg monthly) **or** dapsone 100 mg daily + pyrimethamine 50 mg weekly	Breakthrough infection is commoner with inhaled pentamidine, particularly affecting the upper lobes, or extrapulmonary sites
Herpes simplex virus (➤121)	Recurrent cutaneous herpes	Acyclovir 400 mg 12-hly	Breakthrough infections may be treated with increased dose
Toxoplasmosis (➤124)	Previous toxoplasma encephalitis	Pyrimethamine 25 mg daily, folinic acid 15 mg daily and either sulphadiazine 500 mg 6-hly or clindamycin 300 mg 6-hly	Folinic acid prevents haematological toxicity of pyrimethamine. The benefit of **primary** prophylaxis is being evaluated
Candidiasis (➤121)	Previous candidiasis	Fluconazole 150 mg weekly or 50 mg alt. die.	Breakthrough infections may be treated with increased dose

*A small particle nebuliser is required. The conventional nebuliser commonly used to administer bronchodilators is not suitable.

Table 35 Adverse effects and drug interactions in HIV management

Drug	Adverse effects*	Comments and interactions
Co-trimoxazole	**Neutropenia, hypersensitivity,** nausea and vomiting	Increases serum levels of phenytoin and warfarin
Pentamidine (intravenous)	**Nephrotoxicity, hyper/hypoglycaemia, severe hypotension (with rapid infusion),** hepatitis, hyperkalaemia, pancreatitis, neutropenia, thrombocytopenia, ventricular arrhythmias	Inhaled pentamidine causes cough and wheeze but is otherwise relatively free of adverse effects

continued on p. 119

Table 35 contd

Drug	Adverse effects*	Comments and interactions
Ganciclovir	**Neutropenia, thrombocytopenia**	Additive marrow toxicity with zidovudine. Co-administration with imipenem may cause fits
Foscarnet	**Nephrotoxicity, hypo/hypercalcaemia, hyperphosphataemia, anaemia, hepatotoxicity,** nausea	Maintain hydration and reduce dose in renal impairment. Administration with pentamidine may cause severe hypocalcaemia
Acyclovir	Nephrotoxicity at very high doses	
Zidovudine	**Neutropenia, anaemia**	Additive marrow toxicity with ganciclovir
Didanosine	**Pancreatitis, peripheral neuropathy**	
Pyrimethamine	**Neutropenia, thrombocytopenia,** rash, raised liver enzymes	Haematological toxicity minimised by giving folinic acid 15 mg daily
Sulphadiazine	**Hypersensitivity, crystalluria**	Crystalluria may be avoided by maintaining urine output > 3 l/day and alkalinising urine (sodium bicarbonate, 3 g po 6-hly)
Fluconazole	Nausea, headache, skin rash, hepatotoxicity (rare)	Increases serum levels of cyclosporin A, phenytoin, warfarin and sulphonylureas (oral hypoglycaemics). Rifampicin reduces half-life of fluconazole
Clindamycin	**Antibiotic-associated diarrhoea, rash**	
Primaquine	**Haemolysis in G6PD-deficient patients**	

*More important adverse effects are highlighted in **bold** type.

Specific clinical syndromes in HIV-infected patients

Pulmonary infections in HIV-infected patients

Pneumocystis carinii pneumonia (PCP)

Exposure to *Pneumocystis carinii* is common throughout the world and most children have specific antibodies by age 2. Clinical disease occurs only in the context of severe immuno-deficiency, such as advanced HIV infection, post-transplantation or severe malnutrition. *Pneumocystis carinii* multiplies within the alveolus, damaging the alveolar epithelial cells and causing increased permeability of the alveolar/capillary membrane. This results in low-pressure pulmonary oedema, intrapulmonary shunting, decreased lung compliance and impaired gas exchange.

Risk factors: PCP is unusual in patients with CD4 counts > 200 cells/μl. It is rare in Africa, for reasons that remain unclear. Incidence is reduced by prophylactic treatment (➤118). Breakthrough cases are commoner in patients treated with pentamidine, particularly in the upper lobes where the aerosol does not always penetrate.

Clinical features: Insidious onset over weeks or months with fever, fatigue, weight loss and then cough and progressive dyspnoea. Onset may be particularly subtle in patients on prophylaxis. There may be tachycardia, cyanosis, tachypnoea and confusion. Auscultation may be normal or reveal crepitations. Extrapulmonary pneumocystosis also occurs. Skin, pleura, viscera, eye and lymph nodes can all be involved.

Organism: *Pneumocystis carinii*. This organism, previously a protozoon, has recently been re-classified as a fungus on the basis of DNA homology and membrane sterol content.

Microbiological investigations: Culture is not possible and diagnosis depends on identification of the organism by microscopy, with special stains or immunofluorescent techniques. Suitable materials include induced sputum (produced by inhaling nebulised 3% saline), bronchoalveolar lavage or transbronchial biopsy. If the diagnosis is strongly suspected clinically, treatment is commenced presumptively, and diagnostic tests are arranged as soon as possible thereafter.

Other investigations: Patients are usually hypoxic; Po_2 may be normal at rest but falls rapidly on exercise. CXR is initially normal or shows widespread, diffuse, interstitial shadowing. Focal consolidation suggests bacterial pneumonia but does not rule out PCP. Cystic changes and pneumatocoeles are common, but lymphadenopathy and pleural effusions are rare.

Differential diagnosis: Bacterial pneumonia, pulmonary Kaposi's sarcoma (see below).

Antibiotic management: Co-trimoxazole, 120 mg/kg/day in divided doses orally or iv (i.e. 20 mg/kg/day trimethoprim and 100 mg/kg/day sulphamethoxazole). Adverse effects (➤118) are common, particularly hypersensitivity reactions with severe rash and fever. Alternatively, pentamidine, 4 mg/kg/day in 250 ml 5% dextrose iv over 1 h. Adverse effects (➤118) occur but therapy may usually be continued. The usual time to respond is 4–6 days and patients often deteriorate before they improve. Continued worsening at 4 days or failure to improve by 7 days is an indication to change therapy from co-trimoxazole to pentamidine. Alternative regimens include trimethoprim (20 mg/kg/day) and dapsone (100 mg/day) **or** clindamycin and primaquine. Fluid overload should be avoided. Following recovery, lifelong co-trimoxazole or pentamidine prophylaxis is given.

Supportive management: Steroids improve survival and shorten duration of illness. If Po_2 < 10 kPa, give 80 mg prednisolone daily for 5 days, then 40 mg daily for 5 days and then 20 mg daily for 10 days. High-dose oxygen is given. Mechanical ventilation is required for severe hypoxia or exhaustion. The probability of surviving a first episode of PCP requiring mechanical ventilation is ~40% in experienced centres, and many patients survive for several years thereafter.

Complications: Pneumothorax is not unusual, and can be very difficult to manage. If the pneumothorax is large or there is suspicion of tension, then a chest drain must be inserted, but bronchopleural fistula formation with continued leakage of air is common. The chest drain should be maintained on low-pressure suction to maintain full inflation. Other methods used to close fistulae such as tetracycline pleuradhesis or thoracotomy and repair are not usually successful. It may be necessary to discharge the patient with a chest drain *in situ*, attached to a one-way valve.

Other pulmonary infections

HIV patients are at increased risk of **bacterial pneumonia** (➤22), usually due to *Streptococcus pneumoniae, Haemophilus influenzae* or *Staphylococcus aureus*. Recurrent bacterial pneumonia (> two episodes in 12 months) is now an AIDS-defining diagnosis. Recurrent acute or chronic **sinusitis** (➤15), due to *Streptococcus pneumoniae, Haemophilus influenzae* or *Pseudomonas aeruginosa*, is common. The possibility of rarer organisms should be considered and material obtained for microscopy and culture if infection persists.

Pulmonary tuberculosis occurs with increased frequency in patients with HIV infection. In early infection, typical clinical features of TB, including apical cavitation, are seen. With advanced immunodeficiency, CXR changes are more diffuse and extrapulmonary infection is common. Standard antituberculous therapy should be given, but multidrug-resistant TB has been seen in the US (➤128). Fungal pneumonia due to *Cryptococcus neoformans* usually occurs in the context of disseminated infection.

Kaposi's sarcoma (➤129) may affect the lungs, typically with patchy nodular shadowing and pleural effusions. Bacterial superinfection, particularly with *Staphylococcus aureus*, is common.

Table 36 Common skin infections in HIV-infected patients

Organism	Comments
Staphylococcus aureus	Folliculitis (➤87), bullous impetigo, boils and cellulitis (➤88)
Herpes zoster (➤105)	Occasionally with cutaneous dissemination
Herpes simplex (➤66)	May cause recurrent oral, genital or perianal ulceration. May also present as chronic non-healing ulcer resembling decubitus ulcer. Culture and biopsy are required for diagnosis
Molluscum contagiosum (➤94)	Lesions are larger and more numerous than usual

Skin disease in HIV-infected patients

Infections (Table 36)

Bacillary angiomatosis is a rare cutaneous infection caused by *Rochalimea* spp. (➤237). It presents with disseminated lesions consisting of friable, vascular eruptions resembling granulation tissue, subcutaneous nodules and cellulitis plaques, which may affect any skin or mucosa. Visceral involvement, particularly of liver and spleen (peliosis hepatis), and osteolytic bone lesions occur. Diagnosis is by histology. Infection may be fatal if untreated, but responds well to erythromycin or doxycycline in standard doses for 8 weeks (cutaneous disease) or 16 weeks (visceral disease). Chronic *Rochalimea henselae* bacteraemia has been reported as a cause of malaise, fever and weight loss.

Hypersensitivity reactions

Drug reactions and allergic reactions to insect bites are common. Up to 50% of patients treated with co-trimoxazole for PCP develop a rash. Many patients develop multiple drug allergies. **Scabies** should be excluded in patients complaining of pruritis.

Papulosquamous disorders

Seborrhoeic dermatitis, psoriasis and Reiter's disease with keratoderma blenorrhagica are commoner in patients with HIV. **Seborrhoeic dermatitis** (➤92) causes erythematous plaques with a yellowish greasy scale on the hairy areas of the face, chest, back and groin. It responds to topical steroids and antifungals, such as miconazole/hydrocortisone cream, although stronger steroids are occasionally required. **Psoriasis** often begins after HIV infection and may be complicated by arthritis. It is treated with topical steroids and dithranol, but methotrexate should be avoided as it may cause a sudden deterioration in immune function and death. Psoriasis may improve after starting zidovudine therapy.

The skin is also a common site for **Kaposi's sarcoma** (➤129).

Oral manifestations of HIV infection

Candidiasis

Oral *Candida albicans* infection is common and may be the first indication of immunodeficiency.

Clinical features: Typical white plaques are usually present, but mucosal erythema without exudate, or angular stomatitis, may be due to candidiasis.

Organisms: *Candida albicans*, other *Candida* spp. including *Candida krusei*.

Microbiological investigations: Culture, microscopy of scrapings. Biopsy is required rarely if clinical features are atypical.

Antibiotic management: Fluconazole (150 mg weekly or 50 mg alternate days as prophylaxis). Topical agents such as nystatin or amphotericin lozenges are effective, but oesophageal and genital candidiasis is an indication for systemic therapy. Fluconazole-resistant *Candida albicans* and other *Candida* spp. occur in patients on long-term treatment/

prophylaxis. Increasing the dose of fluconazole or changing to a different imidazole such as itraconazole may be effective; admission for intravenous amphotericin is occasionally necessary.

Gingivitis

Common and sometimes severe with progression to **necrotising stomatitis** with rapid progressive loss of gingival tissue. Urgent dental referral for debridement, application of topical antiseptic and systemic treatment with metronidazole or co-amoxiclav are required.

Oral hairy leukoplakia

Produces white thickening of the buccal mucosa, along the lateral borders of the tongue. It is due to EBV infection (➤243) and is an indicator of poor prognosis and progression to AIDS.

Kaposi's sarcoma (KS) and lymphoma (➤129)

May both affect the mouth.

Gastrointestinal disease in HIV-infected patients

Oesophagitis

Caused by *Candida albicans*, Herpes simplex or cytomegalovirus. All three cause dysphagia and are clinically indistinguishable, although there may be evidence of oropharyngeal candidiasis. Barium swallow will document oesophagitis, which is an AIDS-defining illness. Differential diagnosis is made by endoscopy and biopsy, or by a therapeutic trial of fluconazole, followed by acyclovir. CMV infection responds to ganciclovir, but relapse is common if this agent, which must be given iv, is discontinued. **KS** and **lymphoma** (➤129) both affect the oesophagus and stomach.

Hepatobiliary disease

Right-upper-quadrant (RUQ) pain and tenderness, abnormal liver function tests, and hepatomegaly are common in patients with AIDS, often in the context of previously diagnosed widely disseminated disease such as MAI or KS. Sclerosing cholangitis, often secondary to biliary infection by CMV (➤243) or *Cryptosporidium parvum* (➤263)

is common, causing RUQ pain and marked elevation of alkaline phosphatase. Diagnosis is by ERCP. Endoscopic sphincterotomy may relieve symptoms if there is papillary stenosis.

Diarrhoea

Abdominal cramps, weight loss and large-volume diarrhoea are common, and usually indicate infection. Bacterial pathogens such as *Salmonella* spp. (➤190), *Shigella* spp. (➤192) and *Campylobacter jejuni* (➤196) and protozoa such as *Giardia lamblia*, (➤266) *Entamoeba histolytica* (➤267), *Cryptosporidium parvum* (➤263) and *Microsporidia* (➤264) should be excluded by stool microscopy and culture. Cryptosporidiosis may respond to paromomycin. Malabsorption with severe weight loss may be due to small-bowel infection by MAI (➤128). Diagnosis is made by histology of small-bowel biopsy for acid-fast bacilli.

Diarrhoea, with tenesmus, frequent small-volume stools and rectal bleeding, suggest colitis. The bacteria listed above should be excluded. Sigmoidoscopy may show changes of **CMV colitis** (submucosal haemorrhages, shallow ulcers in the distal colon). Diagnosis is confirmed by biopsy. Treatment with ganciclovir (10 mg/kg/day) is usually effective, and can usually be stopped after resolution of colitis. Concurrent CMV retinitis should be excluded.

No specific pathogens are found in 25–50% of AIDS patients with diarrhoea. If stool examination and sigmoidoscopy are negative, further investigations are unlikely to be helpful.

Neurological disease in HIV-infected patients

Approximately 10% of HIV patients first present with neurological disease. **Seroconversion** (➤115) is frequently associated with neurological symptoms, including meningitis, ataxia and cranial or peripheral neuropathy. Recovery usually occurs over several weeks. During **latent infection** (➤115) there is an increased frequency of demyelinating neuropathy resembling Guillain–Barré syndrome.

In **advanced disease**, neurological disease is common and presents with a number of clinical syndromes (Table 37).

Table 37 Neurological syndromes in HIV+ patients

Clinical syndrome	Causes
Diffuse encephalopathy	**AIDS-dementia complex** (➤see below) CMV encephalitis (➤124) HSV encephalitis (➤124) Hypoxia or metabolic disturbance secondary to sepsis *Toxoplasma gondii encephalitis* (➤124)
Focal cerebral disease	***Toxoplasma gondii* encephalitis** (➤124) **Cerebral lymphoma** (➤130) **Progressive multifocal leucoencephalopathy** (➤124) Tuberculoma (➤128) *Cryptococcus neoformans* abscess (➤125) HSV encephalitis (➤124) VZV encephalitis *Candida albicans* abscess
Meningitis	***Cryptococcus neoformans* meningitis** (➤125) Tuberculous meningitis (➤128) Syphilis (➤127) Metastatic lymphomatous meningitis (➤130)
Peripheral neuropathy	**Sensory polyneuropathy** Iatrogenic toxic neuropathy
Myelopathy	**Vacuolar myelopathy** (➤see below) Acute transverse myelitis due to VZV, lymphoma, toxoplasmosis (➤124) or CMV

It is important to recognise that abnormalities of the CSF, such as mild lymphocytic pleocytosis and moderate elevation of protein, are common in asymptomatic HIV-seropositive patients with relatively intact cellular immunity and preserved CD4 counts.

AIDS dementia complex (ADC)

ADC describes a clinical complex of cognitive, motor and behavioural abnormalities. Neuropathological changes correlate to some extent with the clinical picture, affecting in particular the central white matter, basal ganglia and brain stem. The spinal cord is often affected, with vacuolar myelopathy. These changes are probably due to the direct effects of HIV infection.

Symptomatic ADC occurs in 30–50% of AIDS patients, usually late in their disease. Neuropsychological testing reveals subclinical abnormalities in many more.

Clinical features: Early symptoms of **cognitive deficit** are poor concentration and memory loss, with difficulty completing complex tasks. Progression to severe dementia occurs with, in many cases, an eventual almost vegetative end-stage. **Motor abnormalities** usually lag behind cognitive defects. Poor balance, incoordination and clumsiness are frequent early complaints. Generalised hyper-reflexia and primitive reflexes (e.g. grasp reflex) may develop. Severe ataxia, leg weakness and incontinence are common in later stages. **Behavioural abnormalities** include apathy and lack of initiative or agitation and hyperactivity. Psychiatric illness, including depression and mania, are also common. Fits may occur.

Investigations: The diagnosis is clinical. Neuropsychological testing confirms the diagnosis and quantitates abnormalities. MRI and CT scan show cerebral atrophy with wide sulci and enlarged ventricles. MRI reveals whitematter abnormalities as areas of high signal intensity on T2-weighted images. Scanning is particularly important in the exclusion of other, treatable, conditions. CSF is usually non-specifically abnormal, with a moderately elevated protein and a mild lymphocytic pleocytosis.

Differential diagnosis: Progressive multifocal leucoencephalopathy, CMV encephalitis, HSV encephalitis, hypoxia or metabolic disturbance secondary to sepsis, *Toxoplasma gondii* encephalitis.

Management: Zidovudine is of considerable benefit, with rapid resolution or improvement of symptoms in some patients, although this may not be sustained. Didanosine has also been reported to be effective. Supportive care is very important.

Cytomegalovirus (CMV) encephalitis

Presents in a very similar manner to ADC, although the course is often more rapid. It occurs frequently with concurrent disseminated CMV infection and retinitis. Clinical diagnosis is difficult but can be confirmed by brain biopsy. Ganciclovir is given although the response is often disappointing.

Herpes simplex (HSV) encephalitis

Presents typically (➤78), with rapid onset of headache, fever, confusion and temporal lobe abnormality, or subacutely as a non-specific neurological illness indistinguishable from other causes of diffuse encephalopathy listed above. CSF shows elevated protein and a lymphocytic pleocytosis, but culture for HSV is usually negative. Definitive diagnosis requires brain biopsy, but empirical treatment with acyclovir is often given.

Progressive multifocal leucoencephalopathy (PML)

PML is caused by reactivation of the polyomavirus JC virus (➤246). Approximately 2% of AIDS patients will develop PML, which has also been reported in patients with haematological malignancies or iatrogenic immunosuppression. PML is a disease of patients with advanced immunodeficiency (CD4 count < 100 cells/µl).

Clinical features: Progressive accumulation of focal neurological deficits, typically including hemiparesis, ataxia or aphasia. Fever is absent and there is no clouding of consciousness. Progression is inexorable, over weeks or months, although a relapsing and remitting course has been described rarely. Prognosis is very poor with a median survival of ~16 weeks in one series.

Investigations: CT scan shows multiple non-enhancing lesions with no mass effect scattered throughout the white matter. CSF and EEG are normal or non-specifically abnormal. Brain biopsy is required for definitive diagnosis, primarily to exclude other pathologies.

Differential diagnosis: Cerebral toxoplasmosis (see below), cerebral lymphoma (➤130), tuberculoma.

Management: Supportive. Specific antiviral therapy is not available, although preliminary trials suggest that cytarabine may be helpful in some cases.

AIDS-associated toxoplasmosis

Toxoplasmosis in AIDS is due to reactivation of infection by the protozoan *Toxoplasma gondii*.

Primary infection is usually acquired in childhood by ingestion of infectious oocysts in cat faeces or by eating poorly cooked meat containing tissue cysts. These routes of infection cause an acute infectious mononucleosis similar to primary EBV infection (➤105). Vertical transmission also occurs, and may cause fetal abnormalities (➤110).

After primary infection, cysts of *Toxoplasma gondii* persist in the CNS and multiple extraneural sites. Choroidoretinitis in the immunocompetent patient results from reactivation of tissue cysts later in life. During HIV infection, usually in patients with advanced immunodeficiency, cysts reactivate to cause necrotic inflammatory abscesses scattered throughout the cerebral hemispheres. Toxoplasma encephalitis is the commonest cause of focal neurological deficit in AIDS patients.

Risk factors: The incidence of toxoplasma encephalitis varies depending on rates of seropositivity against *Toxoplasma gondii*. It is particularly common in France, where adult seroprevalence rates are ~80%. Approximately 50% of UK adults are seropositive. Infection usually occurs in patients with advanced immunodeficiency.

Clinical features: Fever, confusion, fits and focal neurological deficit, developing over a few days. In 60%, there are focal neurological signs, including hemiparesis, ataxia, aphasia or visual field defect. *Toxoplasma gondii* also causes **chorioretinitis** (➤85), which may accompany or precede encephalitis. Ophthalmoscopic examination reveals uni- or bilateral diffuse or focal areas of retinal necrosis and haemorrhage.

Organism: *Toxoplasma gondii* (➤264).

Microbiological investigations: Patients are nearly always (97%) seropositive for *Toxoplasma gondii*. Negative serology strongly suggests an alternative diagnosis. Changes in antibody titre and IgM levels are rarely helpful. Serum and/or CSF should be examined for cryptococcal antigen, as *Cryptococcus neoformans* occasionally causes identical CT changes.

Other investigations: CT scan shows multiple hypodense lesions in the cerebral hemispheres—particularly in the basal ganglia and at the hemispheric corticomedullary junction—which develop 'ring enhancement' after injection of iv contrast. Lesions can be solitary and non-enhancing. MRI is more sensitive, and solitary lesions on MRI are unlikely to be due to *Toxoplasma gondii*. Definitive diagnosis is by brain biopsy, but a trial of antitoxoplasma therapy should be initiated before performing biopsy (see Fig. 3). Radiological improvement is usually seen within 2–3 weeks of commencing therapy.

Differential diagnosis: Cerebral lymphoma (➤130), progressive multifocal leucoencephalopathy (➤124), fungal abscess, including *Cryptococcus neoformans* (see below), tuberculoma (➤128).

Antibiotic management: Primary therapy is given for at least 6 weeks. Pyrimethamine, loading dose 200 mg, followed by 1–1.5 mg/kg daily as a single oral dose **plus** folinic acid 15 mg daily **plus** sulphadiazine 1 g 6-hly or clindamycin 600 mg 6-hly. Allergies to sulphadiazine and clindamycin are common (➤119). Clarithromycin (1 g 12-hly) is an al-

ternative. Sulphadiazine causes crystalluria, which presents with flank pain, renal failure and haematuria. To avoid this, maintain urine output >3 l/24 h and urine pH >7 (give sodium bicarbonate 3 g 6-hly po). Steroids may have to be given for cerebral oedema; dose and duration of course should be as low as possible. Anticonvulsants may be required.

After 6 weeks of primary therapy **lifelong maintenance therapy** is commenced: pyrimethamine (25–50 mg 24-hly po) **plus** folinic acid (15 mg 24-hly) **plus either** sulphadiazine (500 mg 6-hly po) **or** clindamycin (300 mg 6-hly po) **or** clarithromycin (500 mg 12-hly po).

Comments: Infection of the spinal cord leading to **transverse myelitis** is described. *Toxoplasma gondii* also causes **pneumonitis**. The value of primary prophylaxis against toxoplasmosis for seropositive AIDS patients is under investigation. Co-trimoxazole prophylaxis against PCP appears to reduce the incidence of toxoplasmosis also.

Cryptococcal meningitis

Cryptococcus neoformans is distributed globally, in contrast to other dimorphic fungi causing systemic infection, such as histoplasmosis and blastomycosis, which are geographically restricted. *Cryptococcus neoformans* is widespread in the environment in bird droppings and infection occurs via inhalation. Whereas this organism does cause pneumonia, most AIDS patients with cryptococcal infection have meningitis.

Risk factors: Rare in patients with CD4 count >100 cells/µl.

Clinical features: Presentation is usually subtle and non-specific with prolonged fever, headache and malaise. Nausea and vomiting occur in ~50%, but neck stiffness and photophobia are unusual, occurring in ~20–30%. Altered mental state is present in ~10–30% and fits or focal signs in <10%. Many patients have a history of recent chest infection which may represent cryptococcal pneumonia. Cryptococcal skin sepsis occurs infrequently. Symptomatic cryptococcal infection elsewhere is rare, although isolation of *Cryptococcus neo-*

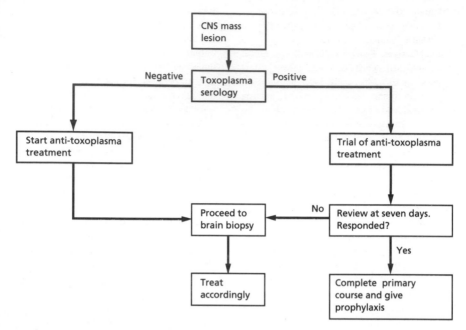

Fig. 3 Management of focal cerebral lesions in HIV+ patients: CT scan and MRI can only suggest the most likely diagnosis in HIV patients with **focal** CNS lesions. For differential diagnosis, ➤123. Patients with toxoplasmosis are rarely seronegative, and usually respond clinically and radiologically to treatment within 7 days. HIV patients with cerebral lymphoma may respond well to radiotherapy. Therefore we recommend the algorithm as given.

formans from blood, urine and GI tract is not uncommon. Persistent asymptomatic genitourinary infection (particularly prostate) is probably a reservoir for relapse after treatment.

Organism: *Cryptococcus neoformans* (➤292).

Microbiological investigations: CSF is negatively stained for capsulate yeasts using **India ink**—positive in ~70% of cases. Serum and CSF **cryptococcal antigen detection** is sensitive and specific, detecting ~99% of cases. The titre usually rises after treatment and then falls. It is unusual for it to become negative even after full clinical response. Routine CSF examination is sometimes normal. Raised opening pressure is common. CSF cell count is <20 in ~60%. CSF glucose may be reduced, but is normal in ~70% and CSF protein may be elevated but is normal in ~50%. CSF fungal culture may be positive.

Other investigations: CXR shows diffuse or focal interstitial infiltrates if there is concurrent cryptococcal pneumonia. Hilar lymphadenopathy is common. Large nodules and cavities are seen rarely. CT head scan is abnormal in 30–50%, but changes seen are non-specific, including cerebral atrophy or occasionally mass lesions with oedema and ring enhancement, indistinguishable from *Toxoplasma gondii* encephalitis.

Differential diagnosis: Cerebral lymphoma (➤130), progressive multifocal leucoencephalopathy (➤124), *Toxoplasma gondii* encephalitis (➤124), tuberculoma (➤128).

Antibiotic management: Amphotericin (0.7 mg/kg/day iv) until stable, then fluconazole 400 mg po for 10 weeks. Thereafter lifelong maintenance is required. Although amphotericin appears to be slightly better as initial therapy, fluconazole (200 mg 6-hly po) is better at preventing relapse, possibly due to better sterilisation of the genitourinary tract.

Comments: Cryptococcal infection occurs in patients with advanced immunodeficiency. Thus, approximately 20% of patients do not survive initial therapy, but those who do have a mean survival >1 year. A very high cryptococcal antigen titre, altered mental state and positive India ink test are associated with worse prognosis. The role of primary prophylaxis is under investigation.

Peripheral neuropathy and myopathy

A predominant **sensory polyneuropathy**, causing numbness, paraesthesiae and dysaesthesiae, mainly in the feet and legs, is common in HIV infection. It is likely to be due directly to HIV infection, but does not respond to zidovudine. Tricyclics, analgesics and carbamazepine may relieve symptoms.

CMV infection causes progressive radiculopathy affecting the sacral and lumbar roots. It occurs in patients with advanced disease and causes flaccid paralysis of the legs with sacral pain and sphincter disturbance. Concurrent CMV retinitis is common. MRI shows thickened spinal roots and CSF contains neutrophils. CMV is often cultured from blood and CSF; ganciclovir should be given.

Certain antiretroviral drugs, including didanosine and zalcitabine, cause **toxic peripheral neuropathy**, which usually resolves after stopping treatment.

Myopathy resembling polymyositis occurs. Zidovudine also causes proximal myopathy rarely.

Syphilis in HIV-infected patients

Syphilis and HIV share a number of risk factors and genital ulcer disease, including syphilis, is thought to enhance transmission of HIV. The two infections may therefore coexist. HIV influences the presentation and management of syphilis in the following ways.

Clinical features: Most HIV patients with primary or secondary syphilis have a typical illness, but neurological disease occurring during secondary syphilis ('early neurosyphilis') is commoner in HIV-infected

persons (>67). The latent period to the development of meningovascular syphilis may be shortened, and uveitis and sensorineural hearing loss occur more frequently.

Diagnosis: False negative specific serological tests (e.g. TPHA) and false positive non-specific tests (e.g. VDRL) have been reported. Changes in titre of VDRL are unreliable as indicators of latency or relapse in HIV-infected persons. The CSF abnormalities attributable to HIV infection and described above (>123) make diagnosis of neurosyphilis difficult. If syphilis is suspected but cannot be confirmed it may be appropriate to monitor clinical course and serology, or to treat presumptively.

Treatment: Treatment failures and neurological relapse are reported in HIV patients with standard regimens. It is recommended that patients are treated wherever possible with penicillin. In patients with syphilis of less than 1 year's duration, and no evidence of neurological involvement, a single dose of benzathine penicillin (2.4 MU im) or procaine penicillin (2.4 MU im daily for 10 days) may be given. In other patients, treatment should be extended (e.g. three doses of benzathine penicillin, 2.4 MU im at weekly intervals, or benzylpenicillin 4 MU 4-hly iv for 14 days).

Cytomegalovirus (CMV) retinitis

Approximately 10% of AIDS patients develop CMV retinitis, usually in the context of severe immunodeficiency (CD4 count < 100 cells/µl).

Clinical features: Unilateral visual field loss, floaters or loss of acuity. Asymptomatic lesions are often discovered at routine fundoscopy. Retinitis appears as fluffy white areas of necrosis and haemorrhage ('cottage cheese and ketchup'). Diagnosis is based on clinical findings and ophthalmoscopic appearances. Without treatment, progression to blindness in both eyes is the rule.

Microbiological investigations: CMV viraemia and viruria are common (>243). Patients are usually CMV seropositive, often to high titres.

Differential diagnosis: *Toxoplasma gondii* retinitis is usually associated with cerebral toxoplasmosis. The lesions are not usually haemorrhagic. Serology may contribute to distinguishing these infections.

Management: Ganciclovir (5 mg/kg 8-hly iv) is given for 14 days as induction therapy. Approximately 80% show stabilisation of ophthalmoscopic appearances, but visual field defects do not usually resolve. Thereafter maintenance therapy (ganciclovir 6 mg/kg iv daily for 5 days/week) is essential, but progression occurs eventually. Ganciclovir causes neutropenia. Dose should be reduced if neutrophil count falls below 1000×10^6/l, and stopped if below 500×10^6/l. Concurrent zidovudine may exacerbate this toxicity. Foscarnet is an alternative agent for treatment of CMV infection (adverse effects ≻119). Induction dose: 60 mg/kg 8-hly iv, maintenance dose 90 mg/kg daily 5 days/week.

Complications: Retinal detachment.

Mycobacterial infection and HIV

Mycobacterium tuberculosis

Tuberculosis (TB) is commoner in the presence of HIV infection. In areas of high TB prevalence such as sub-Saharan Africa, > 50% of patients dying of AIDS have active TB at post-mortem. HIV infection has led to a very significant increase in the prevalence of TB in these areas.

TB in a patient with HIV infection is an AIDS-defining illness.

Clinical features: In the developed world, TB occurs at any time during HIV infection. In patients with relatively preserved cellular immunity (e.g. CD4 count > 300 cells/µl), clinical features are those of typical reactivated TB, with apical cavitation and fibrosis (≻29). In patients with more advanced disease (e.g. CD4 count < 100 cells/µl), pulmonary TB presents atypically with hilar and mediastinal lymphadenopathy and CXR infiltrates in the middle and lower lung fields. Cavitation is rare. Extrapulmonary TB occurs in at least 50%; sites often involved include peripheral lymph nodes, bone marrow, bone, joint, genitourinary tract, liver, spleen, skin and peritoneum. *Mycobacterium tuberculosis* bacteraemia occurs in ~25%. A central nervous system mass lesion ('tuberculoma') has been described. These lesions cause a

wide range of CT appearances and diagnosis is usually made only at brain biopsy.

Diagnosis: Mantoux testing is unhelpful as false negatives are common. Diagnosis depends on obtaining appropriate specimens for microscopy and culture. Special techniques such as lysis centrifugation may be used to detect mycobacteraemia. If TB is strongly suspected clinically, then treatment is commenced whilst waiting 6–8 weeks for the results of mycobacterial culture and antibiotic sensitivity. If acid-fast bacilli are seen, they should be assumed to be *Mycobacterium tuberculosis* until proven otherwise by culture.

Antibiotic management: Standard treatment regimens (≻32) are used although the duration of therapy is usually extended, e.g. isoniazid, pyridoxine, rifampicin, pyrazinamide and ethambutol for 2 months followed by isoniazid, pyridoxine and rifampicin for a further 7 months. Extrapulmonary TB should be treated for 18 months in total. Rifampicin and fluconazole interact, with potential reduction in the serum levels of both drugs. Multidrug-resistant TB has emerged as a problem in AIDS patients in US cities and has become a nosocomial infection hazard. Isolates resistant to rifampicin and isoniazid are seen in patients who stop and start therapy and fail to complete treatment courses. Treatment with alternate drugs including pyrazinamide, ethambutol and rifampicin for 1–2 years may be effective (≻229).

Mycobacterium avium-intracellulare (MAI)

Mycobacterium avium-intracellulare (≻231) causes disseminated infection in patients with advanced immunodeficiency (CD4 count < 100 cells/µl). At least 50% of patients dying of AIDS have post-mortem evidence of MAI, with infection involving bone marrow, lymph nodes and any of the viscera. MAI bacteraemia indicates a poor prognosis, with median survival ~100 days compared with ~300 days for matched patients without MAI bacteraemia.

Clinical features: Fever, malaise, weight loss and anaemia. Diarrhoea and abdominal pain due to colonic infection. Chronic malabsorption with severe weight loss due to small-bowel infection. Extrabiliary obstructive jaundice due to periportal lymphadenopathy. Patients with MAI always have other opportunist infections and/or malignancies, and it is often difficult to attribute symptoms exclusively to one or other pathogen.

Diagnosis: MAI bacteraemia occurs in most patients. Lysis centrifugation blood culture increases the yield of positives. MAI may be seen in or cultured from other tissues such as lymph node, bone marrow, small bowel or liver biopsy. MAI may be found in stools, although this does not always indicate active infection.

Antibiotic management: MAI is resistant to most antituberculous agents, but is usually sensitive to ethambutol and clarithromycin. Treatment with rifampicin or rifabutin, plus ethambutol and clarithromycin, is recommended and may improve symptoms. Primary prophylaxis with rifabutin alone delays onset of MAI bacteraemia, but gives no significant survival benefit.

Comments: Infection with other atypical mycobacteria, such as *Mycobacterium kansasii* and *Mycobacterium xenopi*, has also been reported in AIDS patients.

Cardiac disease in HIV infection

Myocarditis and dilated cardiomyopathy are common post-mortem findings in AIDS patients, but clinical presentation is rare. Symptomatic pericardial effusion occurs infrequently and is usually infectious, due to mycobacteria or *Cryptococcus neoformans*.

Haematological abnormalities in HIV infection

A number of factors cause haematological abnormalities in HIV-infected individuals. These include direct suppression of bone marrow by HIV itself, infiltration of bone marrow by opportunist pathogens or malignancies, drug toxicity, nutritional deficiency and immunodysregulation with autoantibody production.

Anaemia occurs in the majority of patients with AIDS. Most have normochromic, normocytic anaemia, attributable to HIV infection

itself and prolonged ill health with recurrent infections. Iron deficiency is less common, and may result from intestinal Kaposi's sarcoma (>130). Severe anaemia may result from infiltration of bone marrow by MAI. Zidovudine causes macrocytosis in most recipients. It also causes anaemia in a minority; this toxicity is less frequent with low-dose regimens (e.g. 250 mg 12-hly).

Neutropenia is common and frequently due to drugs (e.g. ganciclovir, zidovudine, pyrimethamine, sulphonamides). Bacteraemia is common if neutrophil count falls below $500 \times 10^9/l$. Colony-stimulating factors such as granulocyte–macrophage colony-stimulating factor (GM-CSF) and granulocyte colony-stimulating factor (G-CSF) have been used to sustain the neutrophil count in patients with severe neutropenia or during chemotherapy.

Thrombocytopenia, with platelet-associated immunoglobulin, is common. It is characteristically seen early in HIV infection and often resolves with the onset of AIDS. Bleeding is rare. Zidovudine may be helpful. Steroids (prednisolone 1 mg/kg/day) are usually effective, but the platelet count usually falls as the dose is reduced. Splenectomy may be required and is usually effective.

Malignancies associated with HIV infection

Kaposi's sarcoma, non-Hodgkin's lymphoma and cervical carcinoma are AIDS-defining illnesses.

Kaposi's sarcoma (KS)

KS was previously recognised as an unusual indolent tumour endemic in sub-Saharan Africa and among elderly white men of Mediterranean or East European origin, affecting primarily the legs. It was one of the first conditions to be associated with AIDS and initially was very common. However, the incidence has fallen over the past decade. KS is seen almost exclusively in homosexual men and has been reported only rarely in IVDUs. These two features strongly suggest that some other sexually transmitted agent is a cofactor for the development of KS.

Clinical features: In HIV infection KS is usually an aggressive multifocal tumour. Skin is most frequently involved, with palpable, firm cutaneous nodules, 0.5–2 cm in diameter. Lesions are usually violaceous, although they may be brown or black in pigmented skin. Head and neck are often involved, particularly the buccal mucosa. Lesions tend to progress with time, becoming larger and more numerous. Visceral disease is common and can involve any organ. Gastrointestinal lesions are common and cause haemorrhage. Pulmonary disease typically causes patchy nodular shadowing and pleural effusions. Bacterial superinfection, particularly with *Staphylococcus aureus*, is common. Lymphoedema results from lymph node infiltration.

Diagnosis: Diagnosis is confirmed by biopsy.

Management: Patients with KS have advanced immunodeficiency and usually die from other causes. Therefore specific treatment is not always indicated. Treatment is aimed at palliation and cosmesis. Particular indications include lymphoedema, painful or bulky lesions anywhere, but particularly in the oropharynx, and pulmonary disease, which may progress rapidly. Radiotherapy is the most appropriate therapy for patients with localised disease. Other local therapies include intralesional chemotherapy and cryotherapy. Systemic chemotherapy (e.g. vincristine, etoposide or doxorubicin) is effective in a proportion of patients. Systemic interferon-α has also been shown to be effective in some patients, although adverse effects, including fevers and myalgia, limit its use.

Non-Hodgkin's lymphoma (NHL)

NHL occurs at all stages of HIV infection; ~30% of patients have CD4 counts > 200 cells/μl. The incidence is rising and it has been suggested that this is due to patients avoiding opportunistic infections by taking primary prophylaxis and antiretroviral therapy. CNS lymphomas arise almost exclusively in patients with advanced disease and CD4 count < 50 cells/μl.

Clinical features: Widespread extranodal disease is usual, particularly affecting the gastrointestinal tract, CNS, bone marrow and liver. CNS lymphoma presents with gradual onset of confusion, lethargy, cognitive loss, fits and focal signs such as hemiplegia, aphasia and cranial nerve palsies. CT scan usually shows one or two discrete lesions deep in the white matter, which may be hypodense and weakly contrast-enhancing. Differentiation from *Toxoplasma gondii* encephalitis (➤124) can be very difficult on CT grounds alone, and brain biopsy may be required if there is no response to antitoxoplasma therapy.

Management: Chemotherapy is less likely to be successful in HIV-infected individuals than in non-infected patients with similar tumours. Failure to respond, relapse and severe drug toxicity are all more common. Survival may be better with less aggressive regimens. Patients with relatively good immune function and no previous AIDS-defining illness are good candidates for chemotherapy and may be cured, surviving for several years. Patients with advanced immunodeficiency and cerebral lymphoma may respond to cranial radiotherapy, but most will die within a few months, often from other AIDS-related illnesses.

Cervical carcinoma in HIV infection

Human papillomavirus infection (➤246), abnormal cervical cytology and cervical neoplasia are all more common in HIV-infected women, who should have cervical smears performed at least annually. Many clinics offer baseline culposcopy at the time of HIV diagnosis.

13: Infections in the Immunocompromised Host

Congenital immunodeficiency syndromes

Congenital immunodeficiency syndromes affecting all components of the immune system are described. They are all rare but have served as 'experiments of nature' allowing elucidation of the function of the normal immune system.

Patients with complement deficiency should receive vaccination against *Streptococcus pneumoniae*, *Haemophilus influenzae* and *Neisseria meningitidis*, although these vaccines may not give their usual levels of protection in these patients as the antibody response is poor.

Acquired disorders of immunity

In practice, acquired defects of immunity are far commoner than congenital disorders. These may be **local defects**, due to trauma, burns, fore-

Table 38 Congenital disorders affecting non-antigen-specific ('natural') immunity

Disorder	Examples	Common infectious complications
Neutropenia	Infantile genetic agranulocytosis, autoimmune neutropenia, isoimmune neonatal neutropenia	Recurrent or severe bacterial infection (e.g. staphylococci, streptococci, coliforms, *Pseudomonas aeruginosa*, *Haemophilus influenzae*) and fungi (e.g. *Candida albicans*, *Aspergillus* spp.)
Abnormal neutrophil function (e.g. abnormalities of chemotaxis, adherence, phagocytosis and microbial killing)	Chédiak–Higashi, lazy leucocyte, leucocyte adhesion deficiency, chronic granulomatous disease	
Complement disorders	Inherited deficiencies of C3, C5, C6, C7, C8, factor I, properdin	Severe recurrent infection with capsulate bacteria

Table 39 Congenital disorders of antigen-specific immunity 1: humoral immunity

Disorder	Comments	Common infectious complications
X-linked hypogammaglobulinaemia	Occasionally associated with growth hormone deficiency	Chronic or recurrent bacterial infections. Chronic disseminated enteroviral infection
Common variable immunodeficiency (CVID)	Heterogeneous group of patients with hypogammaglobulinaemia	Chronic respiratory and GI infection
IgA deficiency	Common, affecting 1 : 600 individuals	Frequently asymptomatic. Chronic respiratory and GI infection
IgG subclass deficiency	Usually affects IgG2 or IgG2 and IgG4	Infection with encapsulated bacteria. Poor response to some vaccines
Hyper-IgM syndrome	Failure of B cells to switch from IgM to IgG production	Recurrent pyogenic infection
Transient hypogammaglobulinaemia of infancy	May persist for many months	Diarrhoea. Otitis media

Table 40 Congenital disorders of antigen-specific immunity 2: disorders affecting both cellular and humoral immunity

Disorder	Comments	Common infectious complications
Severe combined immunodeficiency (SCID)	Heterogeneous group of patients with deficient cell-mediated and humoral immunity. Variants include: adenosine deaminase deficiency, purine nucleotide phosphorylase deficiency, MHC class II deficiency, reticular dysgenesis	Chronic recurrent bacterial viral and fungal infections. Often fatal in infancy
DiGeorge syndrome	Embryopathy of 3rd and 4th pharyngeal pouch resulting in thymic aplasia, hypoparathyroidism and congenital heart disease	Chronic and recurrent respiratory and GI infections
Wiskott–Aldrich syndrome	Thrombocytopenia, eczema and immunodeficiency, probably due to mutation in the CD43 antigen	Bacterial and fungal infections. Lymphoma
Ataxia telangiectasia	Cerebellar ataxia, oculocutaneous telengiectasia and immunodeficiency	Chronic sinopulmonary infection. Lymphoma and lymphatic leukaemia also common
Chronic mucocutaneous candidiasis	Frequently associated with endocrinopathies and autoimmune disease	Also more susceptible to bacterial and viral infections
X-linked lymphoproliferative syndrome	Genetic inability to mount immune response to EB virus infection	Chronic EBV infection with hypogamma globulinaemia, pancytopenia and lymphoma

ign bodies, anatomical abnormalities or iv lines, or **generalised defects**, such as:
• malnutrition, advanced age or neoplastic disease;
• viral infections, e.g. increased susceptibility to bacterial infection during measles, or profound immunodeficiency due to HIV infection (➤114);
• chronic diseases, e.g. diabetes mellitus, cirrhosis, alcoholism, renal failure;
• splenectomy;
• iatrogenic due to radiotherapy, cytotoxic chemotherapy and immunosuppression (e.g. steroids, cyclosporin A, cyclophosphamide).

Patients with recurrent severe bacterial infections are common in clinical practice but congenital immunodeficiency is rare. If the history suggests immunodeficiency but factors listed above are not present, the following screening tests are indicated: FBC including differential WBC, quantitation of T-cell subsets, total immunoglobulin levels and IgG subclass levels, complement levels (CH_{50}, C3, C1q, C4). These are best done when the patient is not currently infected. For more specialised tests referral to a clinical immunologist is recommended.

Splenectomy
After splenectomy (whether for haematological malignancy, for trauma, or as the result of sickle-cell disease), patients are at risk from a range of infections, particularly acute severe sepsis due to capsulate bacteria: *Streptococcus pneumoniae*, *Haemophilus influenzae* and *Neisseria meningitidis*. Patients are at increased risk of severe malaria and should take optimum prophylaxis if they travel (➤140). They are also at risk of severe infection with *Capnocytophaga canimorsus* after dog bite (➤90) and of babesiosis (➤263).

The following precautions are recommended:
• Patients must be warned to seek medical help at the onset of symptoms. Their family members should be informed of the early signs of septicaemia and meningitis and patients should be encouraged to wear a medical alert bracelet.

• Patients under 5 years at the time of splenectomy should receive penicillin V prophylaxis until the age of 16 (125 mg 12-hly, modified for age as below). Patients of 5 and over receive prophylaxis for 2 years after splenectomy (6–12 years: 250 mg 12-hly; > 12 years: 500 mg 12-hly). Amoxycillin is an alternative. Erythromycin is given to penicillin-allergic patients (< 2 years: 125 mg 12-hly; 2–8 years: 250 mg 12-hly; > 8 years: 500 mg 12-hly).

• Vaccination against:
  Streptococcus pneumoniae for all > 2 years, repeated once between 5 and 10 years later. Preferably given 2 weeks pre-splenectomy.
  Haemophilus influenzae (single dose).
  Neisseria meningitidis (single dose).
  Influenza (annually).

Common clinical examples of acquired immunodeficiency

Most patients with severe acquired immunodeficiency fall into one of the following categories:
• neutropenia;
• post-solid organ transplant;
• post-bone marrow transplant;
• HIV infection.

The following pages discuss the management of these situations in outline only. Most patients will be managed in specialist centres with established protocols for investigation and treatment of possible infection, drawn up in the light of detailed knowledge of local antibiotic sensitivity rates and immunosuppressive practice, which should be consulted whenever possible. HIV and AIDS are discussed elsewhere in this manual.

Patients with impaired immunity are at risk from a wide range of opportunist organisms, but, in general, the clinical situation and the nature of the immunological defect predict a reasonably reliable short list of likely pathogens. Accurate diagnosis depends critically on obtaining specimens for culture and maintaining close liaison with the microbiology laboratory.

Neutropenia

Neutropenia occurs in patients with haematological malignancy, HIV infection or bone marrow infiltration by malignant disease, but it is most frequently a result of cytotoxic chemotherapy. Risk of infection is inversely related to absolute neutrophil count. Below 0.1×10^9 cells/l, infection is very common; above 1×10^9 cells/l, there is little added risk of infection and patients should be managed as for normal patients with severe infection (➤160). A rapid fall in cell numbers is associated with a higher risk of infection. Neutropenic patients are commonly infected with their own normal flora ('endogenous' or 'autoinfection') and many centres take precautions to reduce exposure to new colonising bacteria (e.g. microbiologically clean food). Some centres nurse patients in HEPA-filtered air (reduces Aspergillus exposure) and a few use full protective isolation precautions (➤6).

Clinical features: Common sites for focal infection include iv lines, the oral cavity, lungs, skin, sinuses, perineal region and urinary tract. Any of these may be accompanied by bacteraemia or this may result 'primarily' by direct translocation of bacteria (commonly aerobic Gram-negative rods) across the barriers between the gastrointestinal tract and the bloodstream. Colonisation and translocation is reduced by preservation of the patient's normal anaerobic and Gram-positive gut flora ('colonisation resistance'). Classical signs of infection such as purulent sputum and CXR changes may be absent. Patients may present with the features of septic shock (➤158). **Neutropenic enterocolitis** (typhlitis) is a serious complication of neutropenia in which the bowel (usually the caecum) becomes ulcerated, oedematous and necrotic. It is associated with Clostridium septicum, which may be grown from blood cultures, and Pseudomonas aeruginosa. Presenting with fever, shock and abdominal pain, usually in the right iliac fossa, it usually requires surgical resection. Pseudomonas aeruginosa bacteraemia is associated with **ecthyma gangrenosum**, which develops as dark red or purple cutaneous macules, which may ulcerate to leave a central ulcer surrounded by an erythematous margin. This was previously considered pathognomonic, but can occur with other Gram-negative bacteraemias.

Table 41 Pathogens common in neutropenic patients

	Common	Less common
Gram-positive organisms	Staphylococcus aureus, Staphylococcus epidermidis, 'viridans' group streptococci	Corynebacterium jeikeum, Bacillus spp., Clostridium spp.
Gram-negative organisms	Escherichia coli, Klebsiella spp., Pseudomonas aeruginosa	Serratia spp., Enterobacter spp., Acinetobacter spp., Bacteroides spp., Capnocytophaga spp.
Viruses	Herpes simplex	Varicella-zoster
Fungi	Aspergillus spp., Candida spp.	Fusarium spp., Trichosporon spp., Torulopsis glabrata

Patients undergoing cycles of chemo-therapy (e.g. for chronic leukaemia) tend to suffer repeated episodes of infection, with each episode involving progressively more antibiotic-resistant pathogens as their normal flora is modified by antibiotic exposure.

Microbiological investigations: Cultures from all available sites (blood via peripheral vein and central line, urine, any focal site) should be taken before starting or altering therapy.

Antibiotic management: The incidence of Gram-negative bacteraemia is reduced by giving prophylactic antibiotics, such as ciprofloxacin or co-trimoxazole, and this is widespread practice. Patients with long-standing iv access (e.g. Hickman catheter) are most commonly infected with *Staphylococcus epidermidis*. Many different regimens to treat sepsis in the neutropenic patient are used in different units and such regimens allow for planned progres-sion of therapy when initial choices fail ☞. Systemic antibiotics are normally begun if the patient's temperature is > 38°C on two occa-sions. A reasonable first-line therapy would be azlocillin **plus** gentamicin, **or** ceftazidime alone. Some centres include vancomycin from the start; others add it if there is no response at 48 h. Metronidazole should be added if there is evidence of perianal sepsis. Patients who fail to respond after 5 days of anti-bacterials and who have no documented bac-terial infection should be started empirically on amphotericin B. Figure 4 outlines the prin-ciples underlying protocols for the manage-ment of neutropenic sepsis. Most centres con-tinue antibiotics for documented bacterial in-fections for 10 days (Gram-positive) or 14 days (Gram-negative), and discontinue agents which are inactive against the isolated organ-isms. Culture-negative cases are normally treated for 5 days after becoming afebrile. Some centres continue all antibiotics until the patient is no longer neutropenic.

Infections associated with solid organ transplantation

Patients receiving organ transplants require con-tinuous immunosuppression and are therefore at risk of infection, which remains a leading cause of death at all times after transplantation. All centres therefore have detailed protocols for prophylaxis and management of infections, which should be consulted. Particular infections are likely to occur at predictable times after transplantation and it is possible to construct a timetable which may direct investigation and presumptive therapy (Table 42). Diagnosis is made more difficult by several features unique to this clinical situation:

• Clinical features may be modified by immunosuppressive therapy.

• Graft rejection may mimic infection, causing fever, myalgia, arthralgia and leucocytosis.

• Similar symptoms may occur as adverse ef-fects of immunosuppressive medication, particu-larly antilymphocyte globulin.

• Transplant recipients are usually predisposed to local infection associated with their original

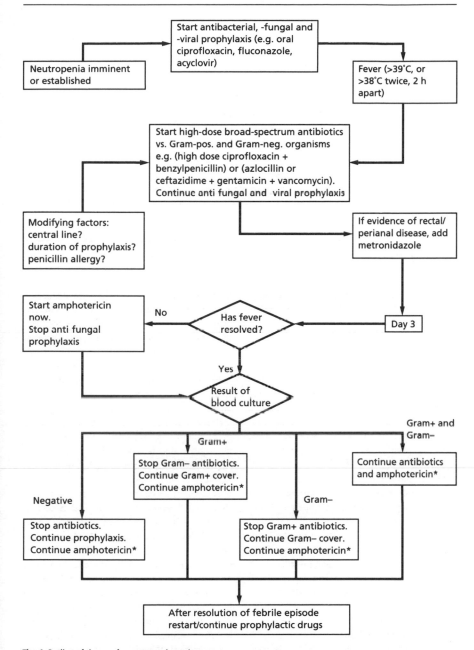

Fig. 4 Outline of therapy for neutropenic sepsis.

*Protocols for duration of amphotericin vary–it is usually continued until neutropenia has resolved. ☎ Close liaison with the microbiology laboratory is essential at every stage. Modification of therapy is often required in the light of antibiotic sensitivity of organisms isolated from blood or surveillance stool cultures.

Table 42 Common infections in solid organ transplant recipients

Time after transplantation	Most common infections
First month	Nosocomial infections: wound infection (➤89), pneumonia (➤22), iv catheter infection Reactivation of pre-existing infection, e.g. tuberculosis (➤29), strongyloidiasis (➤278)
1–6 months	Viral infections, especially CMV, but also hepatitis C (➤52), EBV (➤243) Opportunist infections: *Pneumocystis carinii* (➤119), *Legionella pneumophila* (➤24), aspergillosis, *Listeria monocytogenes*
>6 months	Progressive chronic viral infection, e.g. CMV chorioretinitis, hepatitis B- or hepatitis C-related chronic active hepatitis Opportunist infections: *Pneumocystis carinii* (➤119), *Cryptococcus neoformans* (➤125), *Listeria monocytogenes* (➤178), *Nocardia asteroides* (➤182) (particularly if immunosuppression has been increased to treat rejection) Community-acquired infections: e.g. influenza (➤247), pneumococcal pneumonia (➤22)

Risks of some of these infections may be reduced (for example, by vaccination pre-splenectomy, treatment of strongyloidiasis and resection of polycystic kidneys.

failed organs (e.g. polycystic kidneys remaining *in situ*; *Pseudomonas cepacia* and *Aspergillus* spp. in heart–lung recipients with cystic fibrosis).

CMV IN TRANSPLANT RECIPIENTS
CMV infection is one of the most important infections in solid organ recipients. The risk of clinical disease is highest when infection is acquired by a seronegative recipient from a seropositive donor, although reactivation of infection also occurs in seropositive recipients. Acyclovir prophylaxis reduces the incidence of clinical disease.

Clinical features: During the first 6 months, fever, pneumonia, hepatitis, gastrointestinal ulceration, leucopenia, thrombocytopenia. Encephalitis, transverse myelitis and cutaneous vasculitis occur rarely. After 6 months, progressive chorioretinitis is more common. CMV infection predisposes to superinfection with other opportunist agents and is associated with graft dysfunction and rejection.

Infections associated with bone marrow transplantation

Bone marrow transplantation (BMT) is used to treat haematological malignancy and disorders of haemopoiesis such as aplastic anaemia.

After ablation of their own marrow, patients experience an **initial period (~21 days)** of pro-

found neutropenia, associated with disruption of anatomical barriers by mucositis of the oropharyngeal and gastrointestinal mucosa and the use of indwelling venous catheters. Bacterial and fungal infections are common during this period and should be managed as in neutropenic patients (➤134). Reactivation of herpes simplex virus infection, sometimes with severe cutaneous ulceration, occurs and acyclovir prophylaxis is widely used to reduce this risk. If there is graft failure or rejection, this period of neutropenia may be extended.

After successful engraftment, **between 21 and 100 days,** the major hazard is acute graft-versus-host disease (GVHD), which causes rash, diarrhoea and hepatic dysfunction and is due to donor T cells reacting against host tissue antigens. Differential diagnosis of GVHD and infection can be very difficult. In the absence of GVHD, opportunist infections due to viruses and protozoa may still occur. **Interstitial pneumonia** occurs in ~30% of BMT recipients and has a high mortality. CMV is found in ~50% of cases. *Pneumocystis carinii* is largely prevented by co-trimoxazole prophylaxis. Aspergillosis, adenovirus, HSV and chlamydia are less common causes. Broad-spectrum antibiotics as recommended for neutropenic patients (➤134) should be commenced, and investigations, when possible including bronchoscopy and bronchoalveolar lavage, performed as soon as possible. CMV pneumonia sometimes responds to ganciclovir given with CMV-hyperimmune globulin (➤243).

Infections occuring **after 100 days** affect patients on long-term immunosuppression for chronic GVHD. Bacterial infections, particularly due to *Streptococcus pneumoniae*, *Haemophilus influenzae*, *Neisseria meningitidis*, *Staphylococcus aureus* and *Staphylococcus epidermidis*, are common. Fungal, viral and protozoal opportunist infections occur less frequently. Empirical therapy is the same as in neutropenic patients (➤134) if the neutrophil count is $< 1 \times 10^9$ cells/l, and as for severe infection in normal patients (➤160) if it is $\geq 1 \times 10^9$ cells/l.

14: Travel Medicine

Pre-travel advice

Advice to travellers is based on the countries they intend to visit, current health status (e.g. pregnancy, immunocompromised), type of journey (urban vs. rural), duration of stay and previous medical history (e.g. splenectomy).

Avoiding infection

Antimalarial prophylaxis and vaccinations give only partial protection. Travellers should also be encouraged to take measures to avoid infection.

Avoiding insect-borne infections
• Sleep in a properly screened room and use a knock-down insecticide spray before retiring, or use a mosquito-net which has been impregnated with permethrin.
• Wear long sleeves and trousers after sunset.
• Use an insect repellent containing DEET (*N,N*-diethylmetatoluamide). Preparations containing > 50% DEET (20% in children) should be avoided as neurological toxicity may result from absorption.
• African trypanosomiasis (➤272) is spread by tsetse flies in Africa between 15°N and 20°S. It is very rare in travellers. Those most at risk are travellers to remote rural areas (safari, animal workers). Tsetse flies bite during the day and are attracted to large moving objects and strong dark colours. Wrist- and ankle-length clothing and insect repellent should be worn. Car windows should be kept closed and flies killed with insecticide spray.
• Loiasis (➤284) can be prevented in endemic areas (Cameroon, Central African Republic, Congo, Equatorial Guinea, Gabon, Ghana, Nigeria and Zaïre) by taking diethylcarbamazine 300 mg weekly. This should **not** be prescribed if acute infection is suspected.

Avoiding food- and water-borne infections
• Choose foods which have been freshly prepared and thoroughly cooked with a mini-mum of handling.
• Avoid shellfish, and meat that may be partly cooked.
• Avoid salads, fruit that cannot be peeled, ice and ice-cream.
• Drinking water should be boiled or chemically sterilised. Purification tablets are commercially available and effective unless water is very heavily contaminated. Portable water filters are available but expensive.

Avoiding schistosomiasis
• Schistosomiasis (➤285) is acquired by bathing in fresh water containing snails. Risk is highest in Nile Valley, Lake Victoria, Tigris and Euphrates river systems and in artificial lakes in Africa (e.g. Lake Kariba, Lake Volta). Minimise risk by bathing for short periods in flowing rather than still water, avoiding the early and late parts of the day and rubbing down vigorously with a towel after swimming.

Avoiding blood-borne and sexually transmitted infection
• In parts of the developing world HIV seroprevalence is ~70% in prostitutes. Condoms reduce but do not abolish risk.
• Procedures involving surgery, injections or blood transfusion may transmit HIV or HBV. Travellers should carry an emergency medical pack containing suture materials, needles and syringes, available from pharmacies and travel clinics.

Emergency treatment

Malaria: Standby treatment for malaria (➤272) should be carried by travellers to particularly remote areas.

Traveller's diarrhoea: Travellers are likely to develop diarrhoea (➤48). Fluid and electrolyte replacement is crucial. Bottled drinks, tea or oral rehydration solution (commercial or home-made ➤45) may be used. Fasting is unnecessary, but milk is best avoided.

Table 43 Antimalarial prophylaxis

Area	Regimen
North Africa and Middle East	
Abu Dhabi, Algeria, Egypt (tourist areas), Libya, Morocco, Tunisia, Turkey (most tourist areas)	None*
Azerbaijan (S border), Egypt (El Faiyum only, Jun.–Oct.), Iraq (rural, N, May–Nov.), Syria (N border, May–Oct), Turkey (plain around Adona, Side, SE Anatolia, Mar.–Nov.), Tajikistan (S border)	Cq
Afghanistan (< 2000 m, May–Nov.), Iran (Mar.–Nov.), Oman, Saudi Arabia (except N, E and central provinces, Asir plateau, and western border cities, where very little risk), United Arab Emirates (N rural only), Yemen	CqP
Indian subcontinent	
Bangladesh (except E, no risk in Dhaka), Bhutan (S districts only), India, Nepal (< 1300 m, no risk in Kathmandu), Pakistan (< 2000 m), Sri Lanka (no risk in, and just S of, Colombo)	CqP
Bangladesh (E, including Chittagong Hill tracts)	Mf
Sub-Saharan Africa	
Botswana (N, Nov.–Jun.), Mauritania (S, all year; N, Jul.–Oct.), Namibia (N, Nov.–Jun.), S Africa (NE, low altitude areas of N and E Transvaal, E Natal down to 100 km N of Durban), Zimbabwe (< 1200 m, Nov.–Jun.; Zambezi valley, all year, Mf)	CqP
All other countries of sub-Saharan Africa	Mf
Mauritius (except rural areas where Cq), Cape Verde	None*
Oceania	
Papua New Guinea (< 1800 m), Solomon Islands, Vanuatu	Mf **or** CqMal
Latin America	
Argentina (NW only), Belize (rural except Belize district), Costa Rica (rural, < 500 m), Dominican Republic, El Salvador, Guatemala (< 1500 m), Haiti, Honduras, Mexico (rural), Nicaragua, Panama (W. of canal), Paraguay (rural, Oct.–May).	Cq
Bolivia (rural, < 2500 m; Amazon basin, Mf), Ecuador (< 1500 m), Panama (E of canal), Peru (rural, < 1500 m), Venezuela (rural except coast and Caracas which are malaria free; Amazon basin, Mf)	CqP
Brazil ('legal Amazon' area, Amazon basin, Mato Grosso, and Maranhão; elsewhere very low risk), Colombia (< 800 m), French Guiana, Guyana, Surinam (except Paramirabo and coast), Amazon basin of Bolivia and Venezuela.	Mf
South East Asia	
Bali, Brunei, China (main tourist areas), Hong Kong, Malaysia (except Sabah, Mf; deep forests CqP), Sarawak, Singapore, Thailand (Bangkok and main tourist areas).	None*
Indonesia (other than Bali and cities where low risk; Irian Jaya, Mf), Philippines (rural < 600 m; no risk in Cebu, Leyte, Bohol, Catanduanes), deep forests of Malaysia and Sarawak	CqP
Cambodia (no risk in Phnom Penh; W provinces D), China (Yunnan and Hainan; other remote rural areas, Cq), Irian Jaya, Laos (no risk in Vientiane), Myanmar (Burma), Sabah, Thailand (backpacking in rural areas), Vietnam (no risk in cities or delta area)	Mf
Cambodia (W provinces), Thailand (border areas with Cambodia and Myanmar, but not for routine backpackers)	D

*Risk very low – consider malaria in the event of fever.
See Table 44 for details and key

Table 44 Details of antimalarial regimens

Abbreviation	Preferred regimen	Alternative regimen
Cq	Chloroquine 300 mg (of base) weekly	Proguanil 200 mg daily
CqP	Chloroquine **and** proguanil (doses as above)	Mf
Mf	Mefloquine 250 mg weekly	CqP (except Oceania, where CqMal is best alternative to Mf)
D	Doxycycline 100 mg daily	
CqMal	Chloroquine as above plus Maloprim 1 tablet weekly	

Antidiarrhoeal agents reduce frequency of diarrhoea but do not stop fluid loss into the gut. They should not be given if there is fever or blood in stools, in pregnancy or in children under 12 years. Loperamide is the agent of choice (4 mg initially, thereafter 2 mg after each loose stool, up to 16 mg in 24 h).

Antibiotic treatment is indicated if diarrhoea is severe or prolonged, or is accompanied by fever, prostration or blood in stools. If diarrhoea fails to respond to ciprofloxacin, 500 mg 12-hly for 3 days, it is likely to be protozoal in origin, and metronidazole, 400 mg 8-hly for 5 days should be given. If competent health care is not available, it is sensible for travellers to carry a supply of loperamide, ciprofloxacin and metronidazole, with instructions on their use. Medical advice should be sought as soon as possible.

Antimalarial prophylaxis

Antimalarial prophylaxis (Tables 43 & 44) must be combined with measures to avoid mosquito bites, which are listed above. Recommendations for drug use change with the emergence of new areas of antimalarial resistance; up-to-date information may be obtained from the London School of Tropical Medicine and Hygiene (➤145). For details of individual drugs ➤271. Start 1 week before departure and continue for 4 weeks after return. Remember no prophylaxis is 100% effective. Patients should seek medical advice in the event of fever up to 1 year after return even if they complied fully with prophylaxis.

Antimalarial prophylaxis in pregnancy

Malaria is more severe in pregnancy (➤270) and prophylaxis is essential. Chloroquine and proguanil are safe, but mefloquine is contraindicated in the first trimester. Fansidar is relatively contraindicated. **The best advice to a pregnant woman is not to travel to areas of chloroquine resistance.** If proguanil is given, folate supplements should also be given. Maloprim is contraindicated in the first trimester. If used later in pregnancy, give folate supplements.

Antimalarial prophylaxis for children

Chloroquine, proguanil and mefloquine are used in children subject to the following dosage reductions and age restrictions (Table 45).

Splenectomised travellers (➤132)

Travellers with anatomical or functional asplenia are at high risk of severe or fatal malaria, and optimum antimalarial prophylaxis and bite avoidance are essential. For advice on antibiotic prophylaxis for this group, ➤133. They should receive pneumococcal (➤337), meningococcal (➤142) and Hib vaccination. They are also at risk of babesiosis (➤263) and fulminant septicaemia due to *Capnocytophaga canimorsus* (➤90, 208) after dog bites.

Table 45 Antimalarial prophylaxis in children

		Fraction of adult dose		Mefloquine weekly dose	
Age	Weight (kg)	Chloroquine/ proguanil	Maloprim*	Weight (kg)	Mefloquine tablets (mg)
0–5 wks		$1/_8$	NR		
6–52 wks		$1/_4$	NR		
1–5 yrs	10–19	$1/_2$	$1/_4$	<15	NR
				15–19	$1/_4$ (62.5)
6–11 yrs	20–39	$3/_4$	$1/_2$	20–30	$1/_2$ (125)
				31–45	$3/_4$ (187.5)
≥12 yrs	≥40	Adult dose	Adult dose	>45	Adult dose

NR = not recommended. * Give with folic acid 5 mg 24-hly po.

Immunisation for foreign travel

Polio, tetanus and diphtheria immunisation status should be updated, and a full course or booster given, regardless of destination (➤337). Oral polio vaccine (OPV) may be given simultaneously with other live virus vaccines; ideally they should be separated by at least 3 weeks (➤144).

Travellers to areas of poor hygiene require immunisation against typhoid and hepatitis A.

Typhoid (➤191)

Vaccine, dosage and administration: Three preparations are available. All give ~70% protection (Table 46).

Indications: See Table 56 (➤146) for countries where vaccination is recommended. Also indicated for laboratory workers who may handle specimens containing *S. typhi*.

Contraindications and cautions: All three vaccines are contraindicated in acute febrile illness, after previous severe reaction to the same vaccine or in pregnancy, unless there is a very clear indication. **Whole-cell vaccine** produces local and systemic reactions, the severity of which may be reduced by giving second and subsequent injections as 0.1 ml intradermally. **Oral Ty21a vaccine** is contraindicated in patients on sulphonamides or other antibiotics. If mefloquine is being taken, then these two medications should be separated by at least 12 h. It is contraindicated in immunosuppressed patients and should not be given simultaneously with OPV.

Table 46 Typhoid vaccines

Vaccine (nature)	Primary course	Booster
Whole-cell vaccine (killed *S. typhi*)*	Two doses of 0.5 ml im or deep sc (child 0.25 ml) 4–6 weeks apart	One dose after 3 years
Vi polysaccharide vaccine (purified polysaccharide)**	Single 0.5 ml dose im or deep sc	One dose after 3 years
Oral Ty21a vaccine (live attenuated *S. typhi*)***	One capsule alternate days for three doses	Three-dose course annually

*Not for children under 1 year. **Not for children under 18 months. ***Not for children under 6 years.

The oral vaccine is very sensitive to heat and must be refrigerated and taken with cool liquid only.

Hepatitis A (➤49)

Vaccine, dosage and administration: Passive immunisation with normal human immunoglobulin has been used to protect against HAV. Active vaccination is now available and is preferable to immunoglobulin for patients travelling frequently to endemic areas (Tables 47 & 48).

Immunoglobulin may be given at the same time as HAV vaccine if immediate protection is required.

Indications: See Table 56 (➤146) for countries where vaccination is recommended.

Contraindications and cautions: HAV vaccine is contraindicated in severe febrile illness. It should only be given in pregnancy if there is a high risk of infection. **Normal immunoglobulin** may interfere with the response to live virus vaccines, which should be given at least 3 weeks before or 3 months after an injection of immunoglobulin. This does not apply to yellow fever, since normal immunoglobulin is unlikely to contain antibodies against this virus. For travellers presenting late with insufficient time, this recommended interval may have to be ignored. Active hepatitis A vaccination is an alternative.

Table 47 Hepatitis A vaccine

Vaccine (nature)	Primary course	Booster
Hepatitis A vaccine (killed virus)	Two doses of 1 ml im* 2–4 weeks apart	One dose at 6–12 months

*In deltoid region. Not licensed for children under 16 years.

Table 48 Normal human immunoglobulin

	2 months' protection	3–5 months' protection
Age < 10 years	125 mg	250 mg
Age > 10 years	250 mg	500 mg

Table 49 Yellow fever vaccine

Vaccine (nature)	Primary course	Booster
Live attenuated virus	Single dose 0.5 ml sc	Single dose after 10 years

Yellow fever (➤253)

Vaccine, dosage and administration: Vaccination is only given at designated centres. The International Certificate of Vaccination is valid from 10 days after immunisation for 10 years (Table 49).

Indications: Yellow fever vaccination is a legal requirement for entry to some countries, either for all travellers or for those arriving from endemic areas. Countries currently reported by WHO (June 1994) to have active infection are Angola, Bolivia, Brazil, Cameroon, Colombia, Ecuador, Gambia, Chana, Guinea, Mali, Kenya, Nigeria, Peru, Sudan, Zaïre, but vaccination is required by many more countries. Note that the Indian government regards Zambia as an infected area for the purposes of vaccination requirements. See Table 56 (➤146) for countries where vaccination is required.

Contraindications and cautions: Vaccine is well tolerated with few adverse effects; encephalitis (reversible) occurs rarely and has been reported only in children. Risk is highest for very young children and for this reason vaccination is contraindicated in pregnancy and under 9 months of age unless travel to a high-risk area is unavoidable. Absolutely contraindicated under age 4 months. Vaccine is contraindicated in concurrent febrile illness, immunosuppressed patients, including those on high-dose steroids or chemotherapy or with haematological malignancy or HIV. Contraindicated in patients allergic to eggs, neomycin or polymyxin. Avoid simultaneous administration with cholera vaccine.

Meningococcal vaccine (➤74, 205)

Vaccine, dosage and administration: Vaccine is only available against groups A and C. Most cases occurring in UK are group B, against

Table 50 Meningococcal vaccine

Vaccine (nature)	Primary course	Booster
Meningococcal vaccine (purified polysaccharide)	Single dose 0.5 ml im or deep sc (adults and children >2 months)	Single dose after 2 years (~1 year in young children)

Table 51 Japanese encephalitis vaccine

Vaccine (nature)	Primary course	Booster
Formalin-inactivated virus	Three doses of 1ml sc (child < 3 years, 0.5ml) at 2-week intervals	One dose at 6–18 months; thereafter at 4-year intervals

which the vaccine confers no protection (Table 50).

Indications: Epidemic meningtis occurs in sub-Saharan Africa, particularly during the dry months (Dec.–Feb.) in the 'meningitis belt', which extends between 15°N and 5°N, except in Uganda and Kenya where it reaches the equator. Vaccination is also indicated for travel to New Delhi, Bhutan and Nepal, and is a legal requirement for entry to Saudi Arabia for pilgrims attending the haj. Risk is highest for backpackers and 'rough' travellers, and vaccination should be considered for all such travellers to the developing world. See Table 56 (➤146) for countries where vaccination is recommended. Also indicated in UK for contacts of group A and C cases (in addition to chemoprophylaxis ➤77), in control of local outbreaks and for patients post-splenectomy (➤132) or with complement deficiency (➤131).

Contraindications and cautions: Well tolerated. Contraindicated during febrile illness or if there has been a previous severe reaction to same vaccine. Pregnancy is a relative countraindication.

Japanese encephalitis (➤79, 253)

Vaccine, dosage and administration: An unlicensed vaccine is available for named-patient use only. Protection is ~95%, but does not develop until about 6 weeks after starting immunisation (Table 51). Further information and vaccine supplies from Cambridge Selfcare Diagnostics Ltd (0191 261 5950).

Indications: Rural travel to infected areas for >1 month. Risk is highest during May–June, but is present all year in some areas. See Table 56 (➤146) for countries where vaccination is recommended.

Contraindications and cautions: Curent febrile illness or other infection, heart, kidney or liver disease, diabetes or other hormonal dysfunction, malnutrition, malignancy, hypersensitivity to mouse brain products, pregnancy, history of anaphylaxis or urticaria.

Rabies (➤257)

Vaccine, dosage and administration: Human diploid cell vaccine is expensive but safe (Table 52). For details of other indications for vaccination and post-exposure management ➤258.

Indications: Travellers to enzootic areas who may be unable to obtain post-exposure vaccination or who are particularly likely to be bitten (animal workers, cyclists).

Contraindications and cautions: Local and systemic reactions occur. Anaphylaxis and Guillain–Barré syndrome have been reported.

Table 52 Rabies vaccine

Vaccine (nature)	Pre-exposure prophylaxis	Booster
Human diploid cell vaccine (killed virus)	Three doses of 1 ml im or deep sc* on days 0, 7 and 28	One dose at 2–3-year intervals

* In deltoid region.

Tick-borne encephalitis (TBE) (➤79, 253)

Vaccine, dosage and administration: An unlicensed vaccine is available for named-patient use only. Gives protection against all TBE strains occurring in Europe and Asia

Table 53 Tick-borne encephalitis vaccine

Vaccine (nature)	Primary course	Booster
Killed virus	Three doses of 0.5 ml im, at day 0, 4–12 weeks and 9–12 months	Single dose at 3-year intervals

(Table 53). Further information and vaccine supplies from Immuno Ltd (01732 458101).

Indications: Walkers and campers in warm, deciduously forested parts of Europe and Scandinavia, especially where there is heavy undergrowth and during late spring and summer, are most at risk. TBE occurs in foci throughout the eastern half of Europe, and across Russia, but accurate surveillance data are not available for many countries. Areas of established risk include SE coastal Sweden, around Stockholm and the island of Gotland, S Finland around Turku and the Aland Islands, throughout Poland, Germany, the Czech and Slovak Republics, Switzerland, Austria, Hungary, Slovenia, Croatia and Albania. Very rarely reported from Tuscany, central Italy. Specific immunoglobulin is available from the same supplier for post-exposure prophylaxis.

Contraindications and cautions: Mild local and systemic reactions occur. Contraindicated in acute febrile illness and in allergy to thiomersal or eggs.

Tuberculosis (➤29)
Visitors to Asia, Africa, C and S America who have not had BCG and who are tuberculin-negative should be offered BCG. Contraindicated in immunosuppressed (including HIV), haematological malignancy, pregnancy and intercurrent fever.

Cholera (➤195)
Cholera vaccine gives ~50% protection which lasts 3–6 months, and is no longer recommended for protection of individuals. It plays no part in the control of epidemics. Border officials may rarely ask for evidence of immunisation from travellers arriving from infected areas. Overland travellers should be vaccinated for the purposes of certification. A single dose (0.5 ml im) is sufficient for this purpose.

Plague (➤211)
Plague vaccine is available and may be considered for refugee and rural health workers in enzootic areas. Areas reporting plague to WHO (1994) are indicated on Table 56 (➤146).

Hepatitis B (➤49)
Hepatitis B vaccination is indicated for health care workers and individuals who expect to become resident in endemic areas. For doses ➤50.

Table 54 Timing of vaccinations

Vaccine	May be administered simultaneously	Interval recommended
Inactivated vaccines (except cholera)	All other inactivated vaccines, all live vaccines	
Yellow fever	OPV, hepatitis B	Cholera–3 weeks
Cholera	All inactivated vaccines, all live vaccines except yellow fever	Yellow fever–3 weeks
OPV	All live vaccines, immunoglobulin	Oral typhoid–3 weeks
Oral typhoid (Ty21a)	Yellow fever, immunoglobulin	OPV–3 weeks
MMR	OPV	Other live vaccines–4 weeks
BCG	OPV, immunoglobulin	Other live vaccines–4 weeks
Immunoglobulin	Yellow fever, OPV, all inactivated vaccines	MMR–give 3 weeks before or 3 months after immunoglobulin

Timing of vaccinations

If travellers present late, the spacings in Table 54 should be ignored, but antibody responses may be blunted and consideration should be given to repeating vaccination on return or giving early boosters. A single dose of most vaccines will give some protection. Most travellers can be vaccinated at two visits 4 weeks apart (Table 55).

Table 55 Accelerated vaccination schedule

First visit	Second visit
Yellow fever	Typhoid–dose 2
Typhoid–dose 1	Polio (OPV) booster
Tetanus booster	Meningitis
Hepatitis A vaccine–dose 1	Hepatitis A vaccine–dose 2 or immunogloblin

Sources of information for doctors advising travellers

Publications

• *World Health Organization Weekly Epidemiological Record.*
• *Health Advice for Travellers*, leaflet T4, published by the Department of Health (0800 555777).
• *British National Formulary.*
• *Immunisation against Infectious Disease*, 1992 edition, published by the Department of Health and available from HMSO Publications Centre, PO Box 276, London SW8 5DT (0171-873 9090).

Telephone numbers

• Communicable Disease Surveillance Centre Travel Unit, 61 Conlindale Avenue, London NW9 5EQ (0181 200 6868).
• Scottish Home and Health Department, St Andrew's House, Edinburgh EH1 3DE (0131 556 8400).
• Welsh Office, Cathays Park, Cardiff CF1 3NQ (01222 825111).
• Department of Health and Social Services, Dundonald House, Upper Newtownards Road, Belfast BT4 3FS (01232 63939).

Telephone advice on malaria

• Malaria Reference Lab	0171 636 8636 (prophylaxis only)
• London	0171 387 4411 (treatment)
	0171 637 9899 (travel prophylaxis)
• Birmingham	0121 766 6611
• Glasgow	0141 946 7120
• Liverpool	0151 708 9393
• Oxford	01865 225214
• Recorded advice for travellers	0891 600350

Health problems in returning travellers

Ten per cent of travellers to developing countries suffer from severe, self-limiting diarrhoea, ~1% catch *Giardia lamblia* or *Entamoeba histolytica*, and ~0.1% develop malaria on their return. Other tropical protozoal and helminth infections are extremely rare. The following notes are intended as guidance for some of the commoner problems in the returning traveller.

Fever in the returning traveller

Malaria (treatment ➤268) is common; *Plasmodium falciparum* infection is particularly likely in travellers from Africa within a few days of return. In non-immune patients levels of parasitaemia are often low and one negative film is not conclusive. The typical pattern of cyclical fever is often absent early in disease. (In general, patterns of fever are neither reliable nor useful aids to diagnosis.)

The following **investigations** are recommended in all patients in whom the diagnosis is not clear: three malaria films, full blood count, liver function tests, CXR, three blood cultures, MSU, stools for culture, cysts and parasites, serology for viral infections and rickettsia, USS or CT liver scan for liver abscess.

Apart from positive malarial films or bacterial cultures, the most useful pieces of information are the peripheral white cell count (WBC) and a detailed travel history, since many rickettsial and viral infections have a short and relatively reliable incubation period.

Table 56 Travel guidelines (key, footnotes and sources ➤150)

Country	Hep A, typhoid	Malaria	Yellow fever	Other	Plague/cholera
Afghanistan	R	CqP[1]	3		C
Albania	R		3	T	
Algeria	R	None[2]	3		
Angola	R	Mf	3, Y		C
Anguilla	R				
Antigua/Barbuda	R		3		
Argentina	R	Cq[1]			C
Armenia	R				
Australia			3		
Austria				T	
Azerbaijan	R	Cq[1]			
Bahamas	R		3		
Bahrain	R		3		
Bali	R	None[2]	3	J	
Bangladesh	R	Mf[1] or CqP[1]	3	J	
Barbados	R		3		
Belarus	R				
Belize	R	Cq[1]	3		C
Benin	R	Mf	1	M	C
Bermuda					
Bhutan	R	CqP[1]	3	J, M	C
Bolivia	R	CqP[1] or Mf[1]	3, R, Y		C, P
Bosnia-Herzegovina	R				
Botswana	R	CqP[1]			
Brazil	R	Mf[1]	3, R, Y		C, P
Brunei	R		3	J	
Bulgaria	R				
Burkina Faso	R	Mf	1		C
Burma (Myanmar)	R	Mf	3	J	C
Burundi	R	Mf	3, R		C
Cambodia	R	Mf[1] or D[1]	3	J	C
Cameroon	R	Mf	1, Y	M	C
Canada					
Cape Verde	R	None[2]	3		
Cayman Islands	R				
Central African Rep.	R	Mf	1	M	
Chad	R	Mf	1	M	C
Chile	R				C
China	R	Mf[1] or Cq[1]	3	J	C
Colombia	R	Mf[1]	R, Y		C
Comoros	R	Mf			
Congo	R	Mf	1		
Cook Islands	R				
Costa Rica	R	Cq[1]			C
Croatia	R			T	
Cuba	R				
Cyprus					

continued on p. 147

Table 56 contd

Country	Hep A, typhoid	Malaria	Yellow fever	Other	Plague/ cholera
Czech/Slovak Reps	R			T	
Djibouti	R	Mf	3		C
Dominica	R		3		
Dominican Republic	R	Cq			
Ecuador	R	CqP[1]	3, R, Y		C
Egypt	R	Cq[1]	3		
El Salvador	R	Cq	3		C
Equatorial Guinea	R	Mf	3, R		
Eritrea	R	Mf	3, R	M	
Estonia					
Ethiopia	R	Mf	3, R	M	
Falkland Islands					
Fiji	R		3		
Finland				T	
Gabon	R	Mf	1		
The Gambia	R	Mf	3, R, Y	M	
Georgia	R				
Germany				T	
Ghana	R	Mf	1, Y		C
Greece			3		
Greenland					
Grenada	R		3		
Guam	R			J	
Guatemala	R	Cq[1]	3		C
Guiana, French	R	Mf	1		C
Guinea	R	Mf	3, R, Y		C
Guinea-Bissau	R	Mf	3, R		
Guyana	R	Mf	3, R		C
Haiti	R	Cq	3		
Honduras	R	Cq	3		C
Hong Kong	R	None[2]		J	
Hungary				T	
Iceland					
India	R	CqP	3	J, M	C, P
Indonesia	R	Mf[1] or CqP[1]	3	J	C
Iran	R	CqP[1]	3		C
Iraq	R	Cq[1]	3		C
Israel	R				
Ivory Coast	R	Mf	1	M	C
Jamaica	R		3		
Japan	R			J	
Jordan	R		3		
Kampuchea	R	Mf[1] or D[1]	3	J	C
Kazakhstan	R				
Kenya	R	Mf	3, Y	M	C
Kirgizstan	R				
Kiribati	R		3		

continued on p. 148

Table 56 contd

Country	Hep A, typhoid	Malaria	Yellow fever	Other	Plague/ cholera
Korea (N and S)	R			J	
Kuwait	R				
Laos	R	Mf[1]	3	J	C
Latvia					
Lebanon	R		3		
Lesotho	R		3		
Liberia	R	Mf	1	M	C
Libya	R	None[2]	3		
Lithuania					
Macedonia	R				
Madagascar	R	Mf	3		P
Madeira			3		
Malawi	R	Mf	3		C
Malaysia	R	Mf[1] or CqP[1]	3	J	C
Maldives	R		3		
Mali	R	Mf	1, Y	M	C
Malta			3		
Mauritania	R	CqP[1]	2		C
Mauritius	R	None[2]	3		
Mexico	R	Cq[1]	3		C
Moldova	R				
Monaco					
Mongolia	R				
Montserrat	R		3		
Morocco	R	None[2]			
Mozambique	R	Mf	3		C
Myanmar (Burma)	R	Mf	3	J	C
Namibia	R	CqP[1]	3, R		
Nauru	R		3		
Nepal	R	CqP[1]	3	J, M	C
Netherlands, Antilles	R		3		
New Caledonia	R		3		
New Zealand					
Nicaragua	R	Cq	3		C
Niger	R	Mf	1	M	C
Nigeria	R	Mf	3, R, Y	M	C
Niue	R		3		
Norway					
Oman	R	CqP	3		
Pakistan	R	CqP[1]	3	M	
Panama	R	CqP[1] or Cq[1]	See note[3]		C
Papua New Guinea	R	Mf or CqMal	3		
Paraguay	R	Cq[1]	See note[4]		
Peru	R	CqP[1]	3, R, Y		C, P
Philippines	R	Cqp[1]	3	J	
Pitcairn Islands	R		3		
Poland				T	
Polynesia, French: Tahiti	R		3		

continued on p. 149

Table 56 contd

Country	Hep A, typhoid	Malaria	Yellow fever	Other	Plague/ cholera
Puerto Rico	R				
Qatar	R		3		
Reunion	R		3		
Romania	R				
Russia				J[5]	
Rwanda	R	Mf	1		C
St Helena	R				
St Kitts and Nevis	R		3		
St Lucia	R		3		
St Vincent & Grenadines	R		3		
Samoa	R		3		
São Tomé and Principe	R	Mf	2		C
Saudi Arabia	R	CqP[1]	3	M	
Senegal	R	Mf	1	M	
Seychelles	R				
Sierra Leone	R	Mf	3, R	M	
Singapore	R		3	J	
Slovenia	R			T	
Solomon Islands	R	Mf or CqMal	3		
Somalia	R	Mf	3, R		C
South Africa	R	CqP[1]	3		
Sri Lanka	R	CqP[1]	3	J	C
Sudan	R	Mf	3, R, Y	M	
Surinam	R	Mf[1]	3		C
Swaziland	R	Mf	3		C
Sweden				T	
Switzerland				T	
Syria	R	Cq[1]	3		
Tahiti	R		3		
Taiwan	R		3	J	
Tajikistan	R	Cq[1]			
Tanzania	R	Mf	3		C, P
Thailand	R	Mf[1] or D[1]	3	J	
Togo	R	Mf	1	M	C
Tonga	R		3		
Trinidad and Tobago	R		3		
Tunisia	R	None[2]	3		
Turkey	R	Cq[1]			
Turkmenistan	R				
Turks and Caicos Islands					
Tuvalu	R		3		C
Uganda	R	Mf	3, R	M	C, P
United Arab Emirates	R	CqP[1]			
Ukraine					C
Uruguay	R				
USA					
Uzbekistan	R				
Vanuatu	R	Mf or CqMal			

continued on p. 150

Table 56 contd

Country	Hep A, typhoid	Malaria	Yellow fever	Other	Plague/ cholera
Venezuela	R	CqP[1] or Mf[1]	R		C
Vietnam	R	Mf[1]	3	J	C
Virgin Islands	R				
West Indies	R		3		
West Indies (French)	R		3		
Yemen Arab Rep. (N)	R	CqP	3		
Yemen Arab Rep. (S)	R	CqP	3		
Yugoslavia	R				
Zaïre	R	Mf	1, Y		C, P
Zambia	R	Mf	R		C
Zimbabwe	R	CqP[1] or Mf[1]	3		

R = recommended for personal protection.

See Table 57 for details of malaria prophylaxis.
[1] Depending on area visited and season (➤139).
[2] Risk of malaria very low – consider diagnosis in the event of fever.

Yellow fever: Y = country reporting yellow fever to WHO (June 1994). If a number is indicated, vaccination is an essential entry requirement and a valid certificate is needed. 1 = Immunisation is essential for protection. 2 = Immunisation essential unless arriving from non-infected area and staying for less than 2 weeks. 3 = Immunisation essential if arriving from an infected area where yellow fever is present.
[3] Recommended for all travellers to the province of Darién.
[4] Certificate only required if leaving Paraguay to go to endemic areas.

J = Japanese encephalitis vaccination may be indicated (➤143).
M = Meningitis vaccination may be indicated (➤142).
T = Tick-borne encephalitis vaccination may be indicated (➤143).
[5] Eastern Siberia.

C = country reporting cholera to WHO (1994). Vaccination is not generally indicated (➤144).
P = country reporting plague to WHO (1994). Vaccination is not generally indicated (➤144).

Sources
Health Advice to Travellers, (Leaflet T4) UK Department of Health.
Bradley D. Prophylaxis against malaria for travellers from the United Kingdom. *Br Med J* (1993) 306: 1247–1251.
Bradley D. & Warhurst D. Malaria prophylaxis: guidelines for travellers from Britain. *Br Med J* (1995) 310: 709–714.
Weekly Epidemiological Record, World Health Organisation.

Common presentations (with common diagnoses highlighted in bold type) include those listed in Tables 58–61.

Presentations to recognise:
Severe pneumonia on return from SE Asia: consider melioidosis, due to *Pseudomonas pseudomallei* (➤200). Ceftazidime is the agent of choice.
Cyclical fever 3–6 months after return from malaria-endemic region: relapse of benign malaria: primaquine is required to eradicate hypnozoites (➤268).

Table 57 Details of malaria prophylaxis: for full details and contraindications ➢139–141

Abbreviation	Preferred regimen	Alternative regimen
Cq	Chloroquine 300 mg (of base) weekly	Proguanil 200 mg daily
CqP	Chloroquine **and** proguanil (doses as above)	Mf
Mf	Mefloquine 250 mg weekly	CqP (except Oceania, where CqMal is best alternative to Mf)
D	Doxycycline 100 mg daily	
CqMal	Chloroquine as above plus Maloprim 1 tablet weekly	

Table 58 Acute fever with normal or reduced WBC

Diagnosis	Clues
Malaria (➢268)	Cyclical high fever, response to quinine
Typhoid/paratyphoid (➢191)	Severity of illness, persistent fever, cough
Viral infections (e.g. dengue) (➢254)	Biphasic fever, myalgia, rash
Rickettsia (➢233)	Rash, localised lymphadenopathy, eschar
Acute brucellosis (➢209)	Very rare

Table 59 Acute fever with raised WBC

Diagnosis	Clues
Amoebic liver abscess (➢267)	Liver function often normal, hepatic tenderness often minimal—often diagnosed on USS liver scan
Pyogenic infections (e.g. pneumonia, meningitis, cellulitis)	Localising signs

Table 60 Chronic fever with normal/reduced WBC

Malaria (➢268)
Disseminated tuberculosis (➢29)
Visceral leishmaniasis (➢274)
Brucellosis (➢209)

Table 61 Chronic fever with eosinophilia (➢157)

Schistosomiasis (➢285)
Fascioliasis (➢287)
Visceral larva migrans (➢279)
Filariasis (➢282)

Other causes of significant (>10%) eosinophilia include cat-scratch disease (➢237), *Diphyllobothrium latum* (➢281), trichinosis (➢284), *Taenia* spp. (➢280) and *Echinococcus* spp. (hydatid ➢281).

Diarrhoea in the returning traveller

Certain clinical features allow an educated guess at the cause of diarrhoea.

Diarrhoea of less than 2 weeks' duration

With fever and blood

Shigellosis (➤192), salmonellosis (➤191), *Campylobacter jejuni* (➤196), *Escherichia coli* 0157 (➤188)

With fever, but no blood

Shigellosis, salmonellosis, *Campylobacter jejuni*. Also consider malaria (➤268)

With blood, but no fever

Entamoeba histolytica (➤267). Consider also *Balantidium coli* (➤264), acute schistosomiasis (➤285), *Escherichia coli* 0157 (➤188)

Without blood or fever

Enterotoxigenic and other *Escherichia coli* (➤187), *Staphylococcus aureus* or clostridial food poisoning (➤44), viral diarrhoea (➤258), *Giardia lamblia* (➤266)

Diarrhoea of greater than 2 weeks' duration

Bloody diarrhoea

Entamoeba histolytica, schistosomiasis, carcinoma, inflammatory bowel disease

Steatorrhoea

Giardia lamblia, sprue (➤see below), mesenteric tuberculosis (➤30), other causes of malabsorption unrelated to travel

Wasting and fever

Visceral leishmaniasis (➤274), tuberculous enteritis (➤30)

Diarrhoea and eosinophilia

Schistosomiasis (➤285), strongyloidiasis (➤278), capillariasis (➤279), trichuriasis (➤278)

TROPICAL SPRUE

Malabsorption due to bacterial overgrowth in the small intestine seen in expatriates resident in the tropics.

Epidemiology: Occurs in well-defined areas only, including Indian subcontinent, SE Asia, northern countries of S America, Haiti, Puerto Rico, Cuba and Dominican Republic. Very rare in Africa.

Clinical features: Symptoms develop over months, usually after several years' residence in tropics. Often starts with an attack of acute diarrhoea. Anorexia, weight loss and chronic steatorrhoea. Folate and B_{12} deficiency lead to megaloblastic anaemia. Hypoalbuminaemia may occur. Untreated sprue can persist for decades, even after return to temperate climate.

Investigations: Exclusion of other infections, esp. *Giardia lamblia*. Small-bowel biopsy shows minor degree of villous atrophy and submucosal cellular infiltrate.

Management: Folic acid 5 mg po daily, B_{12} 1 mg im daily for three doses, then monthly, tetracycline 250 mg po 6-hly for several months until full recovery. This regimen is usually highly effective.

Skin lesions in the returning traveller

Fever and a rash immediately on return: Viral infections (e.g. dengue ➤254), meningococcal septicaemia (➤74), other bacteraemias (including *Staphylococcus aureus*), viral haemorrhagic fevers (➤256).

Chronic skin lesions: There include the ulcer of cutaneous leishmaniasis (➤274) and the serpiginous pruritic track of cutaneous larva migrans (➤279). Both are relatively common. Chronic infections of minor skin lesion by non-sporing anaerobes (esp. *Fusobacterium* spp.) and *Corynebacterium diphtheriae* (➤180) occur rarely.

15: Fever

Most patients with fever in hospital or general practice have associated symptoms that make diagnosis straightforward–the majority have viral respiratory infections or uncomplicated bacterial respiratory or urinary infections. Assessment of the acutely ill febrile patient is a familiar problem, and a laborious account is not indicated. However, we emphasise the value of a careful history and repeated full examination.

If the diagnosis is not immediately obvious, particular attention should be paid to special features of history and examination listed below under PUO. First-line investigations include full blood count, MSU and CXR.

Antibiotics should never be started until appropriate cultures have been obtained. Blood and urine (and sputum if produced) should always be cultured.

Although fever is the hallmark of infectious disease, many illnesses cause fever, including trauma and surgery, neoplastic disease, myocardial infarct, cerebrovascular accident, venous thrombosis and pulmonary embolism. A number of non-infectious multisystem diseases may present with clinical features suggesting acute infection. The key features of some of these are outlined in Table 62, with suggestions for diagnostic tests that may help to confirm or exclude them.

Prolonged pyrexia of unknown origin (PUO)

PUO has been variably defined by a number of authors reporting large series of patients. These definitions, which specify a duration of 2 or 3

Table 62 Non-infectious multisystem illnesses causing acute fever ± skin rash

Condition	Relative frequency (hospital practice)	Clinical features	Useful tests
Temporal (giant-cell) arteritis/polymyalgia rheumatica	Common	Age >50, headache, temporal artery tenderness, visual disturbance, myalgia, proximal limb girdle stiffness, jaw claudication	High ESR. Temporal artery biopsy
Sarcoidosis	Common	Pulmonary symptoms, erythema nodosum, bilateral hilar lymphadenopathy, arthritis, granulomata in many tissues	Histology showing non-caseating granulomata. Kveim test. Serum ACE
Erythema multiforme (syn. Stevens–Johnson syndrome)	Common	Hypersensitivity to infection or drugs. Widespread maculopapular or pustular rash with oral and conjunctival ulcers	Clinical diagnosis
Systemic lupus erythematosus	Common. Esp. young women	Facial rash, arthralgia, nephritis, polyserositis, photosensitivity	Clinical diagnosis. Anti-dsDNA antibodies
Wegener's granulomatosis	Rare	Sinusitis, nephritis, cavitating pulmonary nodules	Histology. ANCA
Polyarteritis nodosa	Rare. Commoner in males	Hypertension, angina, nephritis, abdominal pain, variable skin rash, incl. tender subcutaneous nodules and vasculitis (nail-bed and splinter haemorrhages)	Clinical diagnosis. Histology. Angiography

continued on p. 154

Table 62 contd

Condition	Relative frequency (hospital practice)	Clinical features	Useful tests
Polymyositis/ dermatomyositis	Rare. Sometimes associated with malignancy	Muscle pain, tenderness and weakness. Heliotrope rash on eyelids and extensor surfaces	EMG, raised CPK, muscle biopsy. Specific auto-antibody (Jo-1) may be present
Adult-onset Still's disease/systemic-onset juvenile chronic arthritis	Rare	Evanescent salmon-pink rash, worse during high daily fever, arthritis, lymphadenopathy, hepatosplenomegaly	Clinical diagnosis. High serum ferritin. Rheumatoid factor and ANA usually negative
Kawasaki disease	Rare. Occurs in infants and young children	Fever, conjunctivitis, lymphadenopathy, oedema and erythema of hands/feet with rash which may desquamate. Oropharyngeal erythema, fissured red lips. Coronary artery vasculitis	Clinical diagnosis
Sweet's syndrome	Very rare	Tender discrete red/purple cutaneous plaques, arthralgia, myalgia, neutrophilia	Clinical diagnosis. Histology
Familial Mediterranean fever	Very rare in UK. Autosomal recessive inheritance among Jews, Armenians, Arabs, Turks	Recurrent polyserositis: peritonitis, pleurisy, arthritis, skin rash resembling erysipelas, invariably on extensor surface of lower leg and dorsum of foot	Clinical diagnosis

weeks of fever, are nowadays not useful clinically. Advances in culture techniques, serology and imaging have changed the spectrum of diseases that may cause diagnostic delay and confusion. These notes are intended as guidance to the diagnosis of unexplained fever lasting more than 7–10 days.

> Most patients with PUO have a rare presentation of a common illness, rather than a common presentation of a rare illness; occult malignancy, particularly lymphoma, is as common as infection. Patients usually have single rather than multiple causes of fever.

History and examination: The history is of central importance. Apart from the history of the presenting complaint and the patient's previous medical history, direct enquiry should be made about:

• travel (see also fever in the returning traveller ➤145);
• drugs (therapeutic and recreational, including alcohol);
• sexual history, including risk factors for HIV infection;
• family history and history of contacts with similar symptoms;
• occupational exposure, especially animal/agricultural contact;
• pets.

Drug fever (for list ➤156) usually occurs within 7–10 days of starting treatment, although it can begin during long-term treatment with previously well-tolerated drugs. It usually resolves within 12–48 h of discontinuation, although this period may be longer for drugs with long elimination half-lives, such as co-trimoxazole. Ampicillin/amoxycillin rash and fever has been reported up to 3 weeks after the last dose.

Physical examination should be repeated at daily intervals in patients in hospital, looking particularly for changing heart murmurs, chest signs and enlarging lymph nodes. Other areas of particular interest or that tend to be neglected include:

- temporal arteries and scalp;
- fundi;
- sinuses and teeth;
- skin and nails (rashes, stigmata of IE);
- orifices (mouth, ears, rectum, vagina);
- pelvis (gynaecological disease, perirectal abscess);
- hidden or forgotten iv lines and other prostheses/foreign bodies.

Routine investigations: These investigations are likely to have been performed before the label of PUO is applied; it is safer to repeat them, particularly if they were performed early in the course of illness:

- full blood count including differential white cell count;
- ESR and/or C-reactive protein;
- dip-stick testing of urine for blood and protein;
- midstream urine for microscopy and routine bacterial culture;
- microscopy of spun urine deposit for casts (**not** routinely performed by most microbiology labs when processing an MSU);
- sputum, if available, for routine culture;
- blood cultures (send at least 20 ml on three separate occasions);
- biochemical screen including urea, electrolytes, liver function tests and thyroid function tests;
- chest X-ray.

In patients at risk for tuberculosis, or in whom it is suspected for any reason:

- sputum, if available, for AFBs on three occasions;
- early-morning urine for AFBs (send >150 ml on three occasions).

Second-line investigations: Any or all of the following may be indicated, depending on the clinical picture:

- aspiration or biopsy of any lesions discovered. Samples sent for microbiology should not be fixed in formalin;
- immunological screen, including rheumatoid factor, antinuclear antibodies, organ-specific autoantibodies, antineutrophil cytoplasmic antibodies (ANCA), complement levels;
- immunoglobulin electrophoresis;
- coagulation screen (including lupus anticoagulant, fibrin degradation products);
- viral serology, including flu, adenovirus, herpes viruses, mumps, measles and parvovirus;
- bacterial serology, including coxiella, mycoplasma, chlamydia, syphilis, leptospira, legionella and brucella;
- protozoal serology, including toxoplasma;
- fungal serology, including aspergillus.

☎ Most microbiology laboratories will select those serological tests which are most appropriate on the basis of the clinical history. A full and detailed summary on the request form, or preferably a telephone discussion with the microbiologist, is essential.

HIV infection is an unlikely cause of PUO in the absence of a history of risk behaviour. HIV testing may be appropriate, but must only be carried out after the patient has received pre-test counselling (➤117).

Imaging: Advances in imaging have revolutionised the investigation of PUO. We would recommend early ultrasound scan (USS) of the upper abdomen and pelvis in all cases, looking specifically for hepatic lesions (abscess, neoplasm), splenic size, posterior abdominal wall lymph nodes and pelvic sepsis. The following may then be necessary:

- CT scan of the thorax and abdomen — for fluid collections, solid tumours and lymphadenopathy. CT-guided aspiration, or preferably biopsy, may be possible.
- Echocardiography may confirm the presence of vegetations in suspected IE, but a normal echo does not exclude IE.
- Indium-labelled white cell scan (particularly for local collections of pus or to demonstrate inflammatory bowel disease).
- Technetium bone scan.

Table 63 Causes of PUO

Category	Conditions	
Infections	**Infective endocarditis**	Partially treated bacterial endocarditis, coxiella, nutritionally deficient streptococci, fastidious Gram-negative rods, brucella, legionella, fungi, chlamydia
	Collections of pus	Subphrenic, intrahepatic, renal, pelvic (including appendix), pleural, bone, sinuses, spleen
	Systemic bacterial infections	Mycoplasma, syphilis, leptospirosis, Lyme disease, typhoid, coxiella, brucella
	Tuberculosis	(Especially extrapulmonary)
	Viral	E.g. CMV, EBV, hepatitis B
Malignancy	**Visceral**	**E.g. kidney, liver, pancreas**
	Haematological	**Lymphoma**, leukaemia, myeloma
Rheumatological disease	Rheumatoid disease, **SLE**, polyarteritis nodosa, Still's disease, **temporal arteritis** (also ➤153)	
Granulomatous disease	Sarcoidosis, Crohn's disease, granulomatous hepatitis (➤52)	
Drugs	Penicillins, cephalosporins, para-aminosalicylic acid, amphotericin B, antihistamines, barbiturates, phenytoin, quinidine, sulphonamides, iodides, propylthiouracil, methyldopa, procainamide, hydralazine, isoniazid, phenylbutazone, nitrofurantoin	
Hepatic	Cirrhosis, alcoholic hepatitis, chronic active hepatitis, abscess	
Factitious fever	Particularly in health care professionals	

Most frequent causes are indicated in bold type.

Causes of PUO

Any list of causes is incomplete; most large text-books of infectious diseases or general medicine have lists and these should be referred to in conjunction with Table 63.

Fever and rash

The presence of a rash in an acutely febrile patient is always useful diagnostically. Many rashes are characteristic, not only in their appearance but also in their distribution and pattern of progression. Table 64 lists some of the infectious and non-infectious causes of rash in the acutely febrile patient.

Fever and lymphadenopathy

Fever and lymphadenopathy are common manifestations of infection, but also occur in other disorders. The nature of lymphadenopathy may be a helpful aid to diagnosis. Firm, rubbery, mobile, non-tender nodes suggest lymphoma. Hard fixed nodes suggest carcinoma. Tender, asymmetrical, matted or fluctuant nodes suggest infection. Table 65 lists some causes of lymphadenopathy which may need to be excluded.

The clinical characteristics mentioned above are not sufficiently reliable to exclude malignancy. Lymph nodes which fail to regress over a few weeks merit biopsy.

Table 64 Fever and rash

Nature of rash	Possible aetiologies
Purpura	Bacterial infection (e.g. *Neisseria meningitidis*, *Staphylococcus aureus*, *Pseudomonas aeruginosa*), infective endocarditis (➤37), enteroviruses (➤251), rickettsia (➤233 e.g. Rocky Mountain Spotted Fever, typhus), drug hypersensitivity, systemic vasculitis, Henoch–Schönlein disease (➤110)
Vesicles or pustules	Staphylococcal toxins (toxic epidermal necrolysis (➤108), toxic shock syndrome (➤63)), enteroviruses (➤251), Herpes virus infection, varicella-zoster (➤103), disseminated Herpes simplex (➤241), eczema herpeticum (➤93), rickettsialpox (➤235), drug hypersensitivity
Maculopapular	Scarlet fever (➤108), erythema marginatum (➤172), staphylococcal toxins (toxic epidermal necrolysis (➤108), toxic shock syndrome (➤63)), secondary syphilis (➤67), typhoid (➤191), erythema chronica migrans (➤224), viral exanthemata (➤100, e.g. measles, rubella, EBV, adenovirus, enterovirus etc.), primary HIV infection (➤115), drug and food hypersensitivity, Kawasaki disease (➤154), SLE

Table 65 Causes of lymphadenopathy

Category	Conditions
Local infection	Local suppurative disease (staphylococci, streptococci), tuberculosis, atypical mycobacteria, cat-scratch disease
Generalised Infection	EBV, CMV, toxoplasmosis, rubella, secondary syphilis, hepatitis A, malaria, histoplasmosis, coccidioidomycosis, brucellosis, LGV
Malignancy	Lymphoma, leukaemia, carcinoma
Sarcoidosis	
Connective tissue disease	Rheumatoid disease, systemic lupus erythematosus, dermatomyositis
Dermatopathic	Related to local skin disease, particularly eczema
Endocrine	Hyperthyroidism, Addison's disease

Eosinophilia

Table 66 Causes of eosinophilia (➤151 for travel-associated causes)

Category	Conditions
Drugs	Iodides, aspirin, sulphonamides, nitrofurantoin
Parasites	Helminths, but excluding *Enterobius vermicularis*
Tuberculosis	Particularly miliary
Allergy and atopy	Hay fever, asthma, systemic vasculitis, eczema, pemphigus, Churg–Strauss syndrome
Connective tissue disease	Rheumatoid disease, polyarteritis nodosa, dermatomyositis, eosinophilic fasciitis
Malignancy	Carcinomatosis, mycosis fungoides, Hodgkin's disease, chronic myeloid leukaemia, eosinophilic leukaemia
Hypereosinophilic syndromes	Loeffler's syndrome (pulmonary eosinophilia) and Loeffler's endocarditis
Cat-scratch disease	

16: Septic Shock (syn. sepsis syndrome)

Bacteraemia signifies positive blood cultures. **Septic shock**, broadly defined as the development of hypotension and organ failure as a result of severe infection, is an important cause of death in hospital patients, particularly on the intensive care unit. The diagnosis of septic shock remains a clinical one, confirmed by positive blood cultures in only a proportion of cases. It is very useful to have a **clinical definition** which allows identification of patients before they develop positive blood cultures and resistant hypotension. A definition of 'sepsis syndrome' which has been clinically tested and which has achieved widespread acceptance follows:

- hypothermia ($< 35.6°C$) or fever ($> 38.3°C$);
- tachycardia (> 90 beats/min);
- tachypnoea (> 20 respirations/min);
- a presumed site of infection;

and

- evidence of dysfunction of at least one organ:
  altered mental state;
  arterial hypoxaemia ($Po_2 < 10$ kPa);
  elevated plasma lactate; **or**
  oliguria (< 30 ml/h).

Note that hypotension is not included as a criterion as the purpose of this definition is to identify patients early.

Pathogenesis: Septic shock is most often due to Gram-negative bacteraemia, but Gram-positive organisms have become more common in hospital patients with intravenous lines *in situ*. It is not possible to distinguish between Gram-positive and Gram-negative bacteraemia clinically. Shock is the end result of a complex cascade initiated by bacterial endotoxin (➤184), which stimulates the release of inflammatory mediators such as tumour necrosis factor (TNF) and interleukin-1 (IL-1) from host leucocytes. These damage vascular endothelial cells, causing increased capillary permeability, abnormal vasomotor activity and activation of the clotting system, resulting in maldistribution of blood flow and damage to multiple organs, including kidneys, lungs, brain, liver and myocardium.

Risk factors

Sources of sepsis: Extravascular sources include wounds, abscesses, focal infections such as pneumonia, gut perforation or urinary tract infection. Recent trauma or manipulation, such as surgery or IVDU, may be involved. Intravascular sources include infected heart valves in IE (➤37), iv cannulae, infected atheromatous plaques or shunts.

> **Practice point:** Always search for the source of a bacteraemia because it may need specific treatment.

Host factors: Severe underlying illness, such as diabetes, renal failure or hepatic disease, which may compromise the host immune system or cause loss of integrity of epithelial surfaces. Trauma and malignancy are particularly important in this respect. Anatomical abnormalities, such as stones or obstruction in the urinary or biliary tracts, may predispose to infection. Patients at either extreme of age are at increased risk, as are those with indwelling foreign bodies, in particular intravenous medical devices such as central venous cannulae.

Clinical features: There may be a **history of risk factors** as above. **Fever and rigors** commonly occur but elderly, debilitated or immunocompromised patients may not manifest these classical symptoms. **Hypothermia** is common. A **change in mental state**, with apprehension or confusion, may be the first sign of impending sepsis and a search for infection should be considered in any elderly patient who becomes acutely confused. Stupor and coma occur less often. Cough or disturbance of micturition may indicate a **pre-existing nidus of infection**. Careful enquiry and examination for sites of skin sepsis such as boils, infected intravenous lines. Patients should be specifically asked about previous splenectomy and rheumatic and congenital cardiac disease.

On **examination**, there are signs consistent with the clinical features listed above, with or without hypotension ($\leqslant 90$ mmHg). In early shock there is peripheral vasodilatation, decreased systemic vascular resistance and increased cardiac output. The patient is hypotensive, but warm. Later, there is peripheral vasoconstriction, increased systemic vascular resistance and reduced cardiac output. As cardiac output falls, the skin becomes cold, cyanotic and mottled.

Auscultation and chest X-ray may reveal pneumonia or evidence of **acute respiratory distress syndrome** (ARDS), characterised by increased alveolar capillary permeability and pulmonary oedema without left atrial hypertension, leading to hypoxia with reduced lung compliance. ARDS occurs in up to 40% of cases, and is associated with a very high mortality.

Cutaneous manifestations include the signs referred to above due to changes in peripheral perfusion, but also cellulitis, erythema multiforme and, particularly in those who develop disseminated intravascular coagulation, peripheral vasculitic skin lesions progressing to gangrene. Meningococcaemia is associated with a rash that is initially petechial, progressing to a purpuric or ecchymotic rash on limbs and trunk. *Staphylococcus aureus* bacteraemia may cause a very similar rash. *Pseudomonas aeruginosa* bacteraemia is associated with ecthyma gangrenosum, which develops as dark red or purple macules, which may ulcerate to leave a central ulcer surrounded by an erythematous margin. This was previously considered pathognomonic, although it has been reported in association with other Gram-negative bacteraemias.

Organisms: Community-acquired sepsis: coliforms, *Streptococcus pneumoniae*, *Neisseria gonorrhoeae*, *Neisseria meningitidis*, *Staphylococcus aureus*. In hospital patients, particularly with indwelling intravenous lines, *Staphylococcus epidermidis* should also be considered, but septic shock is unusual. In patients with malignancy or abdominal sepsis coliforms, enterococci and anaerobic infections, particularly *Bacteroides fragilis*. In patients with neutropenia, *Pseudomonas aeruginosa* and fungi should also be covered (➤134). Splenectomised patients are at particular risk from capsulated organisms (*Streptococcus pneumoniae*, *Haemophilus influenzae*, *Neisseria meningitidis*). Recent manipulations of particular body sites may suggest particular organisms (Table 67).

Microbiological investigations: Gram stain and culture of urine, pus, sputum or CSF. Blood cultures should be sent as soon as the diagnosis is suspected. At least two venepunctures should be performed in the assessment period and at least 10 and preferably 20 ml of blood should be cultured from each.

Other investigations: Leucocytosis with 'left shift' is often, but not always, present. Thrombocytopenia and disseminated intravascular coagulation with prolonged prothrombin and partial thromboplastin times, reduced plasma fibrinogen and raised fibrin degradation products. Raised serum lactate levels occur in a majority of patients. Most

Table 67 Organisms particularly associated with sepsis after medical manipulation

Manipulated site	Organisms
Dental operation	'Viridans' streptococci, oral anaerobes
GU manipulation	Coliforms, enterococci
Boils	*Staphylococcus aureus*
Septic abortion	Coliforms, anaerobes
IVDU	*Staphylococcus aureus*, enterococci, *Pseudomonas aeruginosa*
IV lines	*Staphylococcus aureus*, coliforms, *Candida albicans*, *Staphylococcus epidermidis*, enterococci

Table 68 Empirical treatment of suspected sepsis syndrome

Clinical situation	Regimen
Adult with community-acquired sepsis	Benzylpenicillin + gentamicin + metronidazole **or** cefotaxime + metronidazole **or** vancomycin + gentamicin + metronidazole
If *Staphylococcus aureus* suspected (cutaneous sepsis, recent flu epidemic, IVDU, iv line)	Substitute flucloxacillin or vancomycin for benzylpenicillin in suggested regimens; cefotaxime gives adequate anti-staphylococcal cover for empirical use
Patients with neutropenia	Azlocillin + gentamicin + vancomycin (+ metronidazole if there is perianal sepsis)

patients with septic shock develop some degree of renal failure, usually due to acute tubular necrosis secondary to hypotension. Abnormal liver function is frequently seen. Chest X-ray may show pneumonia or ARDS. Ultrasound and CT scanning are usually required to exclude local collections of pus.

Differential diagnosis: Specific syndromes causing hypotension and shock include purulent bacterial pericardial effusion, peritonitis, severe pneumonia with hypoxaemia (➤22), mediastinitis (for example, after oesophageal surgery or variceal sclerotherapy), anaphylaxis induced by antibiotics, and toxic shock syndrome (➤63).

Antibiotic management: Depends on likely infectious cause. Many different regimens are suitable—it is important to start as soon as cultures have been taken and to give large doses intravenously (Table 68).

Be guided thereafter by microbiology results. For management of neutropenic sepsis ➤134.

Supportive management: Careful supportive management is as important as administration of adequate antibiotics. Haemodynamic monitoring in the setting of the intensive care unit is often required; a full discussion is beyond the scope of this manual. In patients who are less unwell, or if ICU facilities are not available, proceed as follows:

• Make a full assessment of the patient's condition and the likely aetiology as above.

• Insert a large-bore peripheral venous line and administer saline or colloid. An initial bolus of 1 litre of normal saline given over 30 minutes is appropriate if the patient is hypotensive. Volume replacement is a priority, and should be monitored by central venous line, vital signs and urine output. A mixture of $^2/_3$ crystalloid (e.g. $^2/_3$ N saline and $^1/_3$ 5% dextrose) and $^1/_3$ colloid (human albumin or gelfusin) is appropriate for most situations. Insert a urinary catheter. Observe carefully for fluid overload and be aware of the possibility of acute renal failure.

• Take cultures, then choose and start appropriate antibiotics.

• Give supplementary oxygen by face mask or nasal speculae.

• Remove or drain any obvious source of infection such as a boil or infected iv line.

• Inotropic support with dopamine and/or dobutamine is required for prolonged hypotension.

• Monoclonal antibodies against endotoxin and TNF remain experimental. Steroids are not indicated.

• Monitor and treat DIC ☎.

Complications: Patients who enter the later phase of cold shock have a poor prognosis. Mortality increases with the number of organ systems involved—approaching 100% if four or more organ systems fail. In terminal stages patients become progressively acidotic, with resistant hypotension refractory to treatment with fluids and inotropic drugs.

Section 2:
Microbiology

Bacteria

Classification of medically important bacteria

In the following chapters we have used the classification in Table 69, which provides a practical, memorable and clinically relevant structure.

Table 69 Classification of medically important bacteria

Group		Most important species	Chapter
Gram-positive aerobes	Cocci	*Staphylococcus* spp.	17 (➤165)
		Streptococcus spp.	18 (➤169)
	Rods	*Bacillus* spp.	19 (➤176)
		Listeria spp.	
		Corynebacterium spp.	
Gram-negative aerobic rods	Coliforms (*Enterobacteriacae*)	*Escherichia* spp.	20 (➤184)
		Klebsiella spp.	
		Proteus spp.	
		Salmonella spp.	
		Shigella spp.	
	Vibrios	*Vibrio* spp.	
	Campylobacters	*Campylobacter* spp.	
		Helicobacter spp.	
	Pseudomonads	*Pseudomonas* spp.	21 (➤199)
Fastidious Gram-negative organisms		*Haemophilus* spp.	22 (➤203)
		Neisseria spp.	
		Legionella spp.	
		Bordetella spp.	
Anaerobes	Spore forming	*Clostridium* spp.	23 (➤214)
	Non-spore-forming	*Bacteroides* spp.	
		Fusobacterium spp.	
	Spirochaetes	*Treponema* spp.	24 (➤223)
		Borrelia spp.	
		Leptospira spp.	
Mycobacteria		*Mycobacterium* spp.	25 (➤228)
Mycoplasma		*Mycoplasma* spp.	26 (➤233)
		Ureaplasma spp.	
Chlamydia		*Chlamydia* spp.	
Rickettsia		*Rickettsia* spp.	
		Coxiella spp.	

17: Staphylococci and their Relatives

Staphylococci ('bunch of grapes') are members of the family *Microccaceae*—round, Gram-positive organisms arranged in clumps or packets. All are commensals of human skin. *Staphylococcus aureus* ('golden' colonies) is a major pathogen, causing pyogenic and toxin-mediated infections in humans. More recently, coagulase-negative staphylococci (CNSt) have emerged as potential pathogens, especially in the urinary tract and as opportunists in hospital-ised patients.

Classification (Table 70)

All CNSt used to be grouped as '*Staphylococcus albus*'. Many laboratories now use '*Staphylococcus epidermidis*' to refer to all CNSt and micrococci. Identification (other than *epidermidis* and *saprophyticus*, when needed) is best done with commercial biochemical test kits.

Staphylococcus aureus

Pathogenesis: Produces a wide variety of extracellular enzymes and other products. Some cause general tissue damage, others have specific effects:

- **General**:
  Lysins, leucocidin, staphylokinase, lipase, phospholipase (cell membrane damage). Clumping factor, coagulase (converts fibrinogen to fibrin).
  Protein A (immunoglobulin Fc region-binding).
  Collagen-binding protein, fibronectin-binding protein (adhesion).
  Deoxyribonuclease, proteases, hyaluronidase.

- **Specific**:
  Epidermolytic toxins: staphylococcal scalded-skin syndrome (SSSS) (syn. Ritter's disease, toxic epidermal necrolysis, Lyell's syndrome) (➤108); exfoliative toxin; toxic shock syndrome toxin-1 (TSST-1; also called enterotoxin F) (➤63). **Enterotoxins** types A–E cause food poisoning (➤44); produced by 40% of *Staphylococcus aureus* strains overall.

Epidemiology: Regularly carried by 20–30% normal people in anterior nares, usually one

Table 70 Classification of staphylococci

Genus	Species	Notes
COAGULASE +		
Staphylococcus	**aureus**	Human pathogen.
	intermedius	Animal pathogen; occasionally infects bites
COAGULASE −		
Staphylococcus	**epidermidis**	
	saprophyticus	
	(*capitis, hominis, lugdunensis, schleiferi, haemolyticus, auricularis, warneri, simulans, cohnii,* etc.)	
(*Micrococcus*	*luteus, varians, roseus,* etc.)	
(*Stomatococcus*	*mucilaginosus*)	Mucoid colonies
Peptococcus	*niger* (➤214)	'Anaerobic staph.'

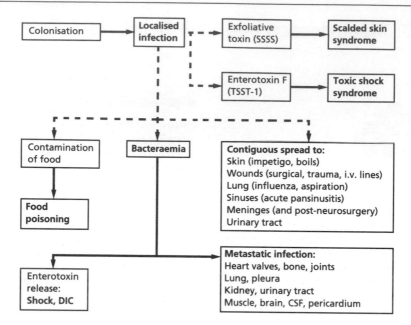

Fig. 5 Pathogenesis of staphylococcal infections.

strain for long periods; ~50% of the remainder carry different strains intermittently. Sometimes carried heavily on axillary and/or perineal skin, but 98% of these individuals also positive in anterior nares. New strains are acquired by direct contact (e.g. hands of staff) and airborne exposure (e.g. from clouds of staphylococci dispersed during bedmaking). Acquisition is enhanced by prior antibiotic therapy. Single nose swab detects 80% of carriers. Staphylococci mainly spread from anterior nares to hands to skin to squames to air. Very few directly from anterior nares to air. Frequent and heavy skin carriage in insulin-dependent diabetics, haemodialysis, iv drug misusers (all with repeated skin puncture). **Bacteriophage ('phage') typing** of strains by patterns of lysis by bank of bacteriophages (➔).

Spectrum of disease: Hallmark of local sepsis is **abscess** formation (➤88).

Impetigo (➤87)

Cellulitis (➤88)

Toxic shock syndrome (TSS) (➤63)

Hospital-acquired bacteraemia, most commonly from iv catheter infection, usually short-lasting with easily treatable focus. Uncommonly associated with metastatic infection.

Community-acquired bacteraemia often long-lasting, sometimes presenting with shock, purpuric rash, meningism. Common metastatic infection, including acute endocarditis (➤37).

Laboratory diagnosis: Clumps of Gram-positive cocci readily seen in pus, but indistinguishable from coagulase-negative staphylococci. Rapid (24 h) growth on common media ⇒ rapid-slide coagulase test (confirm by 4 h tube coagulase test). If bacteraemic, 24–48 h growth from aerobic and anaerobic blood culture bottles. Diagnosis of **TSS** is made by clinical criteria plus isolation of *Staphylococcus aureus* from local site (TSST-1 production confirmed by ➔).

Treatment

• Drain pus, remove foreign bodies whenever possible.

• More than 85% are penicillin-resistant (β-lactamase production) in and out of hospital; locally variable erythromycin and tetracycline resistance rates ~3–10%.

• **(Flu)cloxacillin** drug of choice: 5–7 days'

therapy for mild infections. Co-amoxiclav is a broad-spectrum alternative.

• For **severe infection**: give flucloxacillin for 2–6 weeks, initially iv: consider combining with gentamicin or oral fusidic acid or rifampicin (if penicillin-allergic, consider substituting erythromycin, vancomycin, teicoplanin or cefotaxime for flucloxacillin). Osteomyelitis 6–12 weeks.

• **Bacteraemia**: 14 days' therapy if short-lasting; 4–6 weeks if long-lasting, possibly endocarditis (repeat blood cultures on first few days of therapy). Follow-up to exclude metastatic infection.

• **TSS**: support circulation; identify site of infection and drain if possible; flucloxacillin.

Methicillin-resistant
Staphylococcus aureus **(MRSA)** ①
Resistant to **all** current β-lactam antibiotics (produces penicillin-binding protein PBP 2', which binds β-lactams poorly).

• Many strains, all spread between hospitals by movement of colonised or infected patients and staff. Some strains may have enhanced abilities to spread in hospitals (e.g. 'EMRSA-16' currently epidemic in southern England).

• Often multiply resistant (erythromycin, tetracycline, gentamicin; occasionally rifampicin, fusidic acid, ciprofloxacin, mupirocin).

• Vancomycin or teicoplanin are the only fully reliable agents.

• Most MRSA are as virulent as methicillin-sensitive strains.

• Sepsis occurs in 5–60% of those colonised —more frequently in ICU or surgical patients.

Prevention: Surveillance swabbing of high-risk units and isolation (≻6) of high-risk admissions (ICU, interhospital transfers, recent hospital stays abroad, previously positive). Swab nose, throat, 'manipulated sites' and areas of damaged skin (wounds, iv catheter sites, etc.); results take 3–5 days.

Management: Isolation ① of proven cases and surveillance swabbing of patient and staff contacts. Control is most successful in specialised isolation unit, with controlled ventilation. Consider closure of wards to new admissions while contacts are screened (many laboratories require two or three negative screens

over a 10-day period) ☎. MRSA now endemic in some hospitals, necessitating expensive substitution of vancomycin for flucloxacillin for surgical prophylaxis (≻312). **Clearance of carriers**: Topical mupirocin and antiseptics; may require systemic antibiotic therapy (☎). Most laboratories require three or four negative weekly screens to prove a once-positive patient clear.

Staphylococcus epidermidis

Pathogenesis: Few potential virulence factors; electrostatic attraction to surfaces. Glycocalyx ('slime') production by some strains aids persistent adhesion (by producing 'biofilm').

Epidemiology: Resident normal flora of skin, nasopharynx, lower urogenital tract. Most infections are endogenous, but multiply resistant strains are also acquired by hospital cross-infection. Outbreaks have been recognised: phage-typing is available (☎).

Spectrum of disease: Predilection for foreign body infection (iv and ia catheters, pacemakers, heart valve and arterial prostheses, haemodialysis shunts (all causing bacteraemia); Spitz–Holter valves and CSF shunts (≻78); CAPD catheters (≻54); joint prostheses (≻96)). Isolation from any site without an implant suggests **contamination**. Also: hospital-associated **UTI** in elderly males (≻58); neonatal septicaemia and meningitis (often iv catheter-associated) (≻110); rare native valve endocarditis (≻37). Other coagulase-negative staphylococci occasionally isolated from similar infections, but more often contaminants. *Staphylococcus lugdunensis* has been associated with endocarditis.

Laboratory diagnosis: Clumps of Gram-positive cocci readily seen in pus (indistinguishable from *Staphylococcus aureus*). Rapid (24 h) growth on common media ⇒ negative rapid slide coagulase test (confirm by 4 h tube coagulase test). If bacteraemic, 24–48 h growth from aerobic and anaerobic blood culture bottles. Isolates are more likely to be significant if foreign body present, if multiple bottles from several blood cultures positive, if all cultures positive within 48 h and if same strain (e.g. same sensitivity pattern) isolated from all cultures.

Treatment: Often multiply resistant, and **vancomycin** is the only fully reliable agent for systemic infections (occasional strains teicoplanin-resistant); await sensitivity testing results before choosing alternatives. **Removal of foreign body** often essential, and may be all that is required in iv catheter infection. If treatment is attempted without device removal (e.g. Hickman line infection), the best choice is vancomycin.

Staphylococcus saprophyticus

Common cause of lower UTI in sexually active women (>58). Usually very antibiotic-sensitive.

Stomatococcus mucilaginosus

Oral commensal; similar pathogenicity to CNSt.

18: Streptococci and their Relatives

Streptococci are round or oval Gram-positive organisms that tend to form chains, especially in the tissues and in liquid culture. They are commensals of the mouth, nasopharynx, colon and lower urogenital tract, and several species are major pathogens. Penicillin remains the drug of choice for most streptococcal infections, but problems of antibiotic resistance have become increasingly common recently.

Classification methods

Lancefield grouping: Classification of cell-wall carbohydrate antigens into groups A–V; originally used only for β-haemolytic strains, now used for many streptococcal species. Colonies are tested by latex agglutination kits; rapid grouping of organisms seen in blood culture broths often possible before growth on solid media.

Haemolysis: Classification based on effects of bacterial colonies on blood agar plates:
- **α-haemolytic:** partial lysis of erythrocytes and haemoglobin breakdown ⇒ green pigment (hence 'viridans' group streptococci);

Table 71 Classification of streptococci

Genus	Species	Notes
Streptococcus	**pyogenes**	Lancefield Gp A β haemolytic streptococcus
	(equisimilis, zooepidemicus, equi, dysgalactiae)	Lancefield Gp C β-haemolytic streptococci
		Lancefield Gp G β-haemolytic streptococci
	agalactiae	Lancefield Gp B β-haemolytic streptococcus
	'milleri' group	Lancefield Gp A, C, F, G or none; β- or non-haemolytic. Includes constellatus, anginosus and intermedius
	(mutans, sanguis, mitis, salivarius)	'Viridans' group; many are α-haemolytic. Mitis sometimes known as mitior
	(bovis)	Lancefield Gp D
	pneumoniae	'Pneumococci'; α-haemolytic
	(suis)	Lancefield Gp R (➤74)
Enterococcus	**faecalis**, faecium (durans, avium, etc.)	Lancefield Gp D
Peptostreptococcus	anaerobius, asaccharolyticus, etc.	'Anaerobic streptococci' (➤214)
(Aerococcus (Leuconostoc spp.) (Pediococcus spp.) (Gemella (Lactococcus	viridans) haemolysans) lactis)	These organisms are commensals of mucosal surfaces, and are rarely pathogenic. They have caused endocarditis and meningitis, and are virtually the only Gram-positive bacteria that are regularly vancomycin-resistant

• **β-haemolytic:** complete haemolysis ⇒ clear zones around colonies;
• **non-haemolytic** (sometimes called 'γ-haemolytic'): no effects.
(NB Strains of many bacterial species produce haemolysis on blood agar.)

Identification: Commercial biochemical kits are now commonly used to identify some groups of streptococci (e.g. 'viridans' group) to species level when necessary.

Streptococcus pyogenes ①
(Gp A β-haemolytic streptococci)

Pathogenesis: Exclusively a human pathogen; many structural and extracellular products with few defined roles. (Table 72).

Epidemiology: Found in nose/throat swabs of 10% normal people; occasionally carried on perineum alone. Minor septic lesions and nasal carriage ⇒ heavy airborne dispersal. Also spread by respiratory secretions and hands. Frequent transmission between household and close physical contacts. Occasional food- and milk-borne outbreaks. Typing by cell-wall proteins (M, T and R antigens; ✣); some types associated with particular diseases (e.g. outbreaks of acute glomerulonephritis type 49, rheumatic fever type 5).

Spectrum of disease

Skin sepsis: Cardinal sign is **cellulitis** (➤88). Often blistering ⇒ serous discharge.

Lymphangitis. Frequently mixed infection with *Staphylococcus aureus*. **Important syndromes: impetigo** (localised crusting ➤87); **erysipelas** (well-demarcated cellulitis, especially of face ➤89); **necrotising fasciitis** (necrosis of skin and subcutaneous tissues ➤91). Nowadays surgical wound infection and puerperal sepsis are rare (and both are now most commonly autoinfections).

Pharyngitis and tonsillitis: 'Fiery red' throat (➤17); may progress to quinsy (➤18).

Acute otitis media: Mainly children (➤15).

Vaginitis: All ages.

Bacteraemia: Uncommonly accompanies severe tissue infection; mortality > 20%. Occasional 'toxic shock'-like syndrome (➤63).

Indirect sequelae (all uncommon in developed world):
• **Scarlet fever** ⌧ (➤108), may accompany throat infection with erythrogenic toxin-producing strain.
• **Rheumatic fever** (➤171).
• **Acute diffuse proliferative glomerulonephritis** (➤171).

Laboratory diagnosis: Ready growth on blood agar in 24 h ⇒ dry colonies with wide haemolysis zone. Confirmed by rapid Lancefield grouping. Rising ASO (especially throat infections) and anti-DNase B (especially skin infections) titres useful for confirming diagnosis of indirect sequelae. Immunoassay kits for direct detection in

Table 72 Gp A streptococcal products contributing to pathogenicity

Factor	Role
M cell-wall protein	Fimbriae-associated; antiphagocytic, anticomplement and epithelial adhesion roles. Specific antibodies are protective
Hyaluronic acid capsule	Antiphagocytic; strains with mucoid colonies produce more capsule and may be more pathogenic
DNases A, B, C, D	Basis of anti-DNase B assay
Streptolysins O and S	Haemolytic, cytotoxic; basis of antistreptolysin O (ASO) assay
Hyaluronidase, streptokinase	? Involved in spread through tissues
Erythrogenic toxins	Produced by some strains after phage lysogeny. Rash, fever, cytotoxic effects ⇒ 'scarlet fever'

Others include pyrogenic exotoxin, NADase, serum opacity factor. Nephritogenic strains probably share antigens with human glomerular basement membrane.

throat swabs are rapid, but expensive and less sensitive than culture.

Treatment: Invariably benzylpenicillin-sensitive, but up to 14.4 g/day sometimes needed for clinical response in serious infection (especially with arterial insufficiency). Combine with flucloxacillin for known or suspected mixed infection with *Staphylococcus aureus* (mild–moderate infections can be managed on flucloxacillin alone). Erythromycin (5–8% resistance) or oral cephalosporin best choices in penicillin allergy. Tetracycline resistance common in some areas; co-trimoxazole/ trimethoprim is poorly effective. β-Lactamase production by throat commensals may reduce penicillin activity, therefore co-amoxiclav or erythromycin may be preferable. To clear carriage, 10 days' therapy required. Benzathine penicillin single-dose therapy is convenient in streptococcal pharyngitis (≻17). Topical agents adequate for impetigo in domiciliary practice (≻87). In hospital, isolate patients with *Streptococcus pyogenes* and consider screening contacts (nose, throat, perineum, skin lesions). Isolation ①.

Important definitions:

Rheumatic fever is an immunological reaction to infection by **group A** β-haemolytic streptococci.

Rheumatic heart disease describes the cardiac damage resulting from a previous attack of rheumatic fever. It does not imply ongoing infection. Valvular scarring may continue in the absence of infection, due in part to disturbed blood flow through damaged valves.

Infective endocarditis (syn. subacute bacterial endocarditis) is infection of the heart valves. It is particularly likely to occur on valves previously damaged by rheumatic fever. Infection is commonly due to α-haemolytic 'viridans' streptococci.

CLINICAL SYNDROMES

Poststreptococcal glomerulonephritis (PSGN)
Immune complex-mediated glomerulonephritis may follow pharyngeal or skin/soft tissue infection by some strains (M-type 12 in the UK) of group A β-haemolytic streptococci (Gp A βHS). It is now rare in the UK.

Clinical features: Asymptomatic episodes of nephritis are common. Patients develop haematuria, proteinuria, hypertension, uraemia and oedema 1–2 weeks after a streptococcal pharyngitis (2–3 weeks after skin infection). Nephrotic syndrome occurs occasionally. Approximately 30% do not recall an antecedent infection. Prognosis in children is very good, with < 1% progressing to chronic renal failure. In adults up to 30% may have long-standing renal damage and ultimate renal failure.

Microbiological investigations: Throat/lesion swab may grow Gp A βHS. Serology.

Other investigations: ESR is elevated. Renal biopsy is rarely indicated, but shows diffuse proliferative glomerulonephritis.

Antibiotic management: Prompt antibiotic treatment of streptococcal pharyngitis reduces the risk of PSGN. Treatment should be given for 10 days with penicillin V, amoxycillin or erythromycin. Alternatively, a single dose of benzathine penicillin (1.2 MU im, 600 000 U for children under 25 kg) is effective and ensures compliance. Antibiotics do **not** abort established PSGN.

Supportive management: Renal failure may require specific management.

Differential diagnosis: IgA nephropathy presents with haematuria at the same time as upper respiratory tract infection.

Rheumatic fever (RF)
RF is an immunologically mediated hypersensitivity response following pharyngeal infection by particular strains of Gp A βHS which do not cause skin infection. Incidence has declined dramatically in developed world, but is increasing in the developing countries. Extremely rare in the

UK. Outbreaks reported in the USA among military personnel.

Risk factors: Previous and recurrent exposure to infection by Gp A βHS predisposes to development of RF. Once RF is acquired it may easily be reactivated by subsequent streptococcal infections—~50% of Gp A βHS infections occurring in the first year after an attack of RF are followed by a second attack.

Clinical features: Onset occurs ~3 weeks (range 1–5) after streptococcal pharyngitis, which may not be recalled by the patient. Diagnosis is made on the basis of modified Jones criteria (see Table 73)—RF is suggested by the presence of two major criteria or one major and two minor criteria, **plus** evidence of recent streptococcal infection. Pleurisy and abdominal pain also occur frequently. Normochromic, normocytic anaemia is common.

Prognosis: Immediate mortality is ~5%. About 50% develop rheumatic heart disease (RHD) 10 years after RF. Mitral regurgitation and mitral stenosis are the commonest lesions; aortic stenosis and regurgitation and tricuspid lesions also occur, but pulmonary valve lesions are uncommon. Valvular damage may progress in the absence of recurrent RF. Following an attack of RF patients should receive **continuous** antibiotic prophylaxis to prevent recurrences—see below. Patients with RHD or a history of RF are also at risk for **infective endocarditis** and should receive antibiotic prophylaxis prior to dental and other procedures (➤40).

Microbiological investigations: Throat swab. Antistreptococcal antibodies, in particular ASOT (see above under PSGN).

Antibiotic management: Penicillin should be given to eradicate persistent Gp A βHS infection. Doses as for PSGN above. Aspirin (6–9 g/day) and steroids (prednisolone 40–60 mg daily initially, reducing over ~6 weeks) may be given to control carditis and arthritis. **Secondary prophylaxis must be given** to prevent recurrences. Penicillin V 250 mg 12-hly po, or benzathine penicillin (1.2 MU im monthly). Erythromycin if penicillin-allergic. Prophylaxis should be continued into adult life in all patients, and many would recommend indefinite treatment. **Primary prophylaxis** may also be used to prevent infection in closed communities such as military barracks.

Strict bedrest for at least 2 weeks is usually advised.

Table 73 Modified Jones criteria for diagnosis of RF

Major criteria	Comments
Carditis	'Pancarditis': Endocarditis causing valvular damage with murmur of mitral regurgitation and, less often, apical mid-diastolic murmur (Carey–Coombs murmur) and aortic regurgitation. Pericarditis (5–10%). Congestive cardiac failure (5–10%). Arrhythmia and heart block rare
Arthritis	Large joints mainly affected. Frequently migratory
Chorea ('St Vitus's dance')	Abrupt erratic purposeless movements and emotional lability. After puberty chorea occurs exclusively in women. It is rare after adolescence. Usually lasts 2–4 months
Subcutaneous nodules	Painless subcutaneous nodules (0.5–2 cm) over bony prominences and tendons. Often symmetrical and occurring in crops. Not attached to skin, which is mobile and not inflamed
Erythema marginatum	Bright pink, blanching, non-indurated, non-pruritic, non-painful, serpiginous 'smoke-ring' rash. May persist for several weeks after recovery
Minor criteria	Fever, arthralgia, previous rheumatic fever or rheumatic heart disease, raised ESR or CRP, prolonged P–R interval

Lancefield Gp C and G streptococci

Release many of the same extracellular products as *Streptococcus pyogenes*, and can cause most of the same diseases; more commonly they behave as commensals, or cause milder illness. Gp C are mainly animal pathogens; Gp G infections associated with underlying malignancy.

Streptococcus agalactiae (Lancefield Gp B)

Lancefield Gp B β-haemolytic streptococcus.

Pathogenesis: Largely unknown mechanisms; shares sialic acid capsular antigen with K1 *Escherichia coli* (➤189). Low neonatal/maternal capsular antibody titres correlate with infection. Distinct strains cause bovine mastitis.

Epidemiology: Faecal commensal in ~30% people, colonising vagina in 10–30%. If maternal vagina positive, neonate has 70% risk of becoming colonised. Disease commoner with prolonged rupture of membranes, prematurity, heavy vaginal carriage, certain racial groups; rising incidence for past 30 years. Typing by carbohydrate and protein antigens (➤).

Spectrum of disease

Neonatal sepsis: Causes 30% cases (➤110).

• **Early onset** (first few days): septicaemic illness with meningitis and pneumonia, acquired during passage through maternal vagina. High mortality.

• **Late onset:** meningitis (occasionally other sites, e.g. skin sepsis, osteomyelitis). Less common, better prognosis. Usually acquired by cross-infection in nursery and not associated with prematurity, etc.

Puerperal sepsis (➤62): Infected retained products, endometritis, pelvic sepsis, occasional bacteraemia. Often mixed infections with vaginal non-sporing anaerobes, *Streptococcus milleri*, *Gardnerella vaginalis*, *Mycoplasma hominis*, coliforms, etc.

Adult infections: Frequently colonises bedsores, varicose ulcers, etc.; occasional cellulitis of ischaemic limbs (usually mixed infections, ➤88), bacteraemia, endocarditis (all associated with diabetes, malignancy).

Laboratory diagnosis: Septic infants: send blood culture, two surface swabs (e.g. ear + umbilicus), maternal HVS. Rapid (24 h) growth on blood agar, forming moist colonies with narrow haemolysis zone. Lancefield grouping of colonies by latex agglutination.

Treatment: Less penicillin-sensitive than *Streptococcus pyogenes*; add gentamicin for severe illness for improved bactericidal effect. Evacuation of retained products of conception plus antibiotics (e.g. cefotaxime + metronidazole) for puerperal sepsis.

Streptococcus 'milleri'

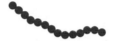

A group of related species causing similar clinical syndromes; mucosal commensals requiring raised CO_2 and humidity for growth on blood agar.

Pathogenesis: Unknown virulence factors.

Epidemiology: Normal flora of mouth, upper respiratory tract, colon and lower urogenital tract. Cause endogenous infections, **often mixed** with other local mucosal commensals (especially non-sporing anaerobes; also coliforms, coagulase-negative staphylococci, coryneforms).

Spectrum of disease: Hallmark is **abscess formation** ± associated bacteraemia; includes intra-abdominal (e.g. perforated diverticulum, appendix abscess, puerperal sepsis), liver (portal pyaemia), lung (aspiration pneumonia, empyema), brain. Also chronic sinusitis, occasionally endocarditis.

Laboratory diagnosis: Tiny Gram-positive cocci in chains, often grow best with anaerobic incubation ⇒ minute colonies (48 h) on blood agar, smelling of toffee. Lancefield grouping of colonies by latex agglutination (most commonly group F).

Treatment: Drain abscesses; broad-spectrum therapy for mixed infections, e.g. iv benzylpenicillin + gentamicin + metronidazole, or oral co-amoxiclav.

'Viridans' and 'non-haemolytic' streptococci

These group names are preferred to *Streptococcus viridans*, which is not a true species.

Pathogenesis: No recognised toxins; strains causing IE often produce complex carbohydrates (dextrans), aiding adhesion to teeth and heart valves.

Epidemiology: Mucosal commensals of mouth, upper respiratory tract; some strains bind to teeth. Replaced by coliforms, pseudomonads, *Staphylococcus aureus* and *Candida* spp. after antibiotic treatment or prolonged tracheal intubation.

Spectrum of disease

Infective endocarditis (≻37).

Gum sepsis, dental caries: Especially *Streptococcus mutans*.

Bacteraemia: With pulmonary symptoms and signs (especially *Streptococcus mitis* in neutropenic patients with oral ulceration, and neonates).

Laboratory diagnosis: Often long chains in broth cultures. Rapid (24 h) growth on blood agar to form tiny α- or non-haemolytic colonies. In IE, 24–48 h growth from aerobic and anaerobic blood culture bottles. Sometimes carry a variety of Lancefield group antigens. Rare strains nutritionally dependent (pyridoxal/cysteine), requiring supplemented media for growth on solid media (☎).

Treatment: Mostly penicillin-sensitive, unless patient given penicillin in past month. Combination with gentamicin improves cidal effect in IE treatment/prophylaxis (≻40).

Streptococcus bovis

Colonic commensal carrying Lancefield Gp D antigen, but bacteriologically very similar to 'viridans' streptococci. Causes IE associated with colonic carcinoma (screen cases with barium enema).

Streptococcus pneumoniae

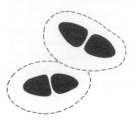

Pathogenesis: Produces various extracellular toxins, but carbohydrate capsule is the most important virulence factor. Heavily capsulate strains form mucoid colonies; those of low serotype (especially types 3, 7 and 1) associated with highest mortality. Protection needs type-specific antibodies and intact phagocytic system. Alcoholics, HIV-1 antibody-positive, elderly, post-splenectomy, post-influenza have greatest risk.

Epidemiology: In normal population, 10–30% nasopharyngeal carriage rate. Typing by capsular swelling with specific antibodies (Quellung reaction; over 80 serotypes ➔).

Spectrum of disease

Community-acquired pneumonia: Commonest cause, up to 80% overall; frequently lobar in pattern. Bacteraemia occurs in 15–25% of patients (≻22).

Acute exacerbations of chronic bronchitis: Often mixed with *Haemophilus influenzae*, *Moraxella catarrhalis* (≻21).

Sinusitis and otitis media (≻15).

Meningitis (≻74).

'Occult bacteraemia': In febrile children.

Rare others: Acute endocarditis, cellulitis.

Laboratory diagnosis: Direct antigen detection in sputum, serum, CSF or urine sometimes useful (detect capsular polysaccharide or common 'C' antigen). Characteristic 'lanceolate' diplococci on Gram stain, but not specific for infection when seen in sputum. In 24–48 h produce α-haemolytic 'draughtsman' colonies (from zonal autolysis) on blood agar. Differentiate from 'viridans' streptococci by optochin sensitivity and bile solubility. May autolyse in blood culture broths (try antigen detection on the broth ☎).

Treatment: Classically, benzylpenicillin is the

drug of choice; erythromycin resistance 5–10%. Avoid tetracycline (resistance up to 20%) and trimethoprim/co-trimoxazole except for acute bronchitis. Occasional strains in UK now less penicillin-sensitive (MIC 0.1–1 mg/l); normally treatable by high doses of conventional therapy. Outbreaks of infection in Spain, South Africa, New Guinea with multiply resistant strains (penicillin MIC > 2 mg/l, also resistant to erythromycin, tetracycline, chloramphenicol); cefotaxime and vancomycin have been successfully used (isolation for these strains: ①).

Prevention: Polysaccharide vaccine available for at-risk groups (➤337); includes 23 capsular serotypes which cause > 90% invasive infections. Combine with penicillin prophylaxis after splenectomy (➤132).

Enterococci

Enterococcus faecalis and *faecium* (and rare others).

Pathogenesis: Various putative virulence factors, including adhesins and enzymes. Commonly superinfect patients receiving cephalosporins.

Epidemiology: Normal flora of colon. Resistant strains spread in hospital by hands and equipment; survive well on surfaces in the environment. Hospital-acquired infections increasingly common.

Spectrum of disease
Urinary tract infection (➤58).

Infective endocarditis (➤37). IE must be excluded whenever enterococci are grown from blood cultures.

IV catheter infection: Also other foreign bodies.

Wound colonisation/infection: Mixed with other faecal flora in wounds, ulcers, abscesses, bedsores. Not usually clinically significant.

Laboratory diagnosis: Tolerant of heat, bile salts and high salt concentrations. Ready (24 h) growth on many media to form small, shiny colonies. Some strains α- or β-haemolytic. Lancefield grouping of colonies by latex agglutination.

Treatment: Benzylpenicillin the drug of choice, but enterococci are naturally among the most penicillin-resistant streptococci (especially *Enterococcus faecium*); not killed by penicillin or vancomycin alone (add gentamicin for synergistic bactericidal effect in infective endocarditis ➤39). More sensitive *in vitro* to ampicillin/amoxycillin than benzylpenicillin, but larger doses of benzylpenicillin can be given so the difference is not clinically significant. Sensitive to vancomycin, teicoplanin; **resistant to cephalosporins**, trimethoprim. Recent outbreaks of 'ampicillin-' and 'high-level gentamicin-resistant' *Enterococcus faecalis* and *faecium* render treatment of serious infection difficult. Thirty to 50% strains in some hospitals are ampicillin- and/or high-level gentamicin-resistant. Occasional vancomycin-resistant and multiply resistant strains. (Isolation for these ①).

19: Aerobic Gram-positive Rods

A mixed bag of mainly facultative anaerobes. Although obligately anaerobic, *Propionibacterium* spp. cause similar clinical syndromes to the coryneforms, and are therefore considered here. Some of these organisms are associated with specific invasive or toxin-associated infections including *Bacillus anthracis*, *Listeria monocytogenes* and *Corynebacterium diphtheriae*. Others are opportunist pathogens. Usage is inconsistent, but we shall use 'coryneforms' and 'diphtheroids' interchangeably for small Gram-positive rods that stain variably, tend to be arranged in angled pairs or palisades, are non-branching, and share various biochemical features. Coryneforms include a number of *Corynebacterium* spp. (e.g. *striatum*, *renale*) and *Listeria* spp., together with a few non-human pathogens.

Table 74 Classification of aerobic Gram-positive rods

Genus	Species	Notes
Bacillus	**anthracis**	Causes anthrax (➤177)
	cereus	Causes food poisoning (➤178)
	(*subtilis, thuringiensis, pumilis, licheniformis*, etc.)	Uncommon opportunistic infections. Environmental organisms, frequently contaminate clinical specimens
Listeria	**monocytogenes**	Grow at low temperature; tumbling motility (➤178)
	(*innocua, ivanovii, seeligeri*, etc.)	Not human pathogens
Corynebacterium	**diphtheriae**	Causes diphtheria (➤180)
	jeikeium	Multiply antibiotic-resistant
	minutissimum	Causes erythrasma
	(*renale, striatum, ulcerans, xerosis*, CDC groups, *pseudotuberculosis*, etc.)	Skin and upper respiratory commensals, rare pathogens
Propionibacterium	acnes, etc.	Obligate anaerobes
(Rhodococcus)	(equi)	Horse and rare human pathogen (➤182)
Arcanobacterium	haemolyticum	Formerly *Corynebacterium haemolyticum*
Lactobacillus spp.		Large group of uncommon pathogens
Erysipelothrix	rhusiopathiae	Causes erysipeloid (➤89)
Nocardia	asteroides (brasiliensis, otitidis-caviarum, 'caviae')	Weakly acid-fast, aerobic

Rothia denticarosa, *Kurthia* spp. and *Bifidobacterium bifidum* are generally mucosal commensals, and very rare causes of local septic lesions in humans.

Bacillus spp.

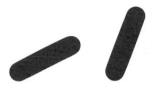

Large, spore-forming Gram-positive rods. Most are obligate aerobes and, with the exception of *Bacillus anthracis*, are common environmental organisms in the UK. Thus they frequently contaminate clinical specimens, and true infection must be carefully distinguished. Considerable colonial, staining (frequently appearing Gram-negative), biochemical and antigenic variation is present within this genus; *Bacillus* spp. are often difficult to identify to species level (✈), and are readily mistaken for other organisms.

Bacillus anthracis ⓘ ⊠
Pathogenesis: Depends on polypeptide capsule (prevents phagocytosis) and plasmid-encoded protein toxins (bind to cell surfaces and block adenyl cyclase ⇒ increased vascular permeability ⇒ shock).

Epidemiology: *Bacillus anthracis* forms spores which may remain infective in soil for decades. Economically important domesticated animal pathogen in many countries of Africa, Asia and Indian subcontinent. Occasional incidents in UK cattle (~two reports p.a.). **Occupational disease** in humans in the UK (mainly hide and wool workers). Acquired from infected herbivore carcasses. In the past anthrax has been associated with tanneries and textile industries in which humans come into contact with animal hide or hair. Vaccination of livestock and industrial disinfection procedures have essentially eradicated this form of disease in the developed world. In the developing world anthrax still occurs, and here is also associated with animal herding.

Spectrum of disease: Causes **anthrax**.

Laboratory diagnosis: One of the few non-motile *Bacillus* spp.; capsule demonstrable by McFadyean's stain. Grows readily (24h) on most media to large, grey colonies with wavy margins ('Medusa head'); ✈. Serology available for epidemiological investigations (✈).

Prevention: Investigation of animal deaths, incineration, isolation, animal vaccination (live, attenuated strain); disinfection of imported animal products; immunisation of exposed workers and vets (repeated toxoid injections). Very rarely spread human to human, but isolate ④.

CLINICAL SYNDROME
Anthrax ⊠ ④
Clinical features: Cutaneous anthrax (syn 'malignant pustule') accounts for most cases. Infection is acquired by inoculation of spores into an abrasion in the skin. After 3–10 days, a painless pruritic papule develops, which then vesiculates and ulcerates, leaving a necrotic ulcer ('eschar'), which may be surrounded by a ring of vesicles. Painful regional lymphadenopathy and local oedema are usual. Malaise, fever and leucocytosis occur in 50% of patients. Untreated mortality is ~20%, usually as a result of bacteraemia. **Inhalational anthrax** is much rarer. It occurs in industry following inhalation of very large numbers of spores, and causes haemorrhage in mediastinal lymph nodes. Patients present with a few days' history of upper respiratory symptoms, followed by rapid deterioration, with dyspnoea, cyanosis, shock and death. CXR shows mediastinal widening and pleural effusion. **Gastrointestinal anthrax** is extremely rare. It occurs after eating meat heavily contaminated with spores and causes abdominal pain and haemorrhagic diarrhoea. **Bacteraemia** is a terminal event common to all these syndromes.

Microbiological investigations: Aspirate fluid from vesicles surrounding pustule, and send blood cultures (**warn lab!**).

Antibiotic management: Antibiotics do not speed healing of the cutaneous lesion, but prevent death due to bacteraemic spread. Penicillin is the drug of choice—iv benzylpenicillin 1.2 g 6-hly, increased in severe infection. Tetracyclines and erythromycin are also effective.

Bacillus cereus

Pathogenesis: Strains causing food poisoning (➤44) either produce heat-stable peptides (emetic syndrome from reheated rice) or enterotoxin (diarrhoea associated with a variety of foods). Production of an enterotoxin and a haemolysin (cereolysin) may be associated with pathogenesis of other infections; produce dermonecrosis in rabbit model. All strains produce phospholipase, which is not believed to have a pathogenic role.

Epidemiology: Widespread in the environment, and present in many foods. Serotyping available (➤). Σ ~130.

Spectrum of disease: Short-lasting **food poisoning** (1–6 h incubation vomiting, or 10–15 h incubation diarrhoeal syndromes). May be isolated from clinical specimens, **frequently as a contaminant** (especially from samples taken from drainage bags, e.g. biliary or wound drainage), but occasionally cause **opportunist infections** in traumatic wounds contaminated with soil, and in the immunocompromised and IVDUs (also burn wounds, iv catheters, bacteraemia, meningitis, CSF shunt infection). Occasional **endophthalmitis** (postsurgical or post-traumatic, also metastatic following bacteraemia).

Laboratory diagnosis: Motile and non-capsulate. Ready (24 h) growth to colonies resembling *Bacillus anthracis*; selective medium available, relying on lecithinase production. Readily isolated, in high numbers, from food vehicles of food poisoning if available (➤ for confirmation of toxigenicity and typing).

Treatment: Food poisoning usually self-limiting. Antibiotic sensitivity unpredictable: often resistant to many β-lactam antibiotics; most strains sensitive to gentamicin, erythromycin and vancomycin.

Prevention: Cold storage and thorough reheating of cooked rice.

Other Bacillus spp. have been isolated from cases of food poisoning, and occasionally from opportunist infections, but are more commonly contaminants. *Bacillus* spp. spores survive washing temperatures, hence they are frequently found in hospital linen, whence patients and specimens (e.g. blood culture broths) may be contaminated.

Listeria monocytogenes and other Listeria spp.

Short Gram-positive rods. Only *Listeria monocytogenes* is considered a human pathogen.

Pathogenesis: Usually acquired by ingestion. Infective dose unknown, but likelihood of infection is clearly dose-related. Listeriolysin O (resembles streptolysin O ➤170) may aid survival within phagocyte. Various toxins, including cytolysin, cell penetration factor, etc. Resistance to infection depends on cell-mediated immunity.

Epidemiology: All *Listeria* spp. are widespread in domestic animal faeces, in the environment and in many foods (meats, dairy produce, vegetables); can multiply at low temperature (from 4°C) to reach high numbers. About 5% faecal carriage rate in normal adults, normally transient following ingestion. May also be transmitted transplacentally, perinatally or by direct contact with infected animals or birds. Some cases/outbreaks have proven source (e.g. coleslaw, pâté, soft cheese, milk), but most are sporadic (plus rare cross-infection in hospital). Rise in UK cases in 1980s, now falling, probably as a result of control measures aimed at pâté and soft cheeses (currently Σ 100). Serotyping (➤) shows most UK cases type 4, with a few type 1/2. No reliable evidence that persistent *Listeria* infection causes recurrent abortion.

Laboratory diagnosis: Grows readily (24 h) on many laboratory media; selective media are useful for isolation from mixed flora (e.g. foods, faeces). Colonies of *Listeria monocytogenes* and a few others are haemolytic and resemble Gp B β-haemolytic streptococci. Differentiation of species reliable by rapid (24 h) commercial biochemical test kits (➤ confirmation for important isolates), but this is only needed from food and environment. **Blood culture** is the most sensitive and specific test for **all** infections, but may be negative in late neonatal infection (LNI). Gram stain is positive in only ~30% CSFs that grow *Listeria*. Culture of conception products positive in early neonatal infection, often negative in LNI. Culture of maternal faeces, urine and HVS is rarely (and serology never) helpful.

CLINICAL SYNDROME
Listeriosis
Clinical features: Most infections occur in three well-defined risk groups: pregnant women, neonates and immunocompromised adults. Disease can occur rarely in adults with no obvious underlying condition.

Pregnancy-associated infection: Of proven infections, 25% cause **abortion and stillbirth**; 70% **neonatal sepsis** (➤110); and 5% maternal infection without fetus being affected. Probably many others go unrecognised; may cause flu-like illness alone. **Early neonatal infections** (ENI: birth–4 days old) usually present with severe systemic sepsis, bacteraemia, meningitis, pneumonia, abscesses: associated with prematurity, maternal fever, obstetric complications (mortality ~50%). **Late neonatal infections** (LNI: from 5 days) are less common and milder (mortality ~10%), and frequently present with meningitis and fever alone.

Adults and the immunocompromised: Meningitis (occasional cerebritis, 'rhombencephalitis' or cerebral abscess with raised CSF white cells but negative culture; cellular reaction may be predominantly lymphocytic) and **bacteraemia**, rare IE (native and prosthetic valves), arthritis, hepatitis. Associated with malignancy, immunosuppression, organ transplants, chronic liver and renal disease, but 10–15% cases have no predisposing illness. Mortality up to 50%.

Microbiological investigations: Isolation of organisms from blood, CSF or other normally sterile site such as joint fluid (see above). In meningitis the CSF findings are indistinguishable from other causes of bacterial meningitis. CSF Gram stain is positive in ~30% that subseqently grow *Listeria monocytogenes* from blood or CSF.

Treatment: Benzylpenicillin or ampicillin/amoxycillin (+ gentamicin for improved cidal effect for first 7–10 days for serious infections). Trimethoprim is an alternative, but chloramphenicol is less effective. Tetracycline and erythromycin are also effective. Treatment should be given for 2 weeks, extended to 3 weeks in severe infection such as parenchymal CNS infection, and 4–6 weeks for endocarditis. **Listeria is always resistant to cephalosporins, hence cephalosporin + benzylpenicillin best used for empirical therapy of neonatal meningitis/septicaemia when Gram stain of CSF negative.**

Prevention of listeriosis
The Department of Health has issued a booklet detailing guidelines to help prevent listeriosis in vulnerable groups. This is also available in a number of ethnic minority languages, and every pregnant woman should be given a copy. Guidelines are summarised below.

Vulnerable groups are defined as pregnant women, neonates and immunocompromised individuals. They should avoid the following **high-risk foods:** soft ripened cheeses (e.g. brie, camembert, blue cheese), all forms of pâté and cooked chilled meals and ready-to-eat poultry unless thoroughly reheated until piping hot before being eaten.

Advice on food storage and handling:
• Keep foods for as short a time as possible, follow storage instructions and observe 'best-by' and 'eat-by' dates.
• Do not eat undercooked poultry or meat products. Reheat cooked chilled meals thoroughly according to instructions on the label. Wash salads, fruit and vegetables that will be eaten raw.
• Make sure refrigerator is working properly and keeping food really cold.
• Store cooked foods in the refrigerator separately from raw foods and cheeses.
• When reheating food, make sure it is heated until piping hot all the way through and do not reheat more than once.
• When using a microwave oven observe the

standing times recommended by the manufacturers to ensure an even distribution of heat before the food is eaten.

• Throw away left-over reheated food. Cooked food which is not to be eaten straight away should be cooled as rapidly as possible and then stored in a refrigerator.

Pregnant women should also avoid contact with sheep at lambing time, and should not handle silage.

Corynebacterium diphtheriae ① ✉

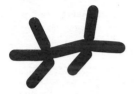

Small, pleomorphic Gram-positive rods, arranged in 'Chinese letters'.

Pathogenesis: Diphtheria toxin coded on *tox* gene inserted into chromosome by lysogenic phage. Iron restriction increases toxin production. Exotoxin is a heat-stable protein consisting of two fragments. Fragment B binds to membrane receptors on target cells in the myocardium, nerves and kidneys. Fragment A enters the cell and abolishes protein synthesis by preventing polypeptide chain elongation at the ribosome. **Local** mucosal necrosis ('pseudomembrane'), and **systemic** absorption ⇒ neuro- and myocardiotoxicity (especially with pharyngeal, rare with skin infection). Laryngeal diphtheria most com-

monly ⇒ respiratory obstruction because of restricted size and rigidity of air passage. No systemic invasion.

Epidemiology: Widespread in the developing world, especially tropics; current major outbreak in CIS and other ex-USSR states. Occasional spread in developed world (e.g. among IVDUs in US cities). Usually spread from case or carrier by nasopharyngeal secretions. Nasal carriers shed the most bacilli and are usually only mildly unwell. Skin infection important in tropics, where it often causes mild local inflammation only and establishes immunity. Since the advent of immunisation, diphtheria is rare in the UK (Σ 5–10, all imported; frequently infections of cutaneous ulcers acquired in Indian subcontinent). No animal reservoir. The organism survives in dust and transmission by fomites occurs.

Spectrum of disease: Causes **diphtheria** (➤181).

Cutaneous infection ('veld sore', 'desert sore') may occur, usually in tropical environments with poor hygiene. Lesions start as tender pustules which break down to leave a punched out ulcer with a grey sloughy base. Sores are highly infectious but systemic toxicity is usually less severe than in pharyngeal infection.

Laboratory diagnosis: Ready growth (24–48 h) on media containing serum to form greyish colonies which are black on tellurite medium. Commercial biochemical test kits reliable for differentiation from commensal coryneforms (further 24 h). Toxigenicity determined by immunoprecipitation in agar (Elek test); this takes only 24 h but is technically demanding

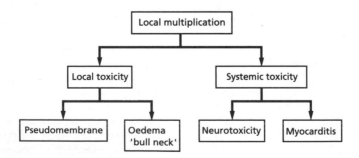

Fig. 6 Pathogenesis of diphtheria.

for laboratories performing it irregularly, ✦. Three main biotypes (*mitis, intermedius* or *gravis*) by staining and colonial appearances; **all** may contain the phage and be toxigenic, but *mitis* less commonly than the others.

Prevention: Has been achieved in the developed world by widespread immunisation with toxoid (➤337). This has also abolished asymptomatic carriage of the organism, although the reason remains unclear. Isolation/prophylaxis of cases and contacts. Patients with non-toxigenic strains should receive antibiotic treatment, and limited screening measures should be considered because contacts may carry toxigenic variants. Discuss therapeutic, diagnostic and public health measures for suspected cases early (☎).

CLINICAL SYNDROME
Diphtheria ✉ ①
A severe pharyngeal infection caused by toxigenic strains of *Corynebacterium diphtheriae*. Death occurs from laryngeal obstruction or the systemic effects of diphtheria exotoxin.

Clinical features:
Incubation time: Two to six days.
Symptoms and signs: Malaise, fever and fatigue. Sore throat (often mild). Thick adherent green-black pseudomembrane on tonsils extending on to the soft palate and uvula. Local lymphadenopathy and oedema ('bull neck'). Nasal infection also occurs, with purulent nasal discharge. Exotoxin causes local pharyngeal paralysis and systemic effects, including myocarditis with signs of heart failure and arrhythmia. Neurological signs include external ophthalmoplegia, dysphagia and peripheral neuritis causing paralysis.
Investigations: Diagnosis depends on clinical suspicion and culture of the organism from the pharynx or wound. ☎ **Always list appropriate travel history and other clinical details on request cards for cases of pharyngitis and skin infection so that appropriate selective indicator media will be inoculated.** Supportive investigations include ECG, which may show abnormality

in the absence of clinical evidence of cardiac involvement. ST–T wave changes and 1° heart block are common Progression to 2° and 3° block are poor prognostic signs.
Management: Antibiotic treatment with benzylpenicillin or erythromycin. Antitoxin (raised in horses) should be given as soon as the diagnosis is seriously suspected. **Mortality increases with delay** between the onset of symptoms and the administration of antitoxin. Isolation ①. Supportive care for respiratory obstruction and systemic effects of exotoxin.
Immunity: Clinical infection does not always induce adequate antibody response against toxin. Patients should be immunised during the recovery phase. The Schick test is a skin test for immunity—it is not routinely used.

Other *Corynebacterium* spp.

Corynebacterium jeikeium (previously 'JK coryneforms')
An uncommon skin commensal causing outbreaks of bacteraemia secondary to iv catheter and wound infection in haematological malignancy wards. Occasionally also on cardiac surgery (causing endocarditis) and neurosurgery (meningitis) wards. Highly antibiotic-resistant; usually sensitive only to vancomycin and teicoplanin. *Corynebacterium* CDC group D2 are bacteriologically similar, but cause UTI, associated with renal stones, and rare bacteraemia.

Corynebacterium minutissimum
Causes an infection of the stratum corneum of the groins, axillae and toe webs (erythrasma ➤92). These areas fluoresce red under Wood's light. Culture is possible from biopsies, but unnecessary.

Corynebacterium ulcerans
Causes bovine mastitis, and zoonotic human pharyngitis and minor skin sepsis (from direct contact or milk), usually without systemic toxic effects. Rare strains produce diphtheria toxin and can cause diphtheria-like illnesses.

Corynebacterium CDC groups A4 and G2
Rarely associated with endophthalmitis and other infections.

Corynebacterium pseudotuberculosis
Pathogen of sheep causing human axillary or cervical lymphadenitis after occupational exposure (especially in Australia).

Most of the above, and many other commensal corynebacteria (including *xerosis*, *bovis*, etc.) are capable of causing bacteraemia and iv catheter and CSF shunt infection, and occasional IE, especially of prosthetic valves. Many isolates are sensitive to penicillin or erythromycin, but vancomycin (or teicoplanin) is the only fully reliable agent while awaiting sensitivity results.

Propionibacterium acnes
Commensal of the skin, mouth, gut and vagina, and is implicated in acne (➤92). It is a rare cause of iv catheter and prosthetic material infection, and very rarely causes IE of prosthetic and native valves. It is a common blood culture contaminant.

Rhodococcus equi
Very rare cause of necrotising pneumonia in immunocompromised patients, which usually responds to erythromycin + gentamicin.

Arcanobacterium haemolyticum
Causes acute pharyngitis in young adults, often associated with a scarlatiniform rash, occasionally with quinsy. Rarely IE or skin sepsis. Responds to erythromycin or oral penicillin.

Lactobacillus spp.
Long Gram-positive rods—commensals of the gastrointestinal tract and vagina—that generally prefer low pH for optimal growth. Some are obligate anaerobes. They may grow to form tiny non- or α-haemolytic colonies on blood agar (24–48 h). Very rare isolates from significant

infections—blood culture, pelvic abscess mixed with other local flora. Dubious role in lower UTI. Occasionally vancomycin- and teicoplanin-resistant.

Erysipelothrix rhusiopathiae
Pathogen of mammals and fish, and causes skin ulcers (rare bacteraemia, IE), especially in butchers and fishmongers (➤89). Usually sensitive to erythromycin or penicillin.

Nocardia asteroides and other spp.
Branched, filamentous. Gram-positive rods, most of which are weakly acid-fast. Aerobic counterpart of *Actinomyces israelii* (➤222) (but most commonly cause invasive infections in the immunocompromised from external sources, rather than focal sepsis from the commensal flora of normal individuals).

Pathogenesis: Common in the environment. Inhalation route, occasionally direct inoculation. Virulence factors unknown.

Epidemiology: Infection by *Nocardia asteroides* almost entirely restricted to patients receiving steroids and other immunosuppressive agents for transplants, haematological malignancy and autoimmune diseases; also HIV. Rare traumatic inoculation to normal patients (usually *Nocardia brasiliensis* or *otitidiscaviarum*); one cause of 'Madura foot' in the tropics (especially *Nocardia madurae*).

Spectrum of disease: Local multiplication ⇒ chronic progressive pulmonary abscesses (⇒ secondary abscesses in brain, liver, mediastinum, bones, etc. in 30%). Often a differential diagnosis of tuberculosis in immunocompromised individuals.

Laboratory diagnosis: Warn laboratory of chronic nature of infection in compromised patient so cultures are prolonged (☎). Culture of invasive specimens (tissue biopsy, BAL) is much more sensitive than sputum or pus alone. Branching filaments may be seen in stains (Gram, ZN), but culture is more sensitive. Strict aerobes, with often slow growth on blood, Sabouraud's and other agars (2–21 days) to waxy, yellowish colonies: ✦. Sometimes isolated fortuitously on Lowenstein–Jensen cultures for mycobacteria.

Treatment: Co-trimoxazole is the most established agent, but patients with AIDS and co-trimoxazole intolerance have responded to various combinations of minocycline, imipenem, co-amoxiclav and amikacin (☎).

20: Coliforms, Vibrios and Campylobacters

Coliforms (syn. enterobacteria, *Enterobacteriaceae*)

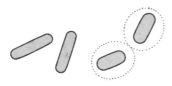

Robust Gram-negative, rod-shaped, facultatively anaerobic organisms that colonise the large bowel of mammals. None produces the enzyme indophenol oxidase, most are motile by flagella. Nowadays most laboratories identify members of this group by commercial biochemical test kits (results take 24 h), but some species are confirmed by antigen content (e.g. agglutination for *Salmonella* spp.). Many different virulence factors can be possessed by members of this group, which is reflected in the wide range of diseases that they can produce, but virtually all are capable of causing UTI and wound infection.

Coliforms rapidly replace the normal largely Gram-positive and non-sporing anaerobic flora of mucosal surfaces of ill patients and those receiving broad-spectrum antibiotics. Granulating surfaces are also frequently colonised. Coliforms are most commonly isolated from these sites in hospitalised patients (including sputum, throat swabs, leg ulcers), and careful clinical assessment is necessary to detect the occasional significant infection amid the abundant cases of colonisation.

Resistance to ampicillin/amoxycillin is now too widespread to recommend these agents for empirical treatment of any coliform, and trimethoprim resistance is rising. Co-amoxiclav and oral cephalosporins remain reliable for 'easy' coliforms (see below); resistance to parenteral or broad-spectrum cephalosporins is uncommon, and resistance to aminoglycosides, imipenem and quinolones is rare overall in *Enterobacteriaceae* from the UK.

Vibrios and campylobacters and their groups are considered with the coliforms (despite bacteriological similarities to the pseudomonads) because of their related clinical significance.

Coliforms may be considered in two groups – '**hard**' and '**easy**' – reflecting their usual pattern of sensitivity to antibiotics, in particular the likelihood they will be or can become cephalosporin-resistant. '**Hard**' coliforms include *Enterobacter* spp., *Serratia* spp., *Citrobacter* spp., *Proteus vulgaris*, *Providencia* spp. and their relatives. '**Easy**' coliforms include *Escherichia coli*, *Proteus mirabilis* and most *Klebsiella* spp.

Lipopolysaccharide/endotoxin and septic shock

Bacterial lipopolysaccharide (LPS or endotoxin; see diagram) is found within the outer cell membrane of most Gram-negative bacteria, and its release plays a major role in infections caused by coliforms, *Neisseria meningitidis*, *Pseudomonas aeruginosa* and *Bacteroides fragilis*. LPS may reach the circulation from bacteria present within the bloodstream (bacteraemia), or be absorbed from abscesses and other local infections (blood cultures negative). It comprises a hydrophobic lipid moiety ('lipid A'), which is buried within the membrane and is highly conserved between different species, a more variable polysaccharide **core**, and a hydrophilic, highly variable polysaccharide **outer region** (O antigen). O antigens are often used to serotype coliform species. Most of the physiological activity of LPS resides in the lipid A; measurable responses follow parenteral administration of minute quantities. Chemical and immunological antagonists of LPS and of the reactions it induces (e.g. TNF and other cytokine release) are under assessment as possible adjuvant treatments for bacterial septic shock; however, the mainstays of all such treatment will remain **circulatory support** and **rapid bacterial killing** by antibiotics. LPS is found uncommonly in the bloodstream of patients presenting with sepsis syndrome (➤158), suggesting that intermittent, local or only early release is important.

Structure of bacterial lipopolysaccharide

Table 75 *Enterobacteriaceae*

Genus	Species	Notes
Escherichia	***coli***	Many strains now recognised and given acronyms (➤187)
	(fergusonii, hermanni, vulneris)	Rare human pathogens
Klebsiella spp.	Sometimes divided into controversial 'species': *oxytoca, pneumoniae, aerogenes, ozaenae, rhinoscleromatis* (➤189)	
Proteus	***mirabilis,*** *vulgaris*	*Proteus vulgaris* is a 'hard' coliform (➤184), clinically similar to *Citrobacter* and *Enterobacter* spp. (➤190)
Salmonella	***typhi, paratyphi A, B and C***	'Enteric' salmonellae. Non-lactose-fermenters (➤190)
	'*enteritidis* gp'	Food-poisoning salmonellae. Over 2200 'species' classified by antigen content. Gut commensals and pathogens, many with broad host range. Non-lactose-fermenters (➤191)
Shigella	***boydii, dysenteriae, flexneri, sonnei***	Exclusively human pathogens. Non-motile. Non-lactose-fermenters (➤192)

continued on p. 186

Table 75 contd

Genus	Species	Notes
Citrobacter	amalonaticus, freundii, koseri	Related groups. Frequently colonise hospitalised patients and occasionally cause nosocomial infections. 'Hard' coliforms (➤184, 193)
Enterobacter	aerogenes, cloacae (gergoviae, sakazakii, 'agglomerans')	
Morganella	morganii	Microbiologically related to Proteus spp.; cause similar infections to Citrobacter and Enterobacter spp. 'Hard' coliforms (➤184)
Providencia	alcalifaciens, rettgeri, stuartii	
Serratia	liquifaciens, marcescens, etc.	Some strains red-pigmented. 'Hard' coliforms (➤184, 194)
Yersinia	pestis	Cause of plague; see under 'fastidious Gram-negative organisms (➤211)
	enterocolitica, pseudotuberculosis, etc.	Cause uncommon gastrointestinal infections (➤194)
(Erwinia)	(herbicola)	Also called Enterobacter agglomerans. Yellow-pigmented
(Hafnia)	(alvei)	Normal gut commensal, very rare pathogen.

Others include Buttiauxella agrestis, Cedecea davisiae and lapagei, Edwardsiella tarda, Kluyvera ascorbata and cryocrescens, Tatumella ptyseos: most have been isolated from the environment and occasionally from animal and human clinical material.

Vibrios and relatives

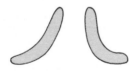

Most are curved, Gram-negative rods, tolerant of high salt ('halophilic vibrios' require high salt-containing media for optimal isolation) and alkalinity, producing indophenol oxidase. Most can cause both **diarrhoea** and **tissue infections**, with the species differing in their tendency to cause one more commonly than the other (Table 76).

Table 76 Classification of vibrios and relatives

Genus	Species	Notes
Vibrio	**cholerae**	Strains carrying the O1 antigen cause cholera (➤194); others ('non-O1' strains) may cause diarrhoea and wound infection
	vulnificus, damsela (alginolyticus etc.)	Wound infection, seawater/shellfish-associated. Rare diarrhoea, seafood-associated (➤196)
	parahaemolyticus, fluvialis, hollisae, mimicus (furnissii)	Diarrhoea, seafood-associated. Rare wound infection, seawater-associated (➤195)
Aeromonas	hydrophila, sobria, caviae (salmonicida)	Wound infection, fresh-water-associated. Probably also rare causes of diarrhoea (➤196)
(Plesiomonas)	(shigelloides)	Antigenically related to Shigella spp.; may cause diarrhoea

Table 77 Classification of campylobacters and relatives

Genus	Species	Notes
Campylobacter	*jejuni, coli (hyointestinalis, lari, upsaliensis,* etc.)	Primarily cause intestinal infections. Most grow selectively well at high temperature (42°C) (➤196)
	fetus	Causes rare septicaemia in immunocompromised patients (➤197)
Helicobacter	*pylori*	Infects gastric mucosa. Strongly urease-positive (➤197)
	(cinaedi, fennelliae, etc.)	May cause proctitis and enteritis in homosexual men, and have been isolated from blood cultures

Campylobacters and relatives

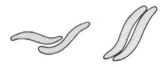

Curved or spiral, motile, Gram-negative rods that generally do not grow in conventional culture conditions: require low O_2 and high CO_2 concentrations, and incorporation of whole blood, haemin, charcoal, etc. in isolation media (Table 77). Produce indophenol oxidase; usually identified by colonial appearance on selective medium, Gram stain, plus a few simple tests.

Escherichia coli

Ubiquitous colonist of the normal colon, and the commonest Gram-negative human pathogen. Best considered as **a group of distinct organisms**, some possessing virulence factors that enable them to cause specific diarrhoeal diseases, urinary tract and systemic infections. Names and abbreviations for these organisms proliferate (see below). All grow rapidly on common laboratory media, most ferment lactose. Typable by somatic 'O', capsular 'K' and flagellar 'H' antigens (➤); some types are associated with possession of particular virulence factors (toxins, epithelial adhesins), and probing for these genes gives specific diagnostic confirmation (➤). Adherence to urinary, intestinal and other epithelia via surface filaments (fimbriae; colonisation factors) is fundamental to pathogenesis.

Enterotoxigenic *Escherichia coli* (ETEC)
Pathogenesis: Three groups of virulence factors:
- **Heat-labile toxin** (LT). Closely related to cholera toxin (➤194).
- **Heat-stable toxin** (ST). At least two types, ST_A (acts via cGMP) and ST_B (uncertain mechanism).
- **Colonisation factors** (CFA I–IV, etc.), adhering to ileum and jejunum. Mannose-resistant haemagglutinins.

ETEC produce a CFA plus one or both of LT and ST.

Epidemiology: Major causes of **diarrhoea in children** < 5 years in developing world; **travellers' diarrhoea** (cause up to 75%; ➤48). Mainly water-borne spread, from faecal contamination. Uncommon in developed world. Rare outbreaks in neonatal units, spread on staff hands and in feeds.

Spectrum of disease: Non-inflammatory acute diarrhoea, sometimes resembling cholera. Incubation period 1–2 days; lasts up to 3 weeks in malnourished children (➤44).

Laboratory diagnosis: Diagnostic investigations not routinely performed in laboratories in developed world nowadays, but variety of tests available for epidemiological research (cytopathic effects in cell culture, immunoassay, DNA probes, animal tests ➤).

Treatment: Symptoms are self-limiting, but duration and severity reduced by ciprofloxacin or trimethoprim. Trimethoprim resistance increasing.

Prevention: Improve sanitation. Breast-feeding is protective. Boil suspect water.

Verocytotoxic *Escherichia coli* **(VTEC)**
Sometimes called enterohaemorrhagic *Escherichia coli* (EHEC).
Pathogenesis: 'Attachment–effacement' to terminal ileum and colon. Produce one or both Vero toxins VT1 and VT2 (also called SLT-I and SLT-II) – very similar to Shiga toxin (*Shigella dysenteriae* type 1 ➤192). This is a ricin-like enzyme with five B subunits which bind to an enterocyte receptor and internalise the single toxic A subunit, which inhibits protein synthesis by inactivating the 60S ribosomal subunit. VT is encoded on a plasmid which is frequently present in type O157 strains (especially O157:H7; occasionally others, e.g. O26, O111). VT also causes vascular endothelial damage, leading to DIC and microangiopathic haemolytic anaemia – see HUS below.
Epidemiology: Increasingly recognised in England and Wales (Σ 473 cases in 1992). Commonest in children < 5 years and the elderly, but affects any age. Found in calf and cattle faeces: widespread outbreaks associated with undercooked beefburgers, unpasteurised milk. Occasional outbreaks in child day care and elderly nursing care centres, probably transmitted on staff hands. Phage-typing available (➤).
Spectrum of disease: Range from mild, **loose stool** to **haemorrhagic colitis** and, in children and adolescents, **haemolytic uraemic syndrome (HUS)** with acute renal failure, microangiopathic haemolytic anaemia and thrombocytopenia. Specialist paediatric renal referral is required. Incubation period of diarrhoea *c.* 4 days, duration 2–9 days.
Laboratory diagnosis: Inform laboratory of haemorrhagic nature of diarrhoea or HUS (☎); faeces inoculated to sorbitol–MacConkey agar. Sorbitol non-fermenting colonies are tested for agglutination with O157 antiserum after 24 h (95% non-O157 *Escherichia coli* do ferment; most O157 do not). Cytotoxicity assays and faecal/colony DNA probes available (➤). Rapid reduction in numbers of VTEC in faeces over first 4 days, and diarrhoeal prodrome may be finished when HUS appears, so serology for O157 antibodies may be useful retrospectively (➤).

Treatment: Supportive; value of antibiotics (e.g. ciprofloxacin) in HUS or haemorrhagic colitis not established.

Enteroinvasive *Escherichia coli* **(EIEC)**
Pathogenesis: Very similar to *Shigella* spp. and contain Shiga-like toxins (➤192). Lipopolysaccharide capsule aids survival of stomach acid and small-bowel enzymes. Penetrate and multiply in colonic epithelial cells ⇒ tissue destruction. Virulent strains can penetrate cells in culture.
Epidemiology: Appears to be exclusively a human disease. Faecal–oral spread, but large infective dose (10^8 bacteria). Occasional outbreaks in developed world in closed communities (e.g. residential homes) with poor hygiene.
Spectrum of disease: Bacillary dysentery-like. Incubation 2–4 days. Occasional penetration to bloodstream in the immunocompromised.
Laboratory diagnosis: Usually non-motile and do not produce gas from glucose fermentation (i.e. like *Shigella* spp.). Ready (24 h) growth on MacConkey agar, then test non-lactose-fermenting colonies with battery of antisera (e.g. O124, O164). Confirm by DNA probes, cell culture penetration tests (➤).
Treatment: Supportive; consider trimethoprim or ciprofloxacin if severe.

Enteropathogenic *Escherichia coli* **(EPEC)**
Pathogenesis: Originally a heterogeneous group. No toxins consistently produced (some 'EPEC' strains produce LT, ST or VT). 'EPEC' should now be reserved for strains that 'attach–efface' to jejunal/ileal epithelial cells, causing microvillar damage, and adhere to Hep-2 cells by non-fimbrial adhesins. Antibodies to these adhesins are protective. Loss of epithelial disaccharidases ⇒ osmotic diarrhoea.
Epidemiology: Now rare in developed world, and many laboratories no longer screen routinely for EPEC (Σ < 1000 now); remains commonest cause of infantile diarrhoea in the tropics. Occasional outbreaks in hospitals, spread on hands of staff and in contaminated infant feeds. Large infective dose (up to 10^{10}). Isolation ②.

Spectrum of disease: Non-inflammatory, watery infantile enteritis. Incubation 8–60 h. Can be long-lasting.

Laboratory diagnosis: Discuss investigations with a microbiologist (☎). Associated (but not specifically) with certain serotypes (e.g. O26, O55, O128ab); after 24 h incubation on MacConkey agar plates, screen lactose-fermenting colonies with agglutinating antisera. Adhesion in cell culture, probes for adhesins (➤).

Treatment: Supportive measures; uncertain value of antibiotics (e.g. trimethoprim, ciprofloxacin). Isolation ②.

Other *Escherichia coli* diarrhoeas
Evidence is growing to support these strains' roles, but little information yet available on management:

• **Enteroaggregative** *Escherichia coli* **(EAggEC):** a cause of probably common, long-lasting inflammatory diarrhoea in children and travellers. EAggEC adhere to colonic mucosa in a 'stacked-brick' pattern, causing haemorrhagic necrosis of villus tips. DNA probes available (➤).

• **Diffusely adherent** *Escherichia coli* **(DAEC):** associated with childhood diarrhoea in the tropics. DNA probe available (➤).

Uropathogenic *Escherichia coli*
Compared with strains colonising the gut, most strains causing cystitis and pyelonephritis (➤58) are positive when probed for Gal–Gal adhesins and P-fimbriae (which adhere to uroepithelium), and they also produce α-haemolysin, belong to only a few O serogroups and demonstrate mannose-resistant haemagglutination. Invasive urinary strains (causing pyelonephritis) belong to a narrower group of O types and additionally are resistant to the killing powers of serum ('serum-resistant').

Treatment: Approximate UK community resistance rates currently: 35% ampicillin/amoxycillin; 15–20% trimethoprim; 4–8% oral cephalosporins, co-amoxiclav, nitrofurantoin; 0–5% aminoglycosides, parenteral or broad-spectrum cephalosporins, quinolones.

Escherichia coli causing wound infection and bacteraemia
These strains are usually serum-resistant. Commonest Gram-negative cause of bacteraemia (➤158). Surprisingly rare cause of iv catheter infection.

Escherichia coli causing neonatal meningitis
Generally carry the K1 capsular antigen, shared with Gp B β-haemolytic streptococcus (➤110, 173).

Klebsiella spp.

Non-motile, Gram-negative rods. Classification into species is disputed within this genus, so '*Klebsiella* spp.' is the best term.

Pathogenesis: Strains causing primary pneumonia (Friedländer's bacillus) usually produce large quantities of antiphagocytic polysaccharide capsular material of serotype 3, and give mucoid colonies on solid media. Some strains from human infections carry plasmid-encoded pili and iron-scavenging systems.

Epidemiology: Many strains are normal commensals of human bowel. Strains associated with hospital outbreaks seem capable of prolonged survival on skin of hands. Capsular serotyping available (➤).

Spectrum of disease: Nosocomial infections, including outbreaks of UTI (➤58), **wound and iv catheter infection, ventilator-associated pneumonia; meningitis and septicaemia in neonates** (➤110). Occasional lower UTI in normal females. Rare community-acquired **primary pneumonia** (Friedländer's ➤25). **Rhinoscleroma:** distinct strains causing chronic upper respiratory infection.

Laboratory diagnosis: Ready growth (24 h) on most laboratory media; identity confirmed by biochemical tests (24 h).

Treatment: Normally 'easy' coliforms (➤184), but **always ampicillin/amoxycillin-resistant**, and *Klebsiella* is the commonest coliform to be clinically resistant to aminoglycosides or quinolones (but still < 5%). Nosocomial outbreaks with parenteral or broad-spectrum cephalosporin-resistant strains (by mutated β-lactamase production) frequent in French hospitals; increasingly recognised in the UK.

Proteus, Morganella and Providencia spp.

Motile, Gram-negative rods producing the enzyme urease. Many strains show 'swarming' of colonies on solid media.

Pathogenesis: No specific virulence factors known. Urease may encourage deposition of urinary calculi.

Epidemiology: *Proteus mirabilis* is a common faecal commensal; other members of the group usually acquired in hospital. Variety of typing schemes available (✦).

Spectrum of disease: UTI (➤58): *Proteus mirabilis* is a common isolate from lower UTI in young females; other members of the group commoner in the abnormal urinary tract, usually acquired in hospital. Sometimes cause pyelonephritis, septicaemia. **Wound and iv catheter infection** and secondary septicaemia.

Laboratory diagnosis: Ready growth in 24 h on most solid media; swarming strains easily recognised, but can swamp other organisms. Confirm identity by biochemical tests (24 h).

Treatment: All are nitrofurantoin-resistant. *Proteus mirabilis* is an 'easy' coliform (➤184) and has a similar sensitivity pattern to *Escherichia coli* (➤187); *Proteus vulgaris*, *Morganella* and *Providencia* are 'hard' coliforms (➤184) and *Providencia* is frequently resistant to aminoglycosides; a quinolone or imipenem may be required.

Salmonella spp.

Motile, Gram-negative rods; non-lactose-fermenters. 'Speciation' within this genus is according to possession of somatic 'O' and flagellar 'H' antigens (over 2200 named species). Not normal human commensals.

Salmonella typhi and paratyphi, A, B and C

Enteric salmonellae; exclusive human pathogens causing septicaemic illnesses (*paratyphi* B is rarely isolated from animals).

Pathogenesis: Infective dose depends upon production of stomach acid, and food vehicle, but usually 10^6–10^9 organisms. Mannose-sensitive adhesins involved in attachment to microvilli of ileum. Epithelium penetrated, and multiplication occurs in epithelial and reticuloendothelial cells ⇒ bacteraemic seeding of many organs (in first 7 days; often asymptomatic). Organisms later released to circulation ⇒ septicaemic presentation, 3 days–6 weeks after ingestion. Gut secondarily infected ⇒ hypersensitivity reaction in Peyer's patches ⇒ ulceration, haemorrhage, perforation.

Epidemiology and transmission: Distributed worldwide. Common in developing countries but rare in developed countries such as UK, due to provision of clean water supply and education of food handlers. Transmission is faeco-oral, either by water (endemic areas) or by contamination of food (non-endemic areas). Risk factors for acquisition of the organism include infancy, hypochlorhydria, abnormal bowel motility and disturbance of bowel flora as occurs following surgery or antibiotic therapy. In contrast to non-typhoidal salmonella infections, asymptomatic carriers (➤46) are a very important source of infection. *Salmonella typhi*: Σ ~175, *S. paratyphi*: Σ ~75 (imported, especially from Indian subcontinent).

Spectrum of disease: Typhoid and paratyphoid (enteric fever) (➤191).

Laboratory diagnosis: Ready growth (24 h) on most solid and blood culture media; a variety of selective media are used for isolation from stool (e.g. desoxycholate-citrate (DCA) or xylose-lysine desoxycholate (XLD) agars; these rely on growth in presence of bile salts, and biochemical reactions giving coloured colonies). Selective broth enrichment of stool for detection of carriers. Agglutination of colonies by specific antisera (e.g. *Salmonella typhi* carries O antigens 9 and 12, H antigen d, and usually also the surface polysaccharide Vi antigen); commercial biochemical test kits are useful (rapid screening of suspect colonies in 4 h, more reliable tests take further 24 h) ✦. Widal serological test only ever useful for epidemiological studies in high-risk populations.

Prevention: Improve sanitation and hygiene; vaccination (➤141). Isolation ②.

CLINICAL SYNDROME

Typhoid and paratyphoid (enteric fever) ✉ ②
Typhoid and paratyphoid, collectively referred to as enteric fever, are systemic, potentially fatal, febrile illnesses due to *Salmonella typhi* and *Salmonella paratyphi* types A, B and C. Paratyphoid is generally a milder illness than typhoid. Rarely other 'non-typhoidal salmonellae' can produce a similar illness.

Clinical features

Incubation time: One to 3 weeks; shorter with larger infecting inoculum.

Symptoms and signs: Insidious onset of fever, myalgia, abdominal pain and severe headache. Classically, fever rises in a stepwise fashion. Cough, constipation and deafness are common. Diarrhoea occurs in < 40% of patients. On examination there may be relative bradycardia, hepatosplenomegaly and rose spots, which are faint, salmon-coloured maculopapular lesions on the trunk, which blanch on pressure. Rose spots occur during the first few days of illness and are easily overlooked. Untreated, fever persists for several weeks. Mortality untreated is ~20%, with death mainly due to intestinal perforation or haemorrhage. Less common complications include psychosis, hepatitis, cholecystitis, pneumonia, pericarditis and meningitis.

Investigations: Leucopenia and abnormal liver function tests are usual. Anaemia occurs secondary to bleeding and due to haemolysis in patients with G6PD deficiency. Diagnosis is confirmed by culture of the organism from blood, stools, urine or bone marrow. Serology (Widal test) is not useful in the diagnosis of the acute attack.

Management: Antibiotic therapy reduces the mortality to < 1%. Chloramphenicol is the drug of choice for developing countries, although resistance has been widely reported, particularly from India, SE Asia and the Middle East. For travellers returning to the UK, ciprofloxacin 750 mg 12-hly po should be given. Alternative agents are amoxycillin and co-trimoxazole. Treatment should be given for 10–14 days; response is typically slow, with resolution of fever over 2–5 days.

Comments: Chronic carriage follows enteric fever in ~5% of cases. Prolonged treatment with ciprofloxacin (750 mg 12-hly po for 1 month) is often successful. Chloramphenicol and amoxycillin are ineffective. Cholecystectomy may be required, particularly if there are gallstones. **Vaccine** produces partial immunity (➤141).

'Salmonella enteritidis' group
Food-poisoning salmonellae, causing gastroenteritis in humans and many other animal species. Certain salmonellae are associated with particular animals (e.g. *Salmonella enteritidis* PT4 and chickens, *dublin* and cattle); others have wider host associations (e.g. *Salmonella virchow* and *typhimurium*).

Pathogenesis: Infective dose depends upon species, production of stomach acid, and food vehicle, but can be $< 10^2–10^9$ organisms. Mannose-sensitive adhesins involved in attachment to microvilli of ileum. Epithelium penetrated, and multiplication occurs in epithelial and reticuloendothelial cells. Incubation period 8–48 h; duration 48–96 h.

Epidemiology: Often transmitted to animals in their feed and spread between them during processing for food (e.g. commercial frozen chicken preparation results in > 50% carcasses positive). Human sporadic cases and common-source outbreaks are zoonoses and originate from inadequately cooked meat, or contamination of food eaten without further cooking. Salmonellae can readily multiply in food at environmental temperatures. Rising reported human cases in England and Wales in past 30 years (Σ 30 654 in 1993); especially brisk increase since 1985 in *Salmonella enteritidis* phage type 4, associated with chicken meat and eggs (Σ 17 258 in 1993).

Different species and phage types are common in other countries. Infection from human case or carrier is uncommon. Phage-typing is available for the common species (→).

Spectrum of disease: Gastroenteritis ⊠ (➤44), sometimes associated with **bacteraemia**, more commonly in the immunocompromised (especially AIDS). By 9 weeks, 90% cases are faecal culture-negative. Prolonged carriage (> 1 year in *c.* 1%) in bile or urine associated with biliary or urinary tract abnormality and with immunodeficiency. **Osteomyelitis** in sickle-cell disease. Rare other focal infections, including arterial aneurysm, joint prostheses. Neonates in developing world may suffer meningitis, osteomyelitis.

Laboratory diagnosis: Ready growth (24 h) on most solid and blood culture media; variety of selective media used for isolation from stool (e.g. DCA and XLD ➤190). Selective broth enrichment of stool for detection of carriers (➤46). Agglutination of colonies by specific antisera (e.g. *Salmonella enteritidis* carries O antigens 1, 9 and 12, H antigen g); commercial biochemical test kits are useful (rapid screening of suspect colonies in 4 h, more reliable tests take further 24 h) →.

Treatment: Salmonella gastroenteritis does not need antibiotic therapy unless patient is systemically ill and bacteraemia is suspected. Salmonellae are frequently fully antibiotic-sensitive in the UK, and extraintestinal infections commonly respond well to many antibiotics active against other 'easy' coliforms (➤184); however, intracellular persistence may lead to incomplete response or later recrudescence. The most reliable agents are quinolones or chloramphenicol.

Prevention: Eradication of salmonellae from farm animals; improved catering practices. Isolation ②.

Shigella spp.

Non-motile, Gram-negative rods that generally do not produce gas from glucose fermentation. All are non-lactose-fermenters except for *Shigella sonnei*, which may do so at 24 h.

Table 78 Diseases due to Salmonella spp.

Syndrome	Features	Species
Enteric fever	Severe systemic infection (see above)	*Salmonella typhi, Salmonella paratyphi* A, B and C
Salmonella gastroenteritis	Usually due to multiplication of organisms in food prior to ingestion. Incubation 8–48 h; duration short and self-limited. Vomiting, diarrhoea, abdominal cramps and fever	Many zoonotic 'non-typhoidal' species, particularly *Salmonella enteritidis*
Bacteraemia with metastatic infection	A constant feature of enteric fever, but transient bacteraemia is probably not uncommon in patients with salmonella gastroenteritis. Metastatic infection may occur in bone/joint (recent joint prosthesis or sickle-cell anaemia predispose), meninges, or very rarely atherosclerotic plaques of large blood vessels and heart valves	All species
Asymptomatic carriage	At 5 weeks, 50% still excrete organism in stools; 9% at 9 weeks. Chronic carriage refers to duration of >1 year. Follows clinical disease or asymptomatic infection. Control of infection (➤46)	All species

Pathogenesis: Small infecting dose (minimum 10–100 organisms). Attachment, then invasion of colonic mucosa; a large plasmid codes for several outer membrane proteins associated with invasion. Escape from phagocytic vacuole by haemolysin activity. Sloughing of necrotic epithelium follows, with underlying inflammation and capillary thrombosis. *Shigella dysenteriae* type 1 produces largest amount per cell of Shiga toxin (➤188) and causes the most severe disease, but other shigellae also release it. Incubation period usually 1–3 days; duration of *sonnei* dysentery usually 48 h with loose stool for several more days. Other species usually more prolonged.

Epidemiology: Worldwide distribution, but only *Shigella sonnei* commonly acquired in the UK (recent increase in reported cases in England and Wales; nearly 10 000 in 1992, 17 000 in 1993). The majority of *flexneri* cases are imported, as are all *boydii* and *dysenteriae* cases (Σ ~900). Faecal–oral spread in areas of poor hygiene (especially direct spread and via contaminated surfaces in infant and junior schools in the UK). Household contacts have high attack rate. Flying insects important in transmission (via food) in developing world. Human long-term carriers are rare, and rarely proven to transmit infection, but 75% cases still culture-positive after 7 weeks. Typing by phage susceptibility and antigen content available (➤).

Spectrum of disease: Bacillary dysentery ▣ (➤44). *Shigella sonnei* tends to produce **mild** disease, often asymptomatic. Systemic spread beyond gut is rare, but commoner in immunodeficiency. *Shigella dysenteriae* type 1 associated with HUS (➤188).

Laboratory diagnosis: Ready growth (24 h) on most solid media; variety of selective media used for isolation from stool (e.g. DCA and XLD ➤190). Selective broth enrichment of stool useful for convalescent cases. Commercial biochemical test kits are useful (rapid screening of suspect colonies in 4 h, more reliable tests take further 24 h); agglutination of colonies by specific antisera allows grouping of non-*sonnei* isolates (➤).

Treatment: Antibiotics not generally indicated for the individual unless immunocom-promised or severely ill with non-*sonnei* dysentery (e.g. ciprofloxacin; 70% resistance to trimethoprim and ampicillin in developing world); their value for curtailing outbreaks is disputed. Outbreak control usually involves excluding symptomatic cases, emphasising lavatory hygiene, and (only rarely) school closure ☎.

Prevention: Improve sanitation. Isolation ②.

Citrobacter spp. and Enterobacter spp.

Motile, Gram-negative rods.

Pathogenesis: No specific virulence factors known.

Epidemiology: Mostly nosocomial pathogens causing opportunist infections sporadically and in small outbreaks; spread on staff hands and occasionally on contaminated wet equipment. Frequently colonise patients given cephalosporins. Various typing schemes available (➤).

Spectrum of disease: Hospital-acquired **wound infection**/colonisation, **UTI, iv catheter infection**; occasional **bacteraemia** secondary to these. Rare **ventilator-associated pneumonia**. *Citrobacter koseri* associated with outbreaks of **meningitis** on neonatal ICUs. *Enterobacter agglomerans* (also called *Erwinia herbicola*) is a frequent environmental commensal (e.g. toilet water), causing occasional opportunist infections of iv catheters, wounds; also bacteraemia and endocarditis in IVDU.

Laboratory diagnosis: Ready growth (24 h) on most laboratory media; confirm identity by commercial biochemical test kits (further 24 h).

Treatment: 'Hard' coliforms (➤184). Many resistant to ampicillin/amoxycillin; often also to trimethoprim, co-amoxiclav. Often carry genetic elements coding for parenteral or broad-spectrum cephalosporinases. Resistance in initially sensitive strains therefore sometimes emerges on treatment, by derepression of class 1 cephalosporinase production or selection for strains that produce large amounts of the enzymes. Aminoglycosides, imipenem, aztreonam, cefpirome and quinolones are more reliable.

> **Practice point:** Avoid cephalosporins in patients infected with 'hard coliforms' (➤184), i.e. *Citrobacter* spp., *Enterobacter* spp., *Proteus vulgaris*, *Providencia* spp. and *Serratia* spp., even if reported as sensitive by the laboratory.

Serratia spp.

Motile, Gram-negative rods. Many produce striking red-pigmented colonies. Clinically similar to *Enterobacter* and *Citrobacter* spp.; especially associated with outbreaks of bacteraemia, meningitis and ophthalmia on neonatal ICUs, where they are spread on staff hands or in contaminated feeds.

Yersinia spp.

Yersinia enterocolitica
Small, Gram-negative coccobacillus.
Pathogenesis: Oral ingestion. Variety of plasmid-associated virulence factors identified, including 'invasin' protein. Invasion of epithelium overlying Peyer's patches ⟹ multiplication in lymphoid follicles ⟹ hyperplasia; can mimic appendicitis. Iron overload increases invasiveness.
Epidemiology: Variety of serotypes associated with pigs, cows, etc.; types 3 and 9 commonest in Europe (✦). Outbreaks associated with milk, ice-cream, pork products. (Σ ~400; probably greatly under-reported). Will multiply slowly at refrigerator temperatures.
Spectrum of disease: Ranges from acute gastroenteritis to invasive colitis and enteritis with inflammatory **diarrhoeas** (➤46) lasting a mean of 2 weeks. **Mesenteric adenitis** in young children and adults. Rare bacteraemia and metastatic spread (osteomyelitis, IE) in the immunocompromised, especially those with diseases of iron accumulation. **Reactive arthritis** (➤96) in 2%, HLA-B27-associated; also Reiter's syndrome and erythema nodosum (➤93).
Laboratory diagnosis: Ready growth (24 h) on many media, but best to use selective medium (CIN agar) incubated at 25°C for isolation from faeces or tissue if diagnosis is suspected (☎). Identified in commercial biochemical kits, incubated at low temperature. Serology useful to confirm cause of recent rheumatological complications (✦).
Treatment: No evidence that course of gastrointestinal illness modified by antibiotics. Usually resistant to ampicillin/amoxicillin; trimethoprim, parenteral or broad-spectrum cephalosporins and quinolones have been used for systemic and focal infections.

Yersinia pseudotuberculosis
Causes mesenteric adenitis with a more chronic picture than *Yersinia enterocolitica*, especially in children and teenagers (Σ 15). Serotype 1 causes most human infections. Diagnosis as for *Yersinia enterocolitica*. Commonly associated with septicaemic illnesses in many animals and birds, and taxonomically very closely related to *Yersinia pestis*, the cause of plague (➤211). There are various other yersinia species which have been isolated from the environment and animals.

Vibrio spp.

Vibrio cholerae
Curved, motile, Gram-negative rods. ✉ ②.
Pathogenesis: Flagellae involved in adhesion to enterocyte. Cholera toxin (enterotoxin) present in O1 strains (also in a few non-O1 strains); comprises one A and five B peptide subunits (related to *Escherichia coli* LT toxin (➤187)). B subunits bind to GM1 ganglioside on enterocyte membrane, and the A subunit is passed through to cytoplasm ⟹ irreversible activation of adenyl cyclase ⟹ inhibition of sodium and chloride uptake and excretion of chloride and bicarbonate ions accompanied by water ⟹ secretory diarrhoea. Both O1 and non-O1 strains produce a variety of other toxins, including mucinase, LT and ST enterotoxins, cytotoxins (Shiga-like) and cytolysins.
Epidemiology: Cholera always an imported infection in most of developed world (Σ ~5). Acquired from faecally contaminated water, vegetables, seafood; direct person-to-person

spread rarely proved. O1 strains divided into classical and eltor biotypes and serologically into O antigen types Inaba, Ogawa and Hikojima. Current seventh cholera O1 pandemic began 1961 in Indonesia—biotype eltor, serotype Inaba. At present cholera is restricted to SE Asia, Indian subcontinent, Middle East, parts of CIS, Africa and South America. Rare indigenous cases reported Texas and Louisiana (Gulf Coast), Yugoslavia, Italy, Spain; acquired from vibrios multiplying in surface waters. Non-O1 cases are usually sporadic or small, common-source outbreaks, but new epidemic O139 strain (cholera toxin-positive) has swept through Indian subcontinent since 1992. Serotyping available (→).

Spectrum of disease: O1 strains typically cause acute-onset **profuse watery diarrhoea** with infection confined to gut (see below). Wide range of severity of illness, with > 90% clinically indistinguishable from other acute diarrhoeal illnesses, and asymptomatic infection common. Non-O1 strains cause spectrum of illness from mild gastroenteritis to fulminant diarrhoea; also rarely associated with **tissue infection**, especially in patients with underlying diseases (e.g. diabetes, arterial insufficiency).

Laboratory diagnosis: Inform laboratory of travel history so appropriate media are inoculated (thiosulphate–citrate–bile salt (TCBS) agar, plus alkaline peptone water enrichment for 5–6 h). Rapid (24 h) production of large yellow colonies on TCBS in acute diarrhoea; sometimes isolated after enrichment when convalescent. Test for indophenol oxidase, and agglutination by O1 antiserum (→). Commercial biochemical test kits are reliable for *Vibrio cholerae* identification (further 24 h).

Prevention: Clean food and water. Chemoprophylaxis (tetracycline 250 mg 6-hly, or co-trimoxazole) should be reserved for household contacts. Vaccination has no role in prevention or control of epidemics (➤144).

CLINICAL SYNDROME
Cholera
Severe secretory diarrhoea caused by *Vibrio cholerae*. ✉ ②

Clinical features

Incubation time: Two to 3 days (range < 1–5).

Symptoms and signs: Sudden onset of profuse painless watery diarrhoea ('rice-water stools') with vomiting. Fever is unusual, except in children. Rapid severe dehydration and circulatory collapse can occur within hours. Fluid loss may be up to 1 l/h, and severely ill patients may lose up to 10% of their body weight in fluid. Mortality (50% in severe untreated cases) is due to fluid loss, and is reduced to < 1% if adequate fluid replacement is given. Complications include metabolic acidosis and renal failure. Asymptomatic and mild cases are common—there may be 10 such cases for every severe case in an epidemic situation.

Investigations: Diagnosis may be confirmed by stool culture. Stool microscopy may be helpful during epidemics.

Management: Rapid aggressive rehydration, either by oral rehydration fluid (➤45), in mild cases, or iv, in severe cases. Slightly hypotonic alkaline solutions containing potassium are favoured for iv use; Ringer lactate solution or WHO iv diarrhoea treatment solution both conform to this specification. If these are not available, normal saline and 1.26% sodium bicarbonate in a ratio of 2:1 (both with potassium 10 mmol/l) should be given. Up to 4 l/h may be required initially. Once fluid deficit has been corrected patients should receive daily (orally or iv) the previous day's output (urine + stool volumes + 500 ml).

Tetracycline, ampicillin and trimethoprim/co-trimoxazole resistance uncommon but increasing in incidence in Africa and Asia; ciprofloxacin reliably active.

Vibrio parahaemolyticus
Curved, motile Gram-negative rods.

Pathogenesis: Adhesion linked to flagella and haemagglutinin; virtually all pathogenic strains are haemolytic on human blood/mannitol agar (Kanagawa phenomenon) (✦). Also cytotoxin (Shiga), mucinase.

Epidemiology: Associated with seafood; common in Japan, Singapore. Σ 20. Serotyping available (✦).

Spectrum of disease: Acute diarrhoea (*c.* 3 days' duration), rarely fulminant (≻46). Rare extragastrointestinal infections associated with local trauma and contamination with seawater/seafood (e.g. cellulitis, endophthalmitis).

Laboratory diagnosis: Grows on TCBS agar; requires high salt concentration (halophilic). Inform laboratory of seafood/travel association and culture suspect foodstuffs. Commercial identification test kits normally reliable with added salt, but confirm by ✦.

Treatment: Antibiotics not normally required for diarrhoea. Usually resistant to ampicillin, antipseudomonal penicillins and oral cephalosporins. For tissue infections use gentamicin or cefotaxime.

Vibrio fluvialis, *hollisae* and *mimicus* (perhaps also *furnissii*) cause clinical illnesses similar to *parahaemolyticus* but have biochemical differences.

Vibrio vulnificus and damsela

Curved, motile, Gram-negative rods.

Pathogenesis: *Vibrio vulnificus* has acidic polysaccharide capsule and is serum-resistant. Also cytolysin (heat-labile), protease, collagenase, iron-binding siderophore.

Epidemiology and spectrum of disease: Tissue infections (sometimes severe, necrotising, bacteraemic), often following local trauma and contamination with seawater/seafood, especially from warm waters (≻90). Commoner in those with diseases of iron accumulation. Rare diarrhoea.

Laboratory diagnosis: Send swabs, tissue, blood culture. Inform laboratory of seawater association. Grow well on TCBS agar; prefer high salt concentration (halophilic), but will grow on blood and MacConkey agars and in blood culture broths. Commercial identification test kits normally reliable with added salt, but confirm by ✦.

Treatment: Often resistant to ampicillin, antipseudomonal penicillins and oral cephalosporins. For tissue infections use gentamicin or cefotaxime. Debride necrotic tissue.

Vibrio alginolyticus

Halophilic vibrio occasionally isolated from minor septic wounds and ear infections after seawater contact.

Aeromonas hydrophila, sobria, caviae and others

Motile, Gram-negative rods with ubiquitous distribution in fresh waters. Wound infection (sometimes severe, necrotising, bacteraemic) and other sepsis often associated with freshwater contamination (≻90). Probably also cause diarrhoea, sometimes bloody, sometimes travel-associated. Other *Aeromonas* spp. are fish and animal pathogens. Aeromonads can penetrate cells in culture, and possess a range of cytotoxins, adhesins and haemolysins with as yet undefined roles. Most are resistant to ampicillin/amoxycillin and antipseudomonal penicillins, and rare strains produce β-lactamases active against parenteral or broad-spectrum cephalosporins; generally reliable agents include aminoglycosides, quinolones and trimethoprim.

Campylobacter jejuni and coli

Curved, motile, Gram-negative rods.

Pathogenesis: Infective dose low; dependent on host factors (especially gastric acid production), but has followed ingestion of 500 organisms. Disease probably involves toxin production (an enterotoxin very similar to cholera toxin, and a cytotoxin), multiplication within jejunal and ileal enterocytes, and penetration of mucosa. Also mesenteric lymph nodes enlarged; acute inflammation of rectal and lower colonic mucosa.

Epidemiology: Commonest proven cause of diarrhoea in England and Wales (Σ 39 383 in 1993). Many additional cases go unreported (estimated 10 × as many). In UK >90% of cases are due to *Campylobacter jejuni* (mainly found in poultry/birds), < 10% *coli* (pigs). A **zoonosis**, with sporadic cases or common-source outbreaks from ingested food (> 60% chicken carcasses are culture-positive; less commonly acquired from other meat, con-taminated/unpasteurised milk, untreated water). Do not multiply in food. Rarely trans-mitted person to person, except infant to in-fant or carers. Rare cause of outbreaks of meningitis and septicaemia in neonatal ICUs. Typing available by O and surface/flagellar antigens (➤).

Spectrum of disease: Incubation period 1–7 days ⇒ **acute enteritis** lasting 2–7 days (➤46). Ex-cretion of organisms continues for about 3 weeks; prolonged carriage very rare in immu-nocompetent people. Occasional reactive ar-thritis or Guillain–Barré syndrome 1–2 weeks after diarrhoea.

Laboratory diagnosis: Appropriate selective/nutritive media are routinely inoculated with faeces by laboratories; grows in 48 h. Bacteraemia very rare.

Treatment: Normally the diarrhoea is self-limit-ing, but early treatment with erythromycin may shorten illness. *Campylobacter coli* more commonly erythromycin-resistant; ciprofloxacin is an alternative.

Prevention: Kitchen hygiene. Isolation of neonates and parturient mothers with diar-rhoea.

Campylobacter hyointestinalis, *lari*, *up-saliensis*, etc. are rare causes of similar diarrhoeal illnesses.

Campylobacter fetus is uncommonly iso-lated from blood cultures in immuno-compromised patients, and causes abortion in sheep and cattle. It carries an antiphagocytic protein 'microcapsule'.

Helicobacter pylori

Curved or spiral, motile, Gram-negative rod. No recognised typing scheme.

Pathogenesis: Colonises gastroduodenal mu-cosa. Intense urease production ⇒ local rise in pH, allowing periepithelial survival in stom-ach.

Spectrum of disease: Causes chronic active gas-tritis and is dominant cofactor in duodenal ulceration; carriage associated with gastric ulceration and gastric cancer.

Laboratory diagnosis: Will grow in low O_2, high CO_2 on media enriched with horse serum.

CLINICAL SYNDROME
Gastritis, duodenal ulcers and Helicobacter pylori

Helicobacter pylori is found in mucus lining the stomach and in areas of gastric meta-plasia in the duodenum. Its presence is strongly associated with gastritis and duode-nal ulceration.

Carriage rate in UK adults > 50 years is > 50%. Rate increases with age. Found in ~90% of patients with *duodenal* ulceration or antral gastritis. Eradication of organism, during/after standard ulcer healing therapy, reduces relapse rate from ~85% to < 20%. It is unclear whether eradication reduces re-lapse rate in *gastric* ulceration.

Diagnosis: The organism may be visualised in and cultured from endoscopic biopsies. It may also be detected by subjecting bi-opsies to the rapid urease test, which may be performed by the endoscopist. In the ^{14}C-labelled urea breath test, *Helicobacter pylori* in the stomach cleave labelled urea, liberating $^{14}CO_2$, which is detected in breath. ^{13}C is used by some departments as it is non-radioactive and is safe for use in children and women of childbearing age, although a mass spectrometer is required to detect it.

Management: No evidence exists to justify eradication of *Helicobacter pylori* in pa-tients with non-ulcer dyspepsia, gastric ulceration or NSAID ulceration. Eradica-tion is indicated in patients with recurrent duodenal ulcer, or who have had compli-cations such as perforation or haemor-rhage.

Bismuth salts and antibiotics are used in combination; regimens including bismuth plus two antibiotics ('triple therapy') are more effective than bismuth plus a single antibiotic ('double therapy'). Metro-nidazole resistance is common (20% of

UK strains). The most effective regimens evaluated to date use colloidal bismuth subcitrate 120 mg 6-hly, metronidazole 400 mg 8-hly plus tetracycline 500 mg 6-hly or amoxycillin 500 mg 6-hly for 2 weeks. Omeprazole plus amoxycillin or omeprazole plus clarithromycin may be as effective.

21: Pseudomonads

Pseudomonas spp. and their relatives.

Often called 'non-fermenters' because, unlike coliforms, they usually derive their energy by oxidative metabolism and fail to ferment glucose. Most are environmental saprophytes, are strict aerobes and produce the enzyme indophenol oxidase. A few are primary pathogens, but most cause opportunist infections in the locally or generally compromised host. Most isolates from this group represent **colonisation** rather than infection, and antibiotic treatment must not be commenced lightly; careful clinical assessment is indicated. Many have unusual antibiotic sensitivity patterns, and are resistant to

common antibiotics and antiseptics. Commercial biochemical test kits are now fairly reliable at identifying pseudomonads, but important isolates should be sent for confirmation to a reference laboratory.

Pseudomonas spp.

Pseudomonas aeruginosa
Motile, slim Gram-negative rods.

Pathogenesis: Produce an enormous range of enzymes and other putative virulence factors. Those associated with specific diseases include: alginate-like polysaccharide with antiphagocytic and antibiotic-trapping properties, and protease-induced mucosal damage in cystic fibrosis; proteases in corneal ulceration and ecthyma gangrenosum; exotoxins and proteases in significant burn infection.

Table 79 Classification of pseudomonads

Genus	Species	Notes
Pseudomonas	*aeruginosa*	Green/blue-pigmented, 'beaten copper' colonies
	pseudomallei, mallei	Primary pathogens, causing infections in the tropics (➤200)
	cepacia	Lung infection in cystic fibrosis (➤201)
	(*putida, fluorescens, picketti, stutzeri, paucimobilis,* etc.)	'Miscellaneous' group, rarely isolated from significant infections. Some pigmented
Acinetobacter	*calcoaceticus, baumannii, 'lwoffii', 'anitratus'*	Skin commensals, occasional nosocomial pathogens (➤201)
Stenotrophomonas	*maltophilia*	Previously in *Pseudomonas*, then *Xanthomonas* genera (➤202)
(*Moraxella*)	(*lacunata, osloensis, phenyl-pyruvica, non-liquifaciens,* etc.)	*Moraxella (Branhamella) catarrhalis* is considered under fastidious Gram-negative rods (➤208)

Other pseudomonads include *Flavobacterium* spp., *Alcaligenes* spp., *Achromobacter* spp., *Agrobacterium* spp., *Weeksella* spp., *Flavimonas* spp., *Chromobacterium violaceum*, etc.

Epidemiology: Found commonly in moist environmental sites and on raw fruit and vegetables. Occasionally isolated from normal faeces ($<10\%$), but rapidly emerges on hospital admission and after antibiotic treatment. Barring occasional common-source outbreaks (e.g. from contaminated antiseptics) and deficient staff aseptic technique, nosocomial infections are usually shown to be with patients' own strains. Hand-borne spread important, especially on neonatal ICU and burns units. Colonisation of large-volume, refilled antiseptic containers (e.g. contact-lens solutions) always likely. A variety of typing methods are available, including serological and pyocine typing (↣).

Spectrum of disease: Frequently colonises moist lesions (e.g. leg ulcers, bedsores, oozing surgical incisions) and the upper airways, especially after antibiotic treatment; occasional progression to superinfection. In the normal patient: **external otitis** (↣16) and **folliculitis** (↣87) (both from exposure to contaminated water). Nosocomial **wound and burn infection, iv catheter sepsis, UTI, ventilator-associated pneumonia** and **secondary bacteraemia. Primary bacteraemia** in neutropenic patients following gastrointestinal colonisation (↣133). May be associated with necrotic skin lesions — ecthyma gangrenosum (↣159). **Pulmonary colonisation/infection** in patients with cystic fibrosis. **Malignant otitis externa** in diabetics (↣16). **Corneal ulceration** with contaminated contact-lens solutions (↣84), and aggressive **panophthalmitis** after penetrating injury (↣85).

Laboratory diagnosis: Ready (24 h) growth on many solid media to form characteristic colonies with ammoniacal odour. Mucoid strains from CF may take 48 h to produce only tiny colonies. Antiseptics (e.g. cetrimide) added to solid agar make useful selective media. Positive indophenol oxidase test gives rapid presumptive diagnosis, with confirmation in further 24 h, usually by commercial test kits.

Treatment: Intrinsically resistant (by broad-spectrum β-lactamase production and impermeable outer cell membrane) to many first-line antibiotics. Generally reliable agents include antipseudomonal penicillins, aminoglycosides, ceftazidime, high-dose ciprofloxacin, imipenem and aztreonam. Ciprofloxacin is the most active quinolone against *Pseudomonas aeruginosa*, and is the only available oral agent.

Prevention: Neutropenic patients should receive bacteriologically clean food. Perform hand hygiene between every patient contact. Avoid antibiotic usage unless clinically necessary. Supply antiseptics in small-volume, disposable containers; alcoholic agents are intrinsically resistant to contamination. Decontaminate medical equipment between each use, and store it dry.

Pseudomonas pseudomallei ♀
Causes melioidosis (see below).

Pathogenesis: Many putative toxins and enzymes produced; survives in reticuloendothelial cells.

Laboratory diagnosis: Gram-negative rods seen in exudates and infected tissue. Culture is not difficult (forms rugose, non-pigmented colonies on many media in 24–48 h), but differentiation from other pseudomonads (including ones that may cause nosocomial infection) may take time (↣) and the organism is a cause of **laboratory-acquired infection**. Variety of serological tests available (↣).

CLINICAL SYNDROME
Melioidosis
A potentially fatal infection caused by *Pseudomonas pseudomallei*. Latent infection with recrudescence after many years can occur. Melioidosis is extremely rare as an imported disease in the UK, but recognition is important as correct antibiotic therapy significantly reduces mortality.

Epidemiology and transmission: Endemic in SE Asia, Oceania and N Australia, where *Pseudomonas pseudomallei* is widely distributed in soil and water. An important cause of community-acquired pneumonia in SE Asia. Individuals exposed to infection may harbour the organisms for many years and develop melioidosis during intercurrent illness or after surgery. This has occurred in many US servicemen returning from Vietnam. Disease is commoner in patients with minor abnormalities of immune function, e.g. diabetes mellitus, renal or hepatic disease.

Clinical features: Asymptomatic infection is common, and can be demonstrated by serology. **Pneumonia** may be severe and acute, with upper-lobe consolidation progressing to cavitation. Chronic presentations also occur and may be mistaken for tuberculosis. **Acute septicaemic melioidosis** presents as a severe septicaemic illness without focal signs, with high fever, constitutional symptoms, hepatomegaly and diarrhoea. Secondary lung involvement is common. **Localised suppurative disease** also occurs, with abscesses in skin, lymph nodes, viscera or brain.

Investigations: Diagnosis is made by culture of the organism from blood, sputum or other infected sites. Serology is not useful in diagnosis of acute cases in endemic regions, but may be helpful, particularly in retrospect, in patients from non-endemic areas.

Management: Ceftazidime as initial therapy (with or without co-trimoxazole) is superior to previous multidrug regimens. Continuation treatment (which may be oral) must be given for several months to prevent relapse. Mortality of acute septicaemic melioidosis remains ~30% despite optimum therapy ☏.

Pseudomonas mallei

Cause of glanders, a respiratory tract and lymphangitic infection of horses in Asia, Africa and the Middle East. Humans may acquire infection in traumatic skin lesions. Microbiologically similar to *Pseudomonas pseudomallei*.

Pseudomonas (Burkholderia) cepacia

Probably to be renamed *Burkholderia cepacia*. A colonist of wet environments and a plant pathogen, distinguishable from the 'miscellaneous' group by its propensity to colonise the damaged respiratory tracts of patients with cystic fibrosis. Various typing schemes available (➤). Pathogenesis unknown, but the organism secretes many enzymes and carries pili which adhere to mucus. Some patients suffer few ill effects, but others develop progressive deterioration of respiratory function, and necrotising pneumonia is seen in 20%. Spread by cross-infection in hospital and clinics; careful disinfection of respiratory equipment is indicated, and some CF units segregate patients carrying *Pseudomonas cepacia*. Frequently multiply antibiotic-resistant; some units use temocillin **plus** amikacin, or temocillin **plus** ceftazidime.

'Miscellaneous' Pseudomonas spp. and 'other' pseudomonads

Generally colonisers of moist environments. They uncommonly colonise patients, and rarely cause opportunist infections. Isolation of these species or *Pseudomonas cepacia* from blood cultures suggests either 'pseudobacteraemia' (contamination of the blood culture system from an environmental source) or iatrogenic infection of the patient (for example, infusion of a contaminated fluid). *Flavobacterium* spp. (yellow or colourless colonies) have caused outbreaks of bacteraemia and meningitis on neonatal ICUs and neurosurgery units.

Acinetobacter calcoaceticus, baumannii, 'lwoffii' and 'anitratus'

Plump, non-motile, indophenol oxidase-negative Gram-negative rods.

Pathogenesis: Unknown mechanisms.

Epidemiology: Commensals of moist skin. Nosocomial infections commoner in hot countries. Spread in hospital on staff hands and contaminated equipment.

Spectrum of disease: Most commonly isolated as colonists of the mucosae of ill, hospitalised patients. All may, like other skin commensals, be opportunist pathogens on **prosthetic materials** and **iv catheters**; nosocomial **UTI, ventilator-associated pneumonia**, etc. common on some units; rare community-acquired pneumonia.

Laboratory diagnosis: In Gram stains may be mistaken for *Neisseria* spp. Ready growth (24 h) on many media to form small, non-pigmented colonies.

Treatment: Community-acquired strains are often resistant only to trimethoprim; nosocomial isolates are often multiply resistant with unpredictable sensitivity patterns.

Stenotrophomonas maltophilia

(formerly *Xanthomonas maltophilia*)

Motile, Gram-negative rods.

Pathogenesis: Unknown virulence factors, but versatile antibiotic resistance mechanisms equip this organism well for superinfection of ICU patients receiving modern antibiotic therapy, especially quinolones or imipenem.

Epidemiology: Environmental coloniser of moist areas. Increasingly recognised to cause outbreaks in ICUs, spread by staff hands and contaminated equipment. Variety of typing methods available (→).

Spectrum of disease: Most commonly only causes colonisation, but may cause **iv catheter** infection and **secondary bacteraemia**, and a variety of **infections in immunocompromised patients**.

Laboratory diagnosis: Slim Gram-negative rod. Ready growth (24–48 h) on many media; green/yellow or non-pigmented colonies smelling strongly of ammonia; usually slowly indophenol oxidase-positive.

Treatment: Often startlingly antibiotic-resistant, including quinolones, aminoglycosides and imipenem; further resistances commonly emerge during therapy. Co-trimoxazole and colistin have been tried for systemic therapy with apparent success.

Moraxella lacunata, osloensis, phenylpyruvica, non-liquifaciens, etc.

Small Gram-negative coccobacilli that colonise oronasopharyngeal mucosae. Indophenol oxidase-positive, and often initially mistaken for *Neisseria* spp. *Moraxella lacunata* sometimes isolated from corneal ulcers; the other species cause occasional opportunist nosocomial infections. Generally quite antibiotic-sensitive.

22: Fastidious Gram-negative Organisms

Gram-negative rods and cocci which share the need for special culture conditions (e.g. nutritative co-factors, blood, serum, CO_2, moisture) and often colonise the mucosae of humans and animals. With a few notable exceptions (such as *Haemophilus influenzae* from sputum and blood cultures) optimal culture will often not routinely be performed for these organisms, so inform the laboratory if a patient falls into an appropriate risk group (☎).

Table 80 Classification of fastidious Gram-negative organisms

Genus	Species	Notes
Haemophilus	***influenzae*** (*parainfluenzae, haemolyticus, parahaemolyticus, haemoglobinophilus, 'aegyptius'*, etc., and see HACEK group below)	Satellitism around *Staphylococcus aureus* colonies on blood agar; require X factor (porphyrins, e.g. haemin) and V factor (coenzyme 1; NAD or NADP) for growth on nutrient agar. 'Para' species require only V factor (➤204)
	ducreyi	Causes chancroid (➤71, 205)
Neisseria	***meningitidis***	Meningococcus (➤74, 205)
	gonorrhoeae	Gonococcus (➤65, 206)
	(*sicca, flava, perflava, subflava, lactamica*, etc.)	*Neisseria lactamica* sometimes mistaken for *meningitidis*
Legionella	***pneumophila*** (*bozemanii, cincinnatiensis, feeleii, gormanii, jordanensis, longbeachae, micdadel, wadsworthii* and others have caused human disease. Some have been classified in the genera *Tatlockia* and *Fluoribacter*) (➤24, 207)	
Human source		
Bordetella	*pertussis* (*parapertussis, bronchiseptica*)	Human respiratory tract infection (➤108, 208)
Moraxella	*catarrhalis*	Human respiratory tract infection. Used to be in the genus *Branhamella*
Gardnerella	*vaginalis*	Has belonged to *Haemophilus* and *Corynebacterium* genera. Gram-variable staining (➤70, 208)
(*Calymmatobacterium*)	(*granulomatis*)	Granuloma inguinale in tropical countries. Genital ulceration (➤72)

continued on p. 204

Table 80 contd

Genus	Species	Notes
(Anaerobiospirillum)	(succiniproducens)	Spiral organism, rarely isolated from blood or faeces
(DF-3)		Causes chronic diarrhoea in the immunocompromised
Capnocytophaga	ochracea	Human oral and systemic sepsis (➤208)
Zoonoses		
Capnocytophaga	canimorsus	Zoonotic wound and systemic sepsis (➤208)
Pasteurella	multocida	Zoonotic wound and systemic sepsis
	(pneumotropica, ureae)	Rare respiratory tract infections
Brucella	abortus, melitensis, suis, ovis, canis, etc.	Zoonotic systemic sepsis (➤209)
Yersinia	pestis	Zoonotic plague (➤211)
(Francisella)	(tularensis)	Zoonotic respiratory, wound or systemic infections (➤212)
(Streptobacillus)	(moniliformis)	Causes rat-bite fever (➤212)
(Bartonella)	(bacilliformis)	Causes Oroya fever in S America. Acquired from sandflies; infects erythrocytes
(Afipia)	felis)	May cause some cases of cat-scratch disease (➤237)
'HACEK' or 'herbie' group		Haemophilus aphrophilus and paraphrophilus and related organisms (➤212)

Haemophilus spp.

Haemophilus influenzae

Small, pleomorphic Gram-negative rods.

Pathogenesis: Invasive strains have polysaccharide capsule which resists phagocytosis unless opsonized; commonly type b (polyribosylribitol phosphate), rarely a, very rarely c–f. Other virulence factors unproven, but include IgA protease, adhesion pili and toxicity for mucosal cilia. Entry to bloodstream occurs from nasopharyngeal invasion.

Epidemiology: Ubiquitous commensals of the upper respiratory tract; capsulate strains carried by up to 5% normal adults and children, and up to 60% in childhood contacts of invasive infections. Childhood infections with type b strains much rarer since introduction of Hib vaccine (➤337). Rare overwhelming infections in patients with asplenia. Capsular typing by agglutination.

Spectrum of disease: Capsulate strains cause meningitis (➤74), epiglottitis (➤18), osteomyelitis (➤97), septic arthritis (➤95), cellulitis (including orbital and periorbital ≻85, 89), and secondary bacteraemia in children < 6 years old (peak incidence 4 months to 2 years). Rare in adults. **Non-capsulate** strains associated with exacerbations of chronic bronchitis (often mixed with *Streptococcus pneumoniae* and *Moraxella catarrhalis* ≻21), sinusitis and otitis media (≻15). Rare cellulitis, meningitis, endocarditis and pneumonia (especially post-influenza) in adults, commoner in the immunocompromised; bacteraemic pneumonia especially common in HIV infection. Invasive strains in adults usually non-capsulate.

Laboratory diagnosis: Poor growth on blood agar; much better (24–48 h) on heated blood ('chocolate') agar, which has greater available X and V factors. Identification 24 h later by test for X and V factor dependence or negative porphyrin production. Direct antigen detection for b-capsulate strains widely available.

Treatment: Ampicillin/amoxycillin resistance (β-lactamase production) currently 25% in capsulate and 10% in non-capsulate strains in UK. Best empirical choices are **oral** tetracycline, trimethoprim, co-amoxiclav, cefaclor, cefixime or ciprofloxacin; **parenteral** broad-spectrum cephalosporin (chloramphenicol is an alternative). Other oral cephalosporins have less activity. Frequently erythromycin-resistant, but clarithromycin and azithromycin are more reliable.

Prevention: Hib vaccine (but weak response in those < 2 years and the immunocompromised ≻337); rifampicin prophylaxis for household contacts of invasive infections (≻77).

Haemophilus aegyptius (Koch–Weeks bacillus) Subtype of *influenzae* associated with epidemic conjunctivitis, which may progress to systemic sepsis (Brazilian purpuric fever). Ampicillin plus chloramphenicol has been used for therapy.

Haemophilus parainfluenzae
Occasionally causes similar infections to non-capsulate strains of *Haemophilus influenzae*.

Haemophilus ducreyi

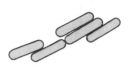

Small Gram-negative rods.
Pathogenesis: Largely unknown.
Epidemiology: Most common in parts of Africa and Asia.
Spectrum of disease: Causes **chancroid** (≻71) or 'soft sore'; painful genital ulceration and regional lymphadenitis. May progress to phimosis and urethral fistula.
Laboratory diagnosis: 'Shoal of fish' arrangement of bacilli in smears from undermined edge of ulcers. Can be isolated with difficulty on selective medium containing serum ☎.
Treatment: Effective new antibiotics include co-trimoxazole, co-amoxiclav and ciprofloxacin; older, cheaper regimens included sulphonamides, streptomycin, erythromycin and tetracyclines.

Neisseria spp.

Neisseria meningitidis ☒ ①
Small, Gram-negative, oval diplococci.
Pathogenesis: Surface pili involved in mucosal adhesion; also produces IgA protease. Polysaccharide capsule essential to avoid phagocytosis; serum antibodies may be protective, and carriage of *Neisseria lactamica* may raise cross-protective antibody. Penetration of mucosa ⇒ bloodstream ⇒ meninges. Possible direct spread through cribriform plate. Host factors then determine whether lipopolysaccharide triggers sepsis syndrome (≻158, 184). Death in fulminant septicaemia (Waterhouse–Friedrichsen syndrome) is from microcirculatory damage and multiorgan failure, not from loss of adrenal function; indeed, circulating corticosteroid levels are usually high.
Epidemiology: Σ 1100. In normal nasopharynx 5–20% carriage rate, mostly non-capsulate strains outside outbreaks. Carriage commoner in closed communities (e.g. barracks,

boarding-schools), and up to 80% during outbreaks. Spread by droplets or direct mucosal contact; household contacts of cases have up to 800 × increased risk of infection. Two-thirds of cases occur in first 5 years of life (predisposing factors ➤74). Serogrouping by capsular polysaccharide, subtyping by outer membrane proteins (➤). Group A strains cause only 2% cases in UK, but associated with epidemics, especially in sub-Saharan Africa. Groups B and C cause 60% and 35% of UK cases respectively. Others include W 135.

Spectrum of disease: Although there is a gradation of presentations between the two, the commonest systemic manifestations can be divided into **meningitis**, comprising two-thirds cases (➤74), and **septicaemia** in one-third cases, with multiple organ failure and purpuric rash (➤158). **Rare presentations** include conjunctivitis (➤82), IE (➤37), arthritis (➤95), pericarditis (➤42), vulvo-vaginitis in children, urethritis, proctitis, pharyngitis, pneumonia. These may occur in isolation or accompany meningitis or bacteraemia, or occasionally with fulminant septicaemia. **Chronic meningococcal septicaemia**, with joint involvement and purulent skin lesions, occurs rarely. Mortality (treated) approaches 100% in fulminant septicaemia, up to 50% in meningitis with septicaemia and rash, and <5% in meningitis and other sites alone.

Laboratory diagnosis: CSF Gram stain is the mainstay of rapid species diagnosis. Meningococci often seen inside polymorphs in CSF, blood smears or pus ('intracellular diplococci'). Gram stains of purpuric skin smears allow rapid confirmation, and differentiation from *Staphylococcus aureus* (☎). Rapid capsular antigen detection rarely any more useful than Gram stain of CSF. Neisserias are sensitive to drying. Require CO_2, moisture, serum/heated blood (e.g. 'chocolate' agar) for optimal growth ⇒ tiny, indophenol oxidase-positive colonies at 24 h, larger at 48 h. Sensitive to liquoid (anticoagulant and anticomplement; added to many blood culture systems); therefore some laboratories supply 'meningitis bottle' optimised

for neisserias. Confirmation by biochemical tests (rapid (4 h) commercial kits available) and antigen content, but biochemically atypical strains are not rare and will need confirmation ➤.

Treatment: Benzylpenicillin remains the drug of choice; cefotaxime or ceftriaxone are as effective, and are usefully broad-spectrum when the diagnosis is uncertain, and they retain activity against the currently very rare penicillin-resistant meningococci (reported largely from Spain). Steroid therapy of additional benefit in children only. Eradicate carriage from cases with rifampicin (➤77).

Prevention: Closure of meningeal defects; rational use of antibiotic prophylaxis and meningococcal vaccine in asplenia and close contacts of cases (➤142). No vaccine currently effective against group B strains (unstable, non-immunogenic capsule).

Neisseria lactamica

Biochemically and antigenically similar to meningococci, but ferments lactose slowly. Rarely causes focal infections, as may the other commensal neisserias.

Neisseria gonorrhoeae

Small, Gram-negative, oval diplococci.

Pathogenesis: Piliated strains more virulent (increased adhesion to urethral epithelium and resistance to killing by serum). Also produce a variety of proteases, including IgA protease.

Epidemiology: Only spread by direct mucosal contact; risk of transmission depends on frequency and duration of intercourse. Infected females and those with rectal or pharyngeal infections are often asymptomatic. Typing possible by outer-membrane proteins or biochemistry ('auxotyping' ➤); certain auxotypes are associated with invasive disease. Neonate infected during passage through cervix. Incidence rose in UK 1960s–1980s, then fell, probably because of increased use of barrier contraception with appearance of HIV. Σ 61 per 100000 population (1990). Σ 300 β-lactamase-producing isolates.

Spectrum of disease: Mucosal infection of urethra, uterine endocervix and sometimes rectum or pharynx (➤65); vulvovaginitis (prepubertal). **Ophthalmia neonatorum** (>83). Secondary **local spread**, including epididymitis, salpingitis, peritonitis. Most with the Fitz-Hugh–Curtis syndrome (perihepatitis) are coinfected with *Chlamydia trachomatis*. **Metastatic spread**, causing acute or chronic bacteraemia, arthritis (>95), skin pustules, rare endocarditis or meningitis.

Laboratory diagnosis: Intracellular Gram-negative diplococci seen in urethral swab of male with urethritis is highly sensitive and specific for gonorrhoea; this is not true for other sites because of their normal flora which contains many similar-looking organisms (commensal neisserias and meningococci, *Acinetobacter* spp., etc.). A delicate, strictly aerobic organism; ideally inoculate selective, nutritive medium (e.g. vancomycin–colistin–nystatin–trimethoprim (VCNT) agar, with lysed blood) with charcoal swabs directly in the clinic; otherwise use transport medium. Forms small colonies in (24–)48 h. In the female, culture of endocervical swab more sensitive than HVS. Bacteriologically very similar to the meningococcus (see above), but differentiated by biochemical reactions and antigen content.

Treatment: Mean penicillin MIC has progressively risen since 1950s; β-lactamase-producing strains appeared in 1976, and remain largely associated with contacts from Far East and Africa. **Drugs of choice in UK** remain single-dose oral ampicillin (3.5 g) or amoxycillin (3 g) **plus** probenecid (1 g). For known or suspected resistance or in penicillin allergy, use **single-dose oral** ciprofloxacin, cefuroxime axetil + probenecid, or **parenteral** cefotaxime, ceftriaxone or spectinomycin. Oral ampicillin/amoxycillin is less effective for pharyngeal or rectal gonorrhoea.

Prevention: Barrier contraception or abstinence. Contact tracing and treatment. Silver nitrate prophylaxis to neonatal eyes in high-prevalence areas.

Legionella pneumophila and other legionellas

Slim Gram-negative bacilli.
Pathogenesis: Inhalation of aerosol containing bacteria ⇒ pneumonia ⇒ bacteraemia in severe cases. Legionella protease involved in pathogenesis. Survive within macrophages. Pathogenesis of Pontiac fever not understood.

Epidemiology: Live in water, especially if warm, often in symbiosis with amoebae; frequently colonise piped water systems and evaporative condensers of air-conditioning cooling towers. Large inocula may be released as aerosols to be inhaled by susceptible people. Pneumonic infection commoner with immunosuppression, age >60, chronic chest disease. In 50% there is an association with travel, especially Spain, Balearics, Greece, Turkey, USA. No human to human transmission; the only bacteria (other than *Coxiella burnetii*) to cause outbreaks of pneumonia out of hospital. Various typing methods for the major species are available (✦): *Legionella pneumophila* causes >95% cases, and serogroup 1 comprises the majority of these. Recently falling incidence in England and Wales (129 cases in 1993).

Spectrum of disease: Legionnaire's disease – pneumonia ± bacteraemia, with 7–10-day incubation period. Mortality 10–85% (mean 15%) depending on underlying illness (>74) **Pontiac fever** – minor influenza-like illness with high attack rate in normal people. Incubation 24–48 h, duration 48–96 h. Rare **localised infection**, e.g. IE (usually of prosthetic valves), haemodialysis shunt infection, hepatitis, sinusitis, wound infection, etc.

Laboratory diagnosis: May be difficult to see in Gram stains of clinical material. Immunofluorescent stains available for direct visualisation in sputum, and urinary ELISA is useful (✦). Will not grow on conventional culture media. Culture sputum, lung/pleural aspirates on buffered charcoal–yeast-extract agar (BCYE), which contains iron and cysteine. Forms 'cut-glass' colonies in 48 h–5 days (occasionally up to 10 days). Blood culture broths can be inoculated to BCYE after 3–5 days' incubation in suspected bacteraemic cases (☎). Confirm in reference laboratory by antigen content (✦). Serum antibodies vs. *Legionella pneumophila* serogroup 1 detectable by FAT, RMAT or ELISA and usually develop during second week of illness, but up to 20% reported seroconversions take >1 month (diagnosis requires fourfold rise, or isolated high titre). Serology not widely available for most other serogroups and species (➤).

Treatment: Erythromycin iv 1 g 6-hly; *in vitro* and animal experiments suggest addition of rifampicin or ciprofloxacin may be synergistic in severe infection. Other antibiotics clinically ineffective.

Prevention: Regular maintenance/disinfection of water systems will reduce (but rarely eliminate) contamination. Legionella multiplication reduced by keeping water <20°C or >60°C.

Bordetella pertussis

Small, Gram-negative rods. ✉ ①.

Pathogenesis: Causes superficial infection of respiratory mucosae. Various recognised virulence factors: three major fimbrial agglutinins (adhesin role, important vaccine components, and useful in typing), 'pertussis toxin' (like diphtheria toxin), adenylate cyclase toxin, tracheal cytotoxin, lymphocytosis factor, endotoxin (differs from usual Gram-negative lipopolysaccharide), filamentous haemagglutinin.

Epidemiology: Not a normal commensal. Child-to-child respiratory droplet transmission. Rarely infects adults, but commoner in unvaccinated populations. Highest mortality in children <1 year. Σ ~400. Vaccine uptake in UK now ~90%. Case fatality rate ~1:200 under 2 months of age, ~1:15 000 in 1–4-year age-group.

Spectrum of disease: Whooping cough (➤108).

Laboratory diagnosis: Best yield from **pernasal swab** without transport medium (☎). No growth on conventional media—needs high blood content with antibiotics (e.g. Bordet–Gengou or charcoal medium) and grows slowly to tiny, glistening colonies (72 h or more). Biochemically unreactive—identified by specific antiserum.

Bordetella parapertussis **and bronchiseptica** are less fastidious in their growth requirements, and rarely cause respiratory illness.

Moraxella catarrhalis (formerly *Branhamella catarrhalis*)

Small, Gram-negative diplococci which colonise and probably infect the respiratory tract. Disputed pathogen; may cause **exacerbations of chronic bronchitis** (➤21), but frequently isolated in mixed culture with *Haemophilus influenzae* and the pneumococcus. Sometimes isolated from otitis media, and rarely alone from severe bacteraemic pneumonia. More than 75% isolates produce β-lactamase, which may inactivate ampicillin/amoxycillin used to treat the mixed infection; often trimethoprim-resistant. Usually reliable agents include co-amoxiclav, erythro/clarithromycin, tetracycline, oral cephalosporins.

Gardnerella vaginalis

Small Gram-variable rod. Vaginal and occasional urethral commensal, usually in small numbers. Adheres to squamous epithelial cells ('clue cells') in bacterial vaginosis (➤70), and occasionally isolated from mixed pelvic and puerperal sepsis (➤62), rarely bacteraemic. Facultative anaerobe, but metronidazole-sensitive.

Capnocytophaga spp.

Small, thin, Gram-negative rods with pointed ends. Slow, CO_2-dependent growth (2–5 days) to form small, yellowish colonies with 'gliding' motility. Generally antibiotic-sensitive except to aminoglycosides and trimethoprim.

Capnocytophaga ochracea

Used to be called DF-1 (dysgonic fermenter—ferments carbohydrates to mainly acetate and succinate). Human oral commensal. Opportunist infections, isolated from mixed bacterial periodontitis in those with disorders of neutrophil chemotaxis, and causes oral ulceration and occasional bacteraemia in neutropenic patients. Very rare empyema, endocarditis, osteomyelitis and various abscesses in the normal host.

Capnocytophaga canimorsus

Used to be called DF-2. Oral commensal of

many animals, especially cats and dogs. Important cause of bite wound infection in normal patients (≻90), which may progress to overwhelming septicaemia in asplenics (≻132), alcoholics and the immunocompromised.

Pasteurella multocida

Small, pleomorphic, Gram-negative coccobacilli.

Pathogenesis: Capsulate, and contains lipopolysaccharide, but detailed mechanisms unknown.

Epidemiology: Naso-oropharyngeal commensal of many animals, some suffering similar infections to those seen in humans. Serotyping available (✦).

Spectrum of disease: Important cause of **bite wound infections** (≻90), including local abscesses, cellulitis and lymphangitis progressing to bacteraemia. Rare pneumonia, empyema.

Laboratory diagnosis: Ready growth (24 h) on usual primary culture media to form small, shiny, indophenol oxidase-positive colonies. Usually confirmed by commercial biochemical test kit (futher 24 h).

Treatment: Usually sensitive to penicillin and tetracycline, and resistant to erythromycin; ≻90 for management of bites.

Brucella spp. ☠

Small Gram-negative coccobacilli and bacilli.

Pathogenesis: Ingested in milk or by handling infected carcasses (must survive stomach acid); inhaled close to aborting animals; occasional direct inoculation from animal contact, or of vaccine strain. Spread via lymphatics and bloodstream, then localisation in reticuloendothelial system, causing granulomas.

Epidemiology: Animal pathogens, causing abortion and prolonged excretion in milk. Cause zoonotic infections in a few, clearly defined circumstances. Distributed worldwide. Particularly common in Mediterranean countries such as Spain, Greece and the Middle East and in S America. **Rarely seen in the UK** (Σ 15), but commonly suspected; the diagnosis

can often be ruled out by taking an accurate history. Transmission occurs by eating infected produce, direct contact with infected tissues and by aerosol inhalation, e.g. in abattoir. Person-to-person spread does not occur. *Brucella melitensis* is associated with goats and sheep. Infection is acquired primarily via goat's milk and cheese, occurs at all ages and affects both sexes equally. *Brucella abortus* is associated with cattle. Infection is an occupational disease of farmers, vets and butchers and therefore affects mainly males. *Brucella suis* is associated with pigs, almost exclusively in the USA. Biotyping available (✦).

Spectrum of disease: Varied presenting features (see below). *Brucella melitensis* is associated with more severe acute infection and more frequent complications than other species. Subclinical infection, which is the usual form taken by *Brucella abortus*, is rare.

Laboratory diagnosis: Slow growth on solid media (48–96 h) to small, shiny colonies, and can take ≻3 weeks even in modern blood culture systems (prolonged incubation ☞). Grow best in serum- and glucose-enriched media, and *abortus* needs added CO_2. Confirm identity in ✦. Serology needs expert interpretation, especially in those exposed in the past (standard agglutination test, mercaptoethanol test, CFT, antihuman-globulin test; confirm by ✦). Worth repeating if negative in strongly suspected cases because seroconversion often late.

Prevention: Vaccination of young cattle; pasteurisation of milk and milk products; testing of herds (milk ring test) and slaughter of positive animals.

CLINICAL SYNDROME

Brucellosis (undulant fever, Malta fever)

A disease of variable severity and duration acquired from domestic animals and caused by *Brucella melitensis*, *Brucella abortus* and *Brucella suis*.

Clinical features: The **incubation period** is variable and difficult to ascertain – usually 5–60 days but often several months. Asymptomatic or mild disease occurs, but is unusual. **Acute brucellosis** presents with rapid onset of high fever, constitutional symptoms, arthralgia, myalgia, headache, back pain, anorexia, constipation, weight loss, rigors and prostration. Fever, leucopenia, lymphadenopathy and hepatosplenomegaly are often found. A transient non-specific skin rash is seen in ~5% of cases. The differential diagnosis of fever, prostration and leucopenia in a returning traveller also includes typhoid, malaria and viral infection, which are much commoner in the UK (➢145). Symptoms may resolve after a few weeks, but a relapsing/remitting course often follows. This clinical picture is referred to as **subacute brucellosis** or **undulant fever**. During this phase arthralgia, fatigue, low-grade fever and depression are common. Physical examination may be normal or reveal moderate splenomegaly. This form of brucellosis may also develop insidiously with no preceding acute febrile illness. Suppurative and immune-mediated complications are most likely to occur during this stage. Most patients recover within 1 year.

Chronic brucellosis describes patients who have been unwell for more than a year. The status of this diagnosis remains controversial. Some of these patients have had inadequate antibiotic therapy or have local suppurative complications, but chronic brucellosis has been used in the past to describe a group of patients, usually at occupational risk of acquiring brucellosis, with symptoms indistinguishable from the chronic fatigue syndrome (➢243), who have no evidence of ongoing infection. If clinical examination, blood, urine and bone marrow culture, liver biopsy, radiology and serology all show no evidence of brucellosis, then the diagnosis of chronic brucellosis should not be made, but serology should be repeated over a period of several months.

Complications of brucellosis: **Arthritis** becomes more common as duration of disease increases. Sacroiliitis, acute monoarthritis (usually affecting the hip, knee or ankle) or a polyarticular rheumatoid-like arthritis has been described. **Vertebral osteomyelitis** occurs occasionally and may be associated with paravertebral abscess. Characteristic radiological changes with lateral osteophyte growth ('parrot's beak sign') are described. **Haematological** abnormalities include anaemia, leucopenia and thrombocytopenia, which may be severe, leading to purpura. **Meningitis** and **encephalitis** occur occasionally. The CSF shows a lymphocytic pleocytosis, with raised protein and normal or slightly reduced glucose. **Uveitis** and **epididymo-orchitis** occur. **Pulmonary involvement** is usually restricted to cough with CXR infiltrates, although pleural effusion has been reported. **Brucella endocarditis** is rare and affects primarily the aortic valve. Most patients have pre-existing valve damage. Endocarditis accounts for most of the mortality associated with brucellosis. **Granulomatous hepatitis, hepatic or splenic abscesses** also occur. Granulomatous disease affecting the **kidney, ureter or bladder** may cause urinary symptoms or obstructive uropathy.

Investigations: Diagnosis is usually suspected on epidemiological grounds and is unequivocally confirmed by isolation of organism from blood, bone marrow or focal lesions. This requires special techniques and prolonged culture and presents a hazard to laboratory staff ☎ ☠. Culture any available biopsies and aspirates of local lesions (warn laboratory of suspected diagnosis), and take two or three blood cultures. Culture is positive in the majority of cases of acute brucellosis, but the yield is lower in subacute infection. Serological tests are more widely used, but are never worth requesting without a history of contact or travel. Persistent negative serology reliably excludes acute brucellosis; the interpretation of low-titre positive results in patients with equivocal chronic disease requires discussion with reference laboratory ☎. In this situation bone marrow aspiration and culture are recommended by some authors.

Management: Doxycycline 200 mg daily + rifampicin 600–900 mg/day for 6 weeks. Rifampicin + co-trimoxazole **or** doxycycline + streptomycin are alternatives. Prolonged treatment may be necessary for focal suppurative disease. Patients with brucella endocarditis almost always need valve replacement.

Yersinia pestis ⊠ ④

Pleomorphic, Gram-negative coccobacillus.

Pathogenesis: Antiphagocytic capsule, lipopolysaccharide and various other toxins involved.

Epidemiology and transmission: Transmitted to humans and animals by flea bites, by direct contact with infected animals (for example, by handling infected animal tissues) or by aerosol from humans or animals with pneumonic plague. Major plague pandemics have occurred throughout history (e.g. the Black Death); the most recent started in China in the mid-nineteenth century and peaked in the early part of this century. *Yersinia pestis* is maintained in geographically restricted enzootic foci throughout all continents, notably western USA (~15 cases p.a. in USA), S America, Africa, Central and SE Asia (particularly Burma, Vietnam and Indonesia). Areas reporting human plague to WHO in 1994 are indicated in Table 56 (➤146). Human disease may be sporadic or epidemic. Sporadic cases occur when humans intrude into enzootic areas, following an epizootic or when rodents and fleas enter houses. Epidemic disease is usually associated with poor living conditions, rodent and flea infestation and overcrowding. Person-to-person respiratory spread causing primary plague pneumonia is particularly likely to establish a chain of epidemic spread.

Spectrum of disease: Bubonic and pneumonic plague (see below).

Laboratory diagnosis: Aspirate buboes, collect sputum and blood cultures. Fluorescent antibody staining used in endemic areas. Methylene blue bipolar-stained bacilli. Capsules visible in tissue smears and after culture at 37°C. Best growth on blood agar anaerobically and at low temperature (27°C) ➤. Serology also available.

Prevention: Depends on rodent and flea control. Contacts of cases should be disinfested of fleas. Contacts of suspected plague pneumonia should be given chemoprophylaxis (tetracycline or a sulphonamide for 1 week). International quarantine regulations apply to passengers arriving from a plague-endemic area. Vaccine is available for immunisation of laboratory and field workers particularly likely to be exposed (➤144).

CLINICAL SYNDROME

Plague (syn. bubonic plague) ⊠ ④

A disease of rodents caused by *Yersinia pestis*.

Clinical features

Incubation time: Two to 6 days (1–6 days for primary plague pneumonia).

Symptoms and signs: Bubonic plague results from percutaneous inoculation of *Yersinia pestis* by flea bite or by contamination of a wound by infected material. Presents with sudden onset of fever, rigors, headache, myalgia, prostration, GI upset and abdominal pain, and tender enlarged regional lymph nodes ('bubo'). Untreated, secondary spread occurs, leading to septicaemia, meningitis and secondary plague pneumonia. In ~10–20% of cases, **primary plague septicaemia** occurs, with bloodstream invasion without primary regional lymphadenopathy. Symptoms are similar to bubonic plague, but recognition is difficult. Mortality is very high as all progress to secondary plague pneumonia. **Primary plague pneumonia** follows respiratory transmission. After an incubation period which may be as short as 1 day patients develop fever, cough, bloody sputum, headache, rigors and prostration. Death may supervene rapidly, and infection may be transmitted to others by respiratory secretions.

Investigations: Diagnosis is often suspected

on epidemiological grounds. Aspirated material from bubo, sputum or CSF may show characteristic organisms on microscopy. Immunological methods for rapid identification of organisms are available. Culture of blood, sputum, bubo material, scrapings from skin lesions or tissue biopsy.

Management: Untreated mortality is high, up to 100% in plague pneumonia. Treatment with streptomycin, tetracyclines or chloramphenicol is highly effective if used within hours of presentation. Penicillin is not effective, and there are no trial data to support the use of parenteral or broad-spectrum cephalosporins or ciprofloxacin, although they are probably effective. Cases of plague pneumonia, and patients with bubonic plague who have cough or CXR changes, should be strictly isolated (☺) until 72 h after the start of antibiotic therapy. Less stringent isolation with drainage/secretion precautions is adequate for cases of bubonic plague.

Streptobacillus moniliformis

Highly pleomorphic Gram-negative rod; one cause of **rat-bite fever**. Upper respiratory commensal of rats causing infections of rat bites and of contaminated skin lesions, also epidemics of systemic illness associated with consumption of contaminated milk (**Haverhill fever**). Usually

causes severe systemic symptoms with fever, polyarthritis and rashes; rare local sepsis unassociated with bites, also IE and pneumonia. Untreated mortality ~10%. Grows readily in blood cultures, and on blood agar with added CO_2, in 48 h to form small, grey colonies; ✛. Sensitive to benzylpenicillin.

HACEK or herbie group

Haemophilus aphrophilus and *paraphrophilus*, *Actinobacillus actinomycetemcomitans*, *Cardiobacterium hominis*, *Eikenella corrodens* and *Kingella kingae* and *denitrificans*—sometimes known as the 'HACEK' or 'herbie' group—are bacteriologically related, rod-shaped human oropharyngeal commensals. *Eikenella* colonies pit solid agar surfaces.

Occasionally isolated from oropharyngeal, lung, pleural and brain abscesses, metastatic osteomyelitis and bite wounds, sometimes in mixed culture with other oral commensals. Rare causes of IE; isolation from blood cultures may require prolonged incubation. Variably benzylpenicillin-sensitive, but co-amoxiclav or parenteral or broad-spectrum cephalosporins are more reliable, with ampicillin plus gentamicin used for IE.

Francisella tularensis ☠

Causes tularaemia. Pleomorphic, capsulate, Gram-negative bacillus. High risk of laboratory-acquired infection ✛.

CLINICAL SYNDROME

Tularaemia ① (syn. rabbit fever, lemming fever, deerfly fever, Ohara disease)
Infection with *Francisella tularensis* is usually acquired from rabbits or hares. It causes a variety of clinical syndromes depending on the route of transmission.

Epidemiology and transmission: Widespread throughout the Northern hemisphere with the exception of the UK; particularly found in N America, Scandinavia, CIS, China and Japan. Many wild animals, including mammals and birds, are infected. Rabbits and hares are most important in human disease. Infection is maintained in the wild by ani-

mal–tick cycle. Human infection is acquired by contact with infected animal carcasses, by tick or mosquito bite, by consuming inadequately cooked rabbit or other infected meat or by inhalation of dust from soil, grain or hay. Laboratory cases occur readily as a result of inhalation. Person-to-person spread is very rare.

Clinical features

Incubation time: Two to 10 days.

Symptoms and signs: Depend on route of acquisition (Table 81). Severe constitutional symptoms (fever, headache, myalgia, cough, vomiting) may accompany all forms. Illness typically lasts 2–3 weeks.

Table 81 Clinical features of tularaemia

Route	Incidence	Clinical form	Clinical features
Percutaneous	~50%	Ulceroglandular	Indolent skin ulcer with regional lymphadenopathy. Pharyngitis, CXR infiltrates, pleural effusion
	~25%	Glandular	As above without the ulcer
Conjunctiva	<5%	Oculoglandular	Blepharitis, severe conjunctivitis with small yellowish nodules and ulcers. Regional lymphadenopathy
Inhalation	<5%	Typhoidal	Severe sepsis without localising features
	<5%	Pneumonic	Dry cough, chest pain, pleurisy, dyspnoea. CXR shows hilar lymphadenopathy or infiltrates
Food-borne	<5%	Oropharyngeal	Pharyngitis and cervical lymphadenopathy

Mortality untreated 10–20%, depending on presentation.
Investigations: Leucocytosis, sterile pyuria and abnormal liver function tests are common. Diagnosis is confirmed by serology.

Culture is hazardous for laboratory staff.
Management: Streptomycin is the drug of choice. Gentamicin and tetracycline are alternatives.

23: Anaerobes

Obligate anaerobes require a reduced oxygen tension for growth, failing to grow on the surface of solid media in 10% CO_2 in air (18% oxygen). They are divided into **sporing** anaerobic (SA: including only *Clostridium* spp.) and **non-sporing** anaerobic (NSA) genera.

Classification of clinically important anaerobes

Nomenclature of the *Bacteroides* genus has recently been revised according to the footnotes in Table 82 (but most laboratories have not yet adopted it).

Table 82 Classification of anaerobes

Gram-positive	Bacilli	Spore-forming	*Clostridium perfringens* ('*welchii*'), *septicum, novyi* ('*oedematiens*'), *tetani, botulinum, difficile,* plus many other non-pathogens
		Non-spore-forming	*Actinomyces israelii* *Propionibacterium* spp. (≻182) *Arachnia propionica* *Bifidobacterium* spp. *Eubacterium* spp.
	Cocci		*Peptococcus niger* ('anaerobic staphylococcus') *Peptostreptococcus* spp. ('anaerobic streptococci')

Gram-negative	Bacilli		*Bacteroides* spp.
			  Gut-associated 'fragilis' group (*fragilis, thetaiotaomicron,* etc.)
			
			  'Pigmented' group (*melaninogenicus,*[1] *asaccharolyticus,*[2] *intermedius,*[1] etc.)
			  'Other' group (*oralis,*[1] *bivius,*[1] etc.)
			Fusobacterium nucleatum, necrophorum, plus many others

	Cocci		*Veillonella* spp.
Spirochaetes and other spiral anaerobes			(≻223)

[1] Transferred to *Prevotella* genus; [2] transferred to *Porphyromonas* genus.

Anaerobes as normal flora

Table 83

Anaerobe group	Skin		Mouth, nasopharynx	Vagina, urethra	Colon
	Above umbilicus	Below umbilicus			
Clostridium spp.		+			+++
Actinomyces spp.			+	+	++
Propionibacterium spp.	++	++			
'Fragilis' (gut) bacteroides					+++
'Pigmented' bacteroides	±*	±ᴬ	++	+	+
'Other' bacteroides	±*	±*	++	+	+
Fusobacterium spp.			+	+	+
Gram-positive cocci	+	+	++	+	++

*Especially in skin follicles of axillae and perineum.

Properties common to obligate anaerobes

Pathogenesis and epidemiology: Many anaerobes are important components of the commensal mucosal flora of humans and animals; *Clostridium* spp. vegetative forms and spores are also common in the environment.

Laboratory diagnosis: Clinical suspicion of anaerobic infection is supported by:

• putrid pus;
• characteristic Gram stain appearances (mixed and 'bizarre' organisms in NSA infections; brick-shaped Gram-positive rods with few pus cells in gas gangrene);
• brick-red fluorescence under long-wave UV light (especially *B. asaccharolyticus*);
• gas–liquid chromatography of pus (for short-chain fatty-acid products of anaerobic fermentation).

Anaerobic involvement should be remembered when patients do not respond to empirical therapy with limited antianaerobic spectra (e.g. parenteral or broad-spectrum cephalosporins, aminoglycosides), and when pus is reported 'culture-negative' (especially if dry swabs were submitted).

Appropriate incubation of all specimens where anaerobes may be clinically relevant is performed routinely nowadays by diagnostic laboratories. Some species are aerotolerant (some surface growth on freshly prepared solid media in air—e.g. *Clostridium tertium*). However, most obligate anaerobes are killed by oxygen; hence liaison between clinician and laboratory (with careful specimen collection and rapid transport, use of controlled anaerobic atmospheres with nutritive selective media) is essential for their reliable isolation ☞. Most clinically important species grow in 48–72 h; full identification can take much longer but, with some important exceptions, this is of dubious clinical relevance. Many clinical laboratories, therefore, report 'anaerobes isolated' from sites where speciation is not useful. Commercial biochemical test kits are now quite reliable for commonly encountered anaerobes, (important isolates ✈). Direct detection of toxin is used for some *Clostridium* infections (*difficile, botulinum*).

Treatment: Drainage/debridement is often the mainstay of therapy, and antibiotic therapy usually needs to cover both anaerobic and aerobic components of mixed infections. Of the clinically relevant anaerobes, only *Actinomyces* spp. and *Propionibacterium* spp. are normally resistant to **metronidazole** (resistance very rare in other genera), but resistance to formerly useful antibiotics, such as tetracycline, erythromycin and most β-lactams, is rising. **Co-amoxiclav, imipenem**

and **piperacillin-tazobactam** are reliable, but aminoglycosides and currently available quinolones have no useful antianaerobic activity. Clindamycin is sometimes useful for common focal infections with mixed anaerobic and Gram-positive facultative bacteria (e.g. lower limb infections in diabetics, chronic sinusitis). Cefoxitin is the only cephalosporin with useful activity.

Spectrum of disease due to anaerobes

Anaerobes cause three types of disease:
• **Toxin-associated**, sometimes with toxic effects remote from the site of bacterial multiplication (e.g. *Clostridium* spp.).
• **Local sepsis involving mixed bacteria** derived from the local mucosal flora (caused by all anaerobic genera). Sometimes 'synergistic' (e.g. *Bacteroides fragilis + Escherichia coli* causing more serious sepsis when present together than separately, as shown in rat peritonitis model).
• **Invasive infections associated with specific pathogens** (e.g. *Clostridium perfringens* causing gas gangrene, *Fusobacterium necrophorum* causing necrobacillosis).

Toxin-associated anaerobic infections

Clostridium perfringens
(Used to be called welchii)

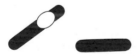

Brick-shaped Gram-positive rod.
Pathogenesis: Lecithinase (α-toxin, produced by all strains; the main virulence factor causing tissue damage in gas gangrene), enterotoxin (type A strains, causing food poisoning; damages intestinal mucosa), β-toxin (type C strains, causing enteritis necroticans) and many others. Predominantly releases saccharolytic enzymes, but some proteases including collagenase, hyaluronidase. Inoculation of spores to damaged tissues with compromised blood supply ⇒ sporulation ⇒ α-toxin release ⇒ myonecrosis with gas production.

Epidemiology: Gut commensal of humans and animals, and common on human skin and in soil, hence many opportunities for contamination of wounds and foods. Gas gangrene commoner in old age, diabetics and after lower limb surgery in arteriopaths. Five types A to E (typed by toxin production), and subtyping available serologically (✛).
Spectrum of disease, diagnosis and treatment: Most commonly isolated from traumatic or surgical wounds contaminated with faeces or soil; sometimes contributes to local tissue infection with mixed flora (i.e. **not** causing gas gangrene). Occasionally grown from blood cultures, usually from skin contamination or as terminal event in dying patient (systemic spread from gut).

Gas gangrene (➤90)**:** Invasive infection, primarily due to α-toxin effects. Patient invariably systemically toxic with severe local pain. Rare cases caused by *Clostridium novyi* (type A strains), *septicum*, *histolyticum* and *sordellii*. Diagnosis is primarily clinical, but Gram stain can be helpful (often mixed with other bacteria, with scant pus cells). Spores rarely seen in clinical material. Blood cultures positive in severe cases ⇒ massive haemolysis. Readily isolated on anaerobic blood agar (24 h), forming large, shiny, clear colonies. Confirm by Nagler reaction (further 24 h): lecithinase (α-toxin) activity on egg-yolk medium, with specific inhibition by antitoxin. Treatment is surgical debridement (plus penicillin or metronidazole). Hyperbaric oxygen may give additional benefit, but gas gangrene antiserum no longer recommended. Prevention by surgical toilet of traumatic wounds, antibiotic prophylaxis and careful skin disinfection (esp. before lower limb amputation).

Food poisoning: ✉ Distinct strains, commonly found in human and animal faeces and in meat; highly heat-resistant spores. Partly heat-resistant enterotoxin preformed in food; especially with high protein content (e.g. meat stews). Sporulation and growth (hence toxin release in food) encouraged by storage at room temperature; additional toxin released in gut by sporulation after passage through stomach. Σ ~1000. Mainly diarrhoea + abdominal pain, may be initial vomiting; 6–12-h incubation, illness lasting 12–48h. Supportive treatment only (➤45). No exclusion from work indicated once asymptomatic, because carriage of toxigenic strains is normally common. Outbreak investigation by typing of isolates from faeces and food (✈).

Necrotising jejunitis: 'Enteritis necroticans' or 'pig-bel' in New Guinea. Type C strain contaminating partly cooked meat in pig feasts. When eaten with vegetable containing trypsin inhibitor (or by malnourished people), the β-toxin ⇒ small intestinal necrosis with 50% mortality.

Nosocomial toxin-associated diarrhoea: Usually antibiotic-associated in elderly patients following overgrowth in gut of *Clostridium perfringens*. Toxigenicity demonstrated in cell culture (as used for *Clostridium difficile*). Therapy supportive + metronidazole.

Clostridium tetani ⊠

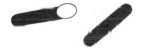

Slender, Gram-positive rod, with terminal spores.

Pathogenesis: Many extracellular products, but virulence factor is **tetanospasmin** (protein with heavy and light polypeptide chains) released by germination of spores in hypoxic tissues. Little or no local invasion needed for toxin release ⇒ axonal transport via motor neurons to CNS, and systemic spread by bloodstream. Inhibits the release of neurotransmitters, including glycine and γ-aminobutyric acid (GABA), resulting in muscle spasms, hyper-reflexia, seizures and autonomic dysfunction.

Epidemiology: Commensal of the gut of humans and animals, and frequently found in environment, especially manured soil. Σ ~20, especially in the elderly (unimmunised, and may have more fragile skin allowing penetration of, for example, rose thorns). Common in developing world, especially in neonates (from umbilical anointment with animal faeces). Rare cases and small outbreaks associated with unsterile surgical cat-

gut or contaminated theatre ventilation systems.

Spectrum of disease: Tetanus (see below).
Laboratory diagnosis: Swarming colonies on selective anaerobic blood agar in 24–48h (often only a film of growth, easily missed).

CLINICAL SYNDROME
Tetanus ⊠
A neurological syndrome characterised by tonic muscle spasms and hyper-reflexia, caused by the exotoxin of *Clostridium tetani*. Tetanus is now rare in the developed world, but it remains common in poor countries where immunisation programmes are not adequate. Immigrants from developing countries and UK residents born before 1961 may not have been vaccinated routinely.

Clinical features: Incubation period is typically 3–21 days, partially depending on the distance between the site of infection and the CNS. In many cases the antecedent wound is trivial or not found. Wound factors that promote spore germination and growth include necrotic tissue, suppuration and the presence of a foreign body. Tetanus may be generalised, localised, cephalic or neonatal.

Generalised tetanus is most common. Trismus (spasm of the masseter muscle causing lockjaw) is the commonest presenting symptom (~75% of cases), causing the *risus sardonicus* ('sardonic smile'). Restlessness, irritability, dysphagia, opisthotonus and seizures occur. Painful reflex spasms, often triggered by noise, light or touch, may be severe enough to cause fractures or rhabdomyolysis.

Localised tetanus is a rare form of tetanus affecting one extremity with a contaminated bite. It may progress to generalised tetanus but the prognosis is good.

Cephalic tetanus occurs in association with head injury or middle ear infection. The incubation period is typically short (1–2 days) and the prognosis is very poor. Isolated cranial nerve lesions (esp. VII), progressing to generalised tetanus, are common.

Neonatal tetanus is widespread in the developing world. It follows infection of the umbilical cord and presents with spasms between 3 and 10 days of age.
Microbiological investigations: Diagnosis made on clinical criteria. Gram stain of swab or pus from lesion rarely useful. Culture worth attempting for confirmation; CSF is normal.
Management: Antitetanus immunoglobulin 150 iu/kg im. Surgical excision of the wound if practical. Benzylpenicillin 2 MU 4-hourly for 10 days. Alternatives include metronidazole. **Intensive care** is usually required. Benzodiazepines may ameliorate spasms and prevent seizures. Paralysis and ventilation may be required. Despite full modern intensive care, the mortality remains 25–50%. Patients who recover may require ventilation for 3–6 weeks.

Prevention of tetanus (Table 84)
Primary prevention is achieved by immunisation with three doses of tetanus toxoid (➤337). A booster is required every 10 years until five doses have been given.
Management of wounds: All wounds should be carefully cleaned. Wounds or burns considered 'tetanus-prone' are:
• all wounds sustained >6 h before adequate surgical toilet is carried out;

• wounds that show a significant degree of devitalised tissue;
• puncture-type wounds;
• wounds contaminated with soil or manure;
• wounds with clinical evidence of sepsis.

Clostridium botulinum ✉
Gram-positive rod with subterminal spores.
Pathogenesis: Spores of *Clostridium botulinum* are ubiquitous in the environment. Germination and toxin production take place when appropriate anaerobic conditions are provided within preserved food. *Spores* can survive boiling at 100°C for several hours, but are killed at autoclave temperatures (121°C) after 5 minutes. *Toxin* is heat-labile and is destroyed by heating to 85°C for 1 minute. Botulism is now extremely rare in the UK because home canning of vegetables is rare. Acid fruits may be bottled safely as low pH inhibits growth. Clostridia producing type E toxin are adapted to low-temperature environments; the spores are less heat-resistant than other types, but toxin production may take place as low as 3°C. They are usually associated with a marine source such as fish or seal meat and are prevalent in Arctic regions.

Botulinum toxin binds irreversibly to peripheral neurons and blocks acetylcholine release at the neuromuscular junction and within the autonomic nervous system.
Epidemiology: *Clostridium botulinum* wide-

Table 84 Antitetanus prophylaxis

Immunisation status	Clean wound	Tetanus-prone wound
Full course or booster within last 10 years	Nil	Nil (a booster dose of toxoid may be given if the risk is thought to be very high, e.g. contamination with stable manure)
Full course or booster more than 10 years ago	Booster dose of toxoid	Booster dose of toxoid **plus** a dose of antitetanus immunoglobulin (250 iu*)
Not immunised or immunisation history not known with certainty	Full course of toxoid	Full course of toxoid **plus** a dose of antitetanus immunoglobulin (250 iu*) in a different site

* Increased to 500 iu if <24 h have elapsed since injury, if there is heavy contamination or following burns.

spread in intestines of humans and animals, plants, soil. Eight serotypes, but only types A, B, E associated with disease in humans. Botulism is usually associated with meat (Latin *botulus* = sausage), fish and, most frequently during this century, with home-preserved vegetables. Last outbreak in UK (1989) from contaminated canned hazelnut purée added to yoghurt; 27 patients affected, 12 needing ICU care, 1 death.

Spectrum of disease: Botulism (see below).

Laboratory diagnosis: ☞ Toxin detection in vomit, food, blood, faeces, etc. by animal testing (✈).

Prevention of botulism: Careful control of commercial canning processes. Preserved vegetables should be boiled for 3 minutes, with stirring prior to use. Infected food may or may not show signs of spoilage. Cans which have 'blown' should never be opened; canned food which smells 'off' should never be tasted, as sufficient toxin to cause disease may be present in very small amounts of food. Honey has been implicated as a source of spores in infant botulism—it should not be fed to children under the age of 1 year.

CLINICAL SYNDROME
Botulism ✉

An acute, descending, symmetrical, paralytic illness affecting primarily cranial and autonomic nerves, due to exotoxin produced by *Clostridium botulinum.*

Clinical features: Botulism is usually **food-borne**—the result of consumption of preformed toxin in contaminated food. Incubation period is 12–72 h depending on the dose. Presenting symptoms include blurred vision, diplopia, dysphagia, generalised weakness, GI upset particularly vomiting, dysphonia, vertigo and urinary retention or incontinence. On examination patients usually have evidence of depressed ventilatory function, specific muscle weakness or paralysis, and ophthalmoplegia. Autonomic involve-

ment may cause ptosis, dry mouth, fixed dilated pupils and constipation. Higher mental functions and sensation remain intact and there is no fever. More rarely **wound botulism** occurs, in which contamination of a wound is followed by endogenous production of toxin, in a similar manner to tetanus (➤217). Symptoms and signs are the same as for food-borne disease. **Infant botulism** is due to colonisation of the infant gut by *Clostridium botulinum.* It affects children under the age of 1 year, and has been associated with consumption of honey, which may contain spores. Presenting signs include weakness, hypotonia, listlessness, constipation, failure to feed and respiratory failure. It is thought to account for a small percentage of cases of sudden infant death syndrome. Gastrointestinal botulism occurs extremely rarely in adults with anatomical abnormalities of the gut.

Microbiological investigations: Diagnosis is based on clinical signs; suspicion is often aroused because of multiple cases in persons who have all eaten the same contaminated food. Confirmation is by demonstration of toxin in food, serum or stools of patients, or culture of the organism from stools (or wound in the case of wound botulism) ✈. Culture of the organism from food is supportive evidence only, as spores are ubiquitous. These investigations may be negative in many cases. In infant botulism, however, the diagnosis may be ruled out if two stool samples obtained during the acute episode are negative for toxin and culture.

Antibiotic management: Antibiotics are usually given (benzylpenicillin) although there is no evidence that they influence outcome. They may be more useful in infant and wound botulism.

Supportive management: Mortality may be reduced to ~15% by expert intensive care; prolonged ventilation for several weeks is usually required. Death is usually due to the complications of prolonged paralysis and ventilation. Recovery may take many months. Trivalent (types A, B and E) botulism antitoxin, prepared in horses, is available and should be given to all suspected cases. Hypersensitivity is common and package instructions relating to test dose and administration must be followed. Antitoxin may be given as a single dose (20 ml im) prophylactically to patients who are suspected of having consumed contaminated food. For patients with established disease, repeated doses are given (20 ml by slow iv infusion, followed by 10 ml 2–4 h later, and further doses at 12–24-h intervals). Antitoxin does not affect toxin already bound to neurons, and is ineffective in infant botulism. Guanidine has been used experimentally to counteract the effects of toxin at the neuromuscular junction.

Clostridium difficile

Gram-positive rod with subterminal, oval spores.

Pathogenesis: Overgrowth of *Clostridium difficile* in gut of patients during or after antibiotic therapy ⇒ toxin release. Two main toxins: A (enterotoxin ⇒ damages villus tips ⇒ 'leaky' gut barrier) and B (cytotoxin ⇒ damages cytoskeleton and cell–cell junctions of enterocytes). Production of both toxins associated with more severe disease. Nontoxigenic strains do not cause diarrhoea. Neonatal enterocytes may lack toxin A receptors; specific antitoxin B IgA in the gut may be protective.

Epidemiology: Normal faecal commensal of neonates and frequent in young children, but rare in adults out of hospital who have not received recent antibiotics. Spores contaminate surroundings of infected (esp. incontinent) patients and survive in environment ⇒ colonise new patients by faecal–oral route; also transmitted on staff hands and unsterilised equipment (e.g. sigmoidoscopes). PMC rarely associated with cytotoxic therapy or gut surgery in the absence of antibiotics. Tenfold increase in reported cases in England and Wales in past decade: Σ > 3000 in 1993, ~15% from antibiotic usage out of hospital. Available typing methods include cell-wall protein electrophoresis and DNA restriction fragment polymorphism analysis (➧). About 50% relapses are reinfections with different strains. True relapses probably due to persistence of spores in gut (but may be reinfections with same strain).

Spectrum of disease: Antibiotic-associated diarrhoea (➢47).

Laboratory diagnosis: Detection of cytotoxin B in stool by cell culture and antitoxin neutralisation (24 h), or variety of immunoassays (for toxins A, B or both; 4–24 h). Some laboratories culture and identify the organism, which is slower (48 h+ on selective medium), expensive and not diagnostically specific, but allows typing for outbreak investigation. Some laboratories test for toxin in all faecal samples, others only when requested or when patients said to be on antibiotics. Avoid sending multiple repeat faecal samples from patients with symptomatic relapse or to assess 'clearance', because continued presence of toxin or organism is common (~ 25%) and not predictive of response or relapse.

Local purulent infections involving mixed bacteria (Table 85)

Table 85 Infections commonly involving non-sporing anaerobes

Region	Condition	
Head, neck, oropharynx	Vincent's infection (necrotising gingivitis)	➢16
	Dental sepsis, periodontal disease	➢16
	Chronic sinusitis	➢15
	Tonsillar and peritonsillar abscess	➢18
	Brain abscess (sinus-associated)	➢79

continued on p. 221

Table 85 contd

Region	Condition	
Pleuropulmonary	Aspiration pneumonia	➤25
	Lung abscess (bronchial obstruction, aspiration)	➤28
	Empyema	➤28
	Bronchiectasis (putrid sputum)	
Intra-abdominal	All large-bowel perforations	➤54
	Appendicitis, diverticulitis, etc.	➤55
	Pyogenic liver abscess	➤56
	Wound infection after colonic surgery	➤89
	Long-standing cholangiostasis, biliary fistulae	➤54
Perirectal	Anorectal abscess (isolation of 'gut' flora is predictive of fistula in ano, 'skin' flora is not)	
	Necrotising fasciitis, 'synergistic gangrene'	➤91
Genital tract (female)	Bacterial vaginosis	➤70
	Bartholin's abscess	➤63
	Tubo-ovarian abscess	➤71
	Septic abortion, retained products, episiotomy infections	➤62
	Postsurgical infection (e.g. post-hysterectomy)	
Genital tract (male)	Scrotal abscess, prostatic abscess	
	Balanoposthitis	
Bone and joint	Osteomyelitis (from faecal contamination, especially after lower limb open fractures)	➤97
	Diabetic lower limbs	➤99
Skin and soft tissue	Ulcers (venous, pressure, diabetic; ulcerating cancers; Meleney's synergistic gangrene)	➤91
	Infected sebaceous cysts	
	Axillary/groin abscesses (including hydradenitis suppurativa)	➤88
	Recurrent breast abscess (not puerperal, which usually involve *Staphylococcus aureus*)	➤88
	Paronychia	
	Bites (human and animal)	➤90

These are autoinfections derived from mucosal normal flora by direct or haematogenous spread, and involve 'non-sporing anaerobes' with local aerobes such as streptococci, coliforms and staphylococci. *Streptococcus 'milleri'* is a frequent companion (➤173).

Very common overall. They present to many clinical specialities, and involvement of anaerobes is often suspected late. Knowledge of normal human anaerobic flora allows the primary source of haematogenously disseminated infections to be inferred (e.g. *Bacteroides* of *fragilis* group = gut source). Little evidence for special 'pathogenicity' for most NSA in this type of infection, except *Bacteroides fragilis* (toxic capsule) and suspected for *Bacteroides asaccharolyticus* (common isolate, but unknown virulence factors).

Invasive, specific pathogen-associated anaerobic infections

These are uncommon, but often serious infections with characteristic clinical signs affecting particular patient groups.

Gas gangrene (➤90, 216)

Clostridium septicum

Produces a cytotoxic and haemolytic α-toxin. Causes 'neutropenic enterocolitis'—presents as abdominal pain + fever during episode of neutropenia. Severe, necrotising colitis (sometimes bacteraemic, and metastatic spread with high mortality). Organism isolatable from blood, necrotic bowel wall or faeces (selection for spore-forming bacteria by heat or alcohol shock). Early colectomy plus antibiotics can be curative (e.g. metronidazole added to a standard regimen for fever in neutropenic patients—➤134). Occasionally also causes bacteraemia in patients with colonic carcinoma, and has been rarely associated with gas gangrene-like illnesses.

Clostridium tertium

Causes bacteraemia in neutropenic patients, from gut or iv catheter source. Aerotolerant organism, which may grow on aerobic culture plates and be misidentified as a *Bacillus* sp. (hence thought to be a contaminant). Usually treated with vancomycin; consider gut resection if necrosis suspected.

Fusobacterium necrophorum

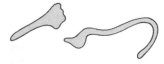

Causes 'necrobacillosis' or 'anaerobic tonsillitis' (Lemierre's syndrome ➤17). Young adults presenting with severe sore throat ⇒ septicaemia ⇒ secondary abscesses (liver, lungs, bone). Also quinsy and internal jugular vein thrombosis from local spread. Grown from blood or pus: bizarrely shaped Gram-negative bacilli. Carry polysaccharide capsule, which may be virulence factor. Sensitive to penicillin or metronidazole.

Actinomycosis

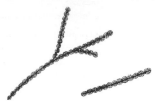

A clinical term describing chronic abscesses and sinuses discharging granular pus ('sulphur granules') containing characteristic microcolonies of Gram-positive branching rods (*Actinomyces israelii*). Begins as a local purulent infection involving mixed bacteria, in which *Actinomyces israelii* attains later predominance: optimal culture will usually isolate several additional organisms even in late stages. Commonest sites include: **oral and neck** (associated with dental disease); **abdominal** (RIF, colon after appendicitis, perforated diverticulum, etc.); **dacryocystitis**; **IUCD and pelvic infection**. Treatment: penicillin/amoxycillin (plus metronidazole for the commonly associated nonsporing anaerobes), or co-amoxiclav for ~6 weeks. Alternatives in penicillin-allergic patients include tetracycline, erythromycin, clindamycin or fusidic acid. Drainage/debridement often needed.

Arachnia propionica is bacteriologically similar to *Actinomyces israelii* and occasionally causes dacrocystitis.

24: Spirochaetes

Slender spiral anaerobic rods. Actively motile with several flagella enclosed within the bacterial outer cell membrane, attached at either end of the cell and wrapping round the cell body. Virulence factors unknown. Lipid-rich outer membrane contributes to sensitivity to detergents and desiccation, and hence only venereal or insect-borne transmission for many species of spirochaete. Pathogenic spirochaetes cannot be cultivated *in vitro* but can be visualised (e.g. dark-ground microscopy of material from syphilitic chancre, or detection of *Borrelia* or *Leptospira* in blood). Serology is important in most spirochaete-associated diseases (often ✛).

Non-venereal treponematoses

Non-venereal infections due to spirochaetes closely related to *Treponema pallidum* occur where environmental conditions allow transmission (Table 87). These organisms are mor-

Table 86 Classification of spirochaetes

Genus	Species	Notes
Treponema	*pallidum*	Syphilis (➤67)
	pallidum ssp. *pertenue, carateum, pallidum* ssp. *endemicum*	Non-venereal treponematoses
Borrelia	*burgdorferi*	Lyme disease (➤224)
	recurrentis and other spp.	Relapsing fever (➤225)
Leptospira	*interrogans*	Leptospirosis (➤226)
(*Anaerobiospirillum* spp.)		Isolated from faeces and blood of some immunocompromised patients with diarrhoea
(*Mobiluncus* spp.)		Associated with bacterial vaginosis (➤70)
(*Spirillum*	*minus*)	One cause of rat-bite fever (➤212)

Table 87 Non-venereal treponematoses

Species	Disease	Environment	Clinical features
Treponema pallidum ssp. *pertenue*	Yaws (syn. frambesia tropica)	Humid tropics. Predominantly a disease of childhood. Skin to skin transmission	Papular skin lesions which may ulcerate. Periostitis and dactylitis. Approximately 10% develop destructive lesions of skin or bone. CNS, CVS and congenital disease do not occur

continued on p. 224

Table 87 contd

Species	Disease	Environment	Clinical features
Treponema pallidum ssp. *endemicum*	Non-venereal endemic syphilis ('bejel', 'njovera')	Arid subtropical or temperate areas. Rural populations where living conditions/hygiene are poor. Mouth to mouth transmission via shared utensils	Initial lesion usually mucous patches in the mouth, followed by skin lesions resembling those of secondary venereal syphilis. Gummata of skin, long bones, nasopharynx occur, but CNS and CVS disease are very rare
Treponema carateum	Pinta ('carate')	Arid tropical Americas. Skin to skin transmission	Confined to skin. Maculopapular pigmented rash, healing to leave depigmented scars

phologically identical to *T. pallidum*, and show only minor antigenic differences. They all cause positive serological tests for syphilis (➤68). All are treated with benzylpenicillin. Mass eradication programmes were mounted against yaws in the 1950–1960s, and it is now less prevalent.

Borrelia spp.

CLINICAL SYNDROME
Lyme disease (LD)
(syn. tick-borne borreliosis)
A multisystem disorder caused by the spirochaete *Borrelia burgdorferi* and transmitted by tick bite.
Epidemiology and transmission: Risk of transmission occurs in areas where ticks are found, during late spring and summer when immature ticks feed. Ticks, mice, deer and other mammals act as a reservoir. It is widely distributed in Europe, China, Japan and Australia. In the USA it is found mainly in the north-east (New England), California, Texas, Wisconsin and Minnesota. It is comparatively rare in the UK (Σ ~30). Infection occurs across southern England from Kent to Devon, in East Anglia, Yorkshire, Cumbria and the Scottish highlands. It is very unlikely in the absence of a history of travel to an endemic area.

Clinical features: Variable, and may be severe or mild, pathognomic or non-specific. They have been arbitrarily divided into three stages, but these may overlap.
Stage 1 (early localised LD): 7 (3–32) days after tick bite, a characteristic rash develops at the site of inoculation in 50–75% of cases. This is an expanding, annular, bright red, hot, painless plaque with central clearing, called **erythema chronica migrans** (ECM). This is often accompanied by local lymphadenopathy and constitutional flu-like symptoms, headache, meningism and arthralgia.
Stage 2 (early disseminated LD) occurs weeks to months after the original tick bite. In some patients, secondary ECM lesions occur elsewhere on the body, usually a few days after the primary lesion. More severe constitutional symptoms and general lymphadenopathy occur. **Neurological** symptoms affect ~15% of patients, including facial palsy and other cranial nerve lesions, aseptic meningitis, peripheral neuropathy or radiculopathy causing pain, sensory loss and weakness in limbs or trunk. Symptoms tend to be migratory and intermittent. Encephalitis, psychosis and focal neurological deficit occur but are rare in the UK. **Cardiac** manifestations occur in ~10% of patients during this stage. A–V block occurs in ~90% of such

cases—it may be complete but is usually reversible. Pericarditis occurs less often and congestive cardiac failure occurs very rarely. **Arthritis** may occur during stage 2 or 3 and affects a large proportion of patients (~50% in the USA). It is usually a recurrent monoarthritis or asymmetrical oligoarthritis affecting large joints, or more rarely a symmetrical seronegative rheumatoid arthritis-like illness. It usually resolves after several years but in a minority the intermittent pattern gives way to chronic arthritis with erosive changes.

Stage 3 (late persistent LD) consists of arthritis, which is relatively frequent, and late neurological complications (neuropsychiatric disease, focal neurological deficits and intermittent incapacitating fatigue), all of which are rare. **Acrodermatitis chronica atrophicans** is a doughy, blotchy discoloration of the skin of the extremities which resembles the changes of peripheral vascular disease, and occurs as an unusual late complication, usually in elderly women.

Infection during pregnancy has been associated with miscarriage but there is no firm link with congenital abnormality.

Diagnosis: Clinical, based on the features described above and a history of travel to an endemic area and possible exposure to ticks. Non-specific findings which may be present include raised ESR, abnormal liver function tests, raised IgM, leucocytosis and microscopic haematuria. In patients with meningitis, CSF findings are typical of aseptic meningitis (➤75); CSF may be examined for the presence of specific antibodies. **Serology** is available, but must be interpreted with care, particularly in the absence of definite clinical evidence of LD and with a good travel history. Serology is not usually positive until some weeks after the onset of illness, and prompt antibiotic therapy may ablate an antibody response. False positives also occur, particularly in rheumatoid disease, infectious mononucleosis and syphilis. Western blotting can be used to improve

specificity. New diagnostic methods such as PCR will be useful. At present, interpretation of test results requires close liaison with the reference laboratory ☎.

Management: Treatment of tick bite alone, with no evidence of ECM, is not recommended except in pregnancy and in known areas of particularly high incidence ☎. Current antibiotic recommendations are shown in Table 88.

Table 88

Stage of disease	Regimen	Comments
Stage 1 (early) and mild cardiac or neurological disease	Doxycycline 100 mg 12-hly po **or** amoxycillin 500 mg 8-hly po (child: 40 mg/ kg/day) **or** erythromycin 250 mg 6-hly po for 21 days	Includes patients with 1° heart block (PR interval < 0.3 s) and Bell's palsy. Treat Bell's palsy for 30 days
Arthritis, more severe neurological or cardiac disease. Stage 3 (late disease)	Benzylpenicillin, 2.4 g 4-hly iv (child 150 mg/ kg/day) **or** ceftriaxone 2 g 24-hly iv (child 75 mg/ kg/day) for 14–21 days	Includes patients with 1° heart block (PR interval > 0.3 s), meningitis, encephalitis or neuropathy

Immunity: After treatment for one episode patients are probably still at risk of infection.

Prevention: Important measures include avoidance of tick bites (➤138) and prompt removal of any ticks attached to skin because transmission requires prolonged attachment of tick for several hours.

CLINICAL SYNDROME
Relapsing fever ✉ ①
Febrile illness transmitted by ticks or lice, characterised by several episodes of clinical relapse. Spirochaetes can usually be seen in

the peripheral blood during attacks, but fibrin strands or leptospires may be mistaken for them.

Risk factors: Louse-borne relapsing fever is a disease of war and starvation, usually occuring as epidemics wherever people are clothed but impoverished. There is no animal reservoir. Tick-borne relapsing fever is a zoonosis maintained in wild rodents. Endemic foci exist in Asia, Africa, the Americas, the Middle East and in some Mediterranean areas, particularly Spain.

Clinical features

Incubation period: Eight (3–32) days.

Symptoms and signs: Fever, headache, prostration and myalgia. Confusion and cough productive of sputum are common. Myocarditis, meningoencephalitis, hepatosplenomegaly, jaundice and hepatic failure may occur. Thrombocytopenia, DIC and a haemorrhagic rash may complicate severe cases. Mortality 2–10% untreated.

Episodes last 4–7 days and if untreated end by crisis with a sudden fall in temperature and occasionally hypotension. Remission lasts a similar period, and is followed by relapse and a further febrile episode. This occurs two or three times in louse-borne disease and up to 10 times in tick-borne disease.

Table 89 Organisms

Species	Transmission	Distribution
Borrelia recurrentis	Louse-borne	Worldwide
Borrelia latychevi	Tick-borne	Iran
Borrelia persica	Tick-borne	Asia
Borrelia hispanica	Tick-borne	Spain
Borrelia parkeri, B. turicatae, B. hermsii	Tick-borne	N America
Borrelia venezuelensis	Tick-borne	S America

Microbiological investigations: Parasitaemia, with extracellular spirochaetes, can be demonstrated by examination of thick blood films as for malaria. Animal inoculation and serology are also available.

Other investigations: Neutrophilia and mild anaemia are common during episodes.

Antibiotic management: Tetracycline 500 mg 6-hly for 7 days. Erythromycin is also effective. Herxheimer-type reactions to treatment are common, with sudden deterioration in clinical condition.

Leptospira interrogans

CLINICAL SYNDROME

Leptospirosis ⊠ ② (syn. Weil's disease, canicola fever)

A spirochaetal infection of variable severity acquired by contact with urine of infected mammals.

Epidemiology and transmission: Distributed worldwide. Occurs in the UK,' although uncommon (Σ ~60, ~three deaths). Tropical fresh water provides the best environment for spirochaete survival. Most often associated with renal infection in rats and dogs, but any mammal may be implicated. Transmission occurs by contact of skin or mucous membranes with urine, tissues or urine-contaminated water. There is usually an exposure history. Risk factors include occupations (e.g. agriculture, sewage workers) and recreational exposures (e.g. fishing, canoeing). Multiple serovars of *Leptospira interrogans* are responsible for disease, including icterohaemorrhagiae (rats), canicola (dogs) and hardjo (cattle).

Pathogenesis: Extensive damage to capillary endothelial cells, and in severe cases widespread visceral haemorrhages, renal failure and hepatocellular failure.

Clinical features

Incubation time: Seven to 12 days (range 2–26 days).

Symptoms and signs: Variable severity but only rarely asymptomatic. Usually a self-limited febrile illness with headache, prominent severe myalgia, rigors, arthralgia, neck stiffness and prostration. Generalised abdominal pain, epistaxis, mild haemoptysis and GI upset also occur. On examination, conjunctival suffusion and a transient truncal rash, which may be macular, maculopapular, purpuric or urticarial, hepatomegaly, meningism, and mild confusion.

Leptospirosis is classically described as a biphasic illness, although this probably only occurs in a minority of cases. During the initial phase, which lasts 4–7 days, leptospires are present in blood. This is followed by an asymptomatic period lasting 1–5 days, followed by a recurrence of fever lasting 4–30 days, during which organisms are present in urine. Neurological symptoms such as meningism are common during this stage. In a minority of patients the initial phase develops into a severe illness with jaundice, renal failure, widespread haemorrhages, shock and confusion. Most deaths are due to renal failure, and dialysis may be required but permanently impaired renal function is rare in patients who recover. Adrenal haemorrhage and severe pulmonary haemorrhage occur rarely.

Investigations: Diagnosis is often suspected on epidemiological grounds. Culture is difficult, and diagnosis is usually confirmed by serology. Microscopy of blood or urine is unreliable outside reference laboratories ➤. Anaemia, thrombocytopenia and neutrophilia are common. The WBC is usually 5–15000 × 10⁹/1. Proteinuria and microscopic haematuria are common. Uraemia, abnormal liver function tests and disordered coagulation occur in sicker patients. CSF shows a pleocytosis, initially polymorphs, but later mainly mononuclear, with normal glucose and normal or elevated protein. CXR infiltrates are common.

Management: Antibiotic therapy shortens duration of illness, particularly if given early. Doxycycline and benzylpenicillin are both effective. Supportive therapy for severe complications may be necessary.

Prevention: Depends on limiting exposure to infective water and animals. If this cannot be achieved, e.g. for sewer workers or military personnel, chemoprophylaxis with doxycycline (200 mg weekly) is effective but rarely indicated. Vaccination against specific serovars for persons at occupational risk has been used in some countries.

25: Mycobacteria

Slowly multiplying Gram-positive bacilli and coccobacilli containing waxes (mycolic acids) in their cell walls, which are responsible for resistance to decolorisation by acid or alcohol after staining by dyes such as carbol fuchsin (acid-fast bacilli, AFB; acid- and alcohol-fast bacilli, AAFB). They are sensitive to alcohols and aldehydes, but resistant to many other disinfectants and to drying.

Diagnostic notes

All processing of sputum and specimens for mycobacterial diagnosis is performed in containment level 3 laboratory. Different diagnostic laboratories vary in whether mycobacterial investigations are performed routinely or only on request for particular specimens. **Always warn the laboratory if mycobacterial involvement is suspected clinically.** Slow growth makes direct microscopical detection in clinical specimens of prime importance—the most sensitive method is auramine phenol (AP)-stained smears, examined in fluorescence microscope. Ziehl–Neelsen staining (with hot carbol-fuchsin; ZN) now usually not used in primary diagnosis. Microscopical morphology can sometimes suggest involvement of MOTT rather than tubercle

bacilli, but this is non-specific. Rapid methods for detection of mycolic acids (e.g. mass spectroscopy) or DNA (e.g. PCR) under assessment. DNA probes can be combined with short-incubation broth culture to give rapid species diagnosis (especially in HIV). Most mycobacteria (including *Mycobacterium tuberculosis*) take up to 8 weeks to grow on primary isolation, but often only 2–3 weeks on subculture. So-called 'rapid growers' (*chelonei* and *fortuitum*) take up to 7 days to grow on subculture. *Mycobacterium leprae* has never been cultivated *in vitro*. Most mycobacteria will grow somewhat on a variety of nutritive media, but Lowenstein–Jensen (LJ) medium commonly used, containing eggs, glycerol, salts, malachite green and selective antibiotics.

Preliminary identification of mycobacteria in diagnostic laboratories is by optimal growth temperature, speed of growth, colonial and bacterial morphology, and pigment production in light or dark under aerobic conditions; confirmation and sensitivity testing: ➔.

Significance of positive mycobacterial culture

Tubercle bacilli always clinically significant. Isolation of MOTT requires careful assessment,

Table 90 Classification of mycobacteria

Genus	Species	Notes
Mycobacterium	**tuberculosis, bovis,** africanum (microti). BCG	Tubercle bacilli, causing tuberculosis (➤29)
	leprae	Causes leprosy (➤230)
	avium-intracellulare, kansasii, marinum, ulcerans, scrofulaceum, xenopi, szulgai, malmoense, haemophilum, chelonei, fortuitum, etc.	'Atypical' mycobacteria, or 'mycobacteria other than TB' (MOTT). Environmental saprophytes causing a variety of opportunist infections (➤128)
	(gordonae, terrae, flavescens, smegmatis)	Also 'atypical' mycobacteria. Environmental saprophytes, very rare pathogens

because some are frequent contaminants (e.g. *xenopi, kansasii* and *gordonae* common in water). Often necessary to demonstrate persistent positivity of smears/cultures before starting treatment. Possibility of significant MOTT infection much higher in immunocompromised patients: ~10% mycobacterial infection in transplant recipients is non-tuberculous.

Mycobacterium tuberculosis

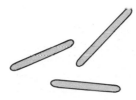

Slender bacilli. ✉. Isolate ① open cases (chest, urine, wound).

Pathogenesis: No recognised toxins or histolytic enzymes, but **cord factor** (glycolipid) found in more virulent strains ⇒ mitochondrial damage. Other glycolipids involved in **survival within macrophages** by inhibiting phagolysosome formation. Acquired most commonly by inhalation from open pulmonary case. Rare cases from inoculation to skin (e.g. prosector's wart in morbid anatomists). First exposure ('primary infection') with rapid bacterial multiplication but little tissue destruction ⇒ control of infection by cell-mediated immunity at primary site (e.g. Ghon focus in lung), local lymph nodes (making a '**primary complex**'), or after dissemination throughout body. Collection of activated macrophages is called an epithelioid granuloma; may contain multinucleate giant cells and have central caseous necrosis, later calcified. Failure to control primary infection (commoner in certain ethnic groups, children, immunocompromised hosts) ⇒ **miliary tuberculosis**. Subsequent reinfection or reactivation ⇒ slower multiplication and spread (controlled by cell-mediated immunity), but greater tissue damage (caused by delayed-type hypersensitivity). This is **postprimary tuberculosis** (➤29).

Epidemiology: Rising prevalence in UK since 1990 (Σ ~6000, ~300 deaths) having declined 10% per year for many decades before. Commoner in immigrants from developing countries (e.g. 20–30 × incidence in immigrants from Indian subcontinent, with higher prevalence of extrapulmonary TB), HIV (30% lifetime risk of TB infection with HIV (➤127), but currently under 5% TB cases notified in UK have HIV), socio-economic deprivation, malnourishment, alcoholism. Problems of multiply drug-resistant tuberculosis among HIV-positive and IVDU populations in US cities (33% resistant to one drug, 19% to rifampicin plus isoniazid in New York, 1992) not yet seen in UK.

Spectrum of disease: Tuberculosis (➤29).

Laboratory diagnosis: See diagnostic notes above, and ➤31 for tuberculin testing. Culture is essential to allow sensitivity testing. Decontamination of sputum to kill non-mycobacteria (e.g. by incubation with sodium hydroxide), followed by culture. Normally sterile samples (e.g. CSF) cultured directly after concentration by centrifugation. Buff, dry, heaped colonies. Liquid media (e.g. Kirchner) more sensitive. Automated culture systems economical in areas of high prevalence. Suitable specimens include sputum, BAL; urine; CSF; gastric lavage; pleural fluid or biopsy; peritoneal fluid; tissue biopsies; bone marrow; liver biopsy.

Treatment: ➤32.

Prevention and control: ➤34.

Mycobacterium bovis

Similar to *M. tuberculosis*, but produces weaker growth on LJ medium. Causes bovine tuberculosis; classically involving infection of the human ileocaecum or cervical lymph nodes (scrofula) from oral ingestion of milk from infected herds. Milk contamination interrupted by pasteurisation and testing of herds. Much *Mycobacterium bovis* infection in developed world is now imported, reactivation, or pulmonary-acquired from human cases. Σ ~40. Resistant to pyrazinamide, but therapy otherwise as for *Mycobacterium tuberculosis*.

Mycobacterium africanum

Causes some cases of TB in equatorial Africa.

Mycobacterium microti

The vole tubercle bacillus is now a very rare isolate from human infections.

Mycobacterium leprae

Epidemiology and transmission: Leprosy is widespread throughout the world, wherever there is poverty and overcrowding. WHO estimates > 12 million cases worldwide, in Africa, Asia and Latin America. Transmission is thought to occur most often by respiratory droplet spread from untreated lepromatous leprosy patients, whose nasal secretions contain large numbers of bacilli. Exposure to *Mycobacterium leprae* is much commoner than clinical disease.

Pathogenesis: Manifestations of disease are determined by host immunity. Persons with strong cell-mediated immunity (CMI) against the organism develop tuberculoid leprosy (TT), in which there is a vigorous granulomatous response and very few bacilli are found in lesions. Those with weak or absent CMI against *Mycobacterium leprae* develop lepromatous leprosy (LL) with no granulomatous response and massive infiltration of skin and nerves by mycobacteria. Between these extremes there is a continuum from borderline tuberculoid (BT) through borderline (BB) to borderline lepromatous (BL). Patients with BB or BL tend to downgrade to LL with time. *Mycobacterium leprae* predominantly affects nerves and skin; tissue damage may be caused by infiltration of organisms or by the host granulomatous response.

Spectrum of disease: Leprosy.

CLINICAL SYNDROME
Leprosy ✉ ①
A chronic granulomatous disease due to *Mycobacterium leprae*.
Clinical features: Clinical disease develops insidiously after a prolonged incubation period (~2–5 years for TT, 8–12 years for LL). **TT** is characterised by one to three localised asymmetrical hypopigmented macules with sharp, raised edges. Lesions are usually anaesthetic due to damage to nerves within the skin, and there may also be thickening of the peripheral nerve related to the lesion. **LL** has a more insidious onset. Lesions are very numerous, ill-defined, widely distributed and tend to be symmetrical. The skin is thickened but not usually anaesthetic until late in disease. Thickening of facial skin and loss of the outer third of the eyebrow ('madarosis') cause the typical 'leonine' facies. Widespread thickening of multiple peripheral nerves occurs; those most often affected, and which should be deliberately palpated if leprosy is suspected, include the ulnar, median, radial, common peroneal, posterior tibial and greater auricular nerves. Nasal stuffiness, anosmia and epistaxis are common. Septal perforation and collapse of the bridge of the nose may occur. Bony lesions, glomerulonephritis and amyloidosis also occur. Patients with borderline leprosy present a spectrum of clinical features between these two extremes.

Deformities result from a combination of anaesthesia, paralysis and hypohidrosis (due to autonomic neuropathy) leading to misuse, trauma, secondary infection and tissue loss. **Ocular involvement** causes blindness in ~10% of leprosy patients. Mechanisms include keratitis, iritis, corneal anaesthesia and exposure due to lagophthalmos secondary to facial nerve involvement.

Reactions are episodes of acute inflammation of skin, eyes or nerves which affect ~25% of leprosy patients. **Reversal reactions** (type 1 reaction) occur in patients with borderline leprosy, usually after therapy has begun, and cause acute inflammation of nerves and skin lesions, often with sudden loss of nerve function. **Erythema nodosum leprosum** (ENL, type 2 reaction), occurs in LL, causing a characteristic skin lesion, iritis, episcleritis and neuritis. ENL usually starts during the second year of therapy. Both of these reactions should be treated with anti-inflammatory agents (see below) but antimycobacterial treatment should not be discontinued.

Investigations: Diagnosis is clinical. In BL and LL, acid fast bacilli may be demonstrated in slit skin smears. Biopsy may also be helpful.

Management: For 'paucibacillary' disease (TT or BT, with negative slit skin smear), rifampicin and dapsone are given for 6 months. For 'multibacillary' disease (positive slit skin smear, BL or LL), rifampicin, dapsone and clofazimine are given for at least 2 years. Reactions are treated with clofazimine, thalidomide and steroids. Patients require education to avoid trauma to anaesthetic limbs. Plastic surgery may be required to correct or compensate for deformities. Isolation ① is recommended for smear-positive patients until adequately treated ☎.

Mycobacterium avium-intracellulare
(also known as the MAI complex)

Present in moist environments, and causes tuberculosis in birds and animals. Closely related to a variety of other animal pathogens. Present in ~50% patients dying of **AIDS** (➤128), also rarely in **organ transplant recipients and others with deficient cell-mediated immunity**. Disseminated and pulmonary infection, lymphadenitis. Seen and isolated by conventional AFB techniques in many specimens from such patients: sputum, marrow aspirate, intestinal biopsy, faeces. Granulomata rare; usually only AFB-stuffed macrophages are seen. Frequent chronic bacteraemia detectable by special blood culture techniques (e.g. lysis centrifugation, mycobacterial broths; ☎). Treatment with complex, multidrug regimens may improve symptoms, but rarely eliminates the pathogen or improves survival (➤129); *in vitro* sensitivity or resistance not always matched by *in vivo* response. Typing available (✈).

Local lymph node infection ('scrofula', especially unilateral cervical) is also rarely seen in immunologically normal children; usually treatable by excision alone.

Mycobacterium kansasii

Elongated, beaded bacilli, frequently found in piped water supplies (so beware of contamination of specimens). Causes pulmonary infections in elderly patients with pre-existing lung damage (emphysema, bronchiectasis, pulmonary fibrosis, silicosis, etc.) and sometimes in those with deficient cell-mediated immunity, including AIDS; clinically indistinguishable from TB. Effective regimens include rifampicin, isoniazid and ethambutol for 12–24 months; ciprofloxacin and clarithromycin also used.

Mycobacterium marinum

Elongated, beaded bacilli – the 'fish tubercle bacillus'. Associated with skin granulomas and ulcers after contact of abrasions with water ('swimming-pool granuloma', 'fish fancier's finger'). Rare associated lymphangitis. Diagnosis by microscopy and culture of biopsies of advancing edge of lesions (grows only at low temperature). Usually self-limiting, but responds to co-trimoxazole, tetracycline, ciprofloxacin, or rifampicin plus ethambutol. Modern swimming-pool maintenance eliminates contamination.

Mycobacterium ulcerans

Very slow growth, at low temperature only. Causes 'Buruli' or 'Bairnsdale' ulcer; chronic, progressive, undermining skin ulceration in tropical countries. Necrosis of underlying dermis. Geographically localised, especially to wetlands, where it is probably present on vegetation. Eventually self-heals (associated with appearance of cell-mediated immunity to the organism), but excision speeds resolution. Possible additional value of antibiotics (e.g. rifampicin plus clofazimine, or co-trimoxazole).

Mycobacterium scrofulaceum

Is ubiquitous in the environment, and occasionally causes unilateral lymph node infection in children, treatable by excision. Very rare pulmonary infections (as *Mycobacterium kansasii*). Treatment as for MAI.

Mycobacterium xenopi, szulgai and malmoense

Rare causes of pulmonary (as *Mycobacterium kansasii*) and lymphatic infection. *M. xenopi* commonly contaminates piped water systems, and *M. malmoense* may require up to 10 weeks' incubation on solid media. Unpredictable response to therapy (☎).

Mycobacterium haemophilum

Rarely associated with skin nodules in organ transplant recipients. Rifampicin, doxycycline and co-trimoxazole have been used in therapy.

Mycobacterium chelonei (or chelonae) and fortuitum

'Rapid growers', present in moist environments, most commonly causing localised, chronic infection of injection abscesses and traumatic wounds. Usually respond to drainage and curettage. Very rare pulmonary and disseminated infections. *M. chelonae* is relatively resistant to glutaraldehyde and has contaminated bronchoscope washer-disinfectors, causing diagnostic confusion when bronchial aspirates are stained for AFB. Both resistant to conventional TB chemotherapy, but *M. fortuitum* usually sensitive to ciprofloxacin, macrolides, co-trimoxazole or imipenem. *M. chelonei* often more resistant, but tobramycin, amikacin, erythromycin and clarithromycin have been used (☎).

26: Mycoplasmas, Chlamydiae and Rickettsiae

Mycoplasmas

The smallest prokaryotic organisms able to grow in cell-free culture media. Multiply by binary fission, often producing branching filaments which fragment to produce single pleomorphic cells. Several species have specialised structures at one or both ends of the cell by which they attach to respiratory or genital mucosa.

Classification of pathogenic mycoplasmas
(Table 91)

Laboratory diagnosis: Culture is not routinely performed. Serology is available. Patients with atypical pneumonia due to *Mycoplasma pneumoniae* may develop cold agglutinins, which were used in the past as surrogate for specific serology. Haemolytic anaemia may occur as a complication.

Treatment: Tetracyclines or macrolides are used. See individual syndromes.

Comments: In patients with **hypogammaglobulinaemia**, mycoplasmas (particularly *M. hominis* and *U. urealyticum*) may cause suppurative arthritis, subcutaneous abscesses, persistent urethritis and cystitis. Sternal would infections due to *M. hominis* have occurred in heart and lung transplant patients.

Chlamydiae

Small non-motile Gram-negative bacteria which are obligate intracellular parasites. Unlike viruses they contain both DNA and RNA, ribosomes and a cell wall and they divide by binary fission. They do not have peptidoglycan and cannot produce ATP, for which they depend on the host cell (hence 'energy parasites').

Metabolically inert infectious particles ('elementary bodies') are 300–350 nm in diameter. Once inside the host cell the organisms become metabolically active and increase in size to 800–1000 nm diameter ('reticulate bodies').

Classification of chlamydiae (Table 92)

Laboratory diagnosis: Organisms can be cultured in eggs or tissue culture but this is not routinely performed. Sensitive ELISA or immunofluorescent techniques are used routinely to demonstrate chlamydial antigens in respiratory or genital secretions. Serology is also used, although this does not routinely distinguish between species.

Treatment: Tetracyclines or macrolides are used. See individual syndromes.

Rickettsiae (Tables 93 & 94)

Rickettsiae are obligate intracellular Gram-negative parasites. Most are zoonoses spread to humans by arthropods. Rickettsiae replicate within the cytoplasm of endothelial cells and smooth-muscle cells of capillaries, arterioles and

Table 91 Classification of pathogenic mycoplasmas

Genus	Species	Notes
Mycoplasma	pneumoniae	Atypical pneumonia (➤22). Rarely associated with acute neurological complications, haemolytic anaemia, pericarditis, Stevens–Johnson syndrome and erythema nodosum
	hominis	Non-gonococcal urethritis (➤66). Respiratory infections in neonates (esp. low birth weight)
Ureaplasma	urealyticum	Non-gonococcal urethritis. Rare neonatal meningitis

Table 92 Classification of chlamydiae

Genus	Species	Serovars	Notes
Chlamydia	trachomatis	A, Ba, B, C	Trachoma (➤83)
		D–K	Inclusion conjunctivitis (➤83)
			Ophthalmia neonatorum ⊠ (➤83)
			Genital infections (➤66)
			Respiratory infection in neonates (➤113)
		L1–L3	Lymphogranuloma venereum (➤72)
	psittaci		Psittacosis (➤23)
	pneumoniae (formerly 'TWAR' agent)		Pharyngitis, atypical pneumonia (➤22)

small arteries causing necrotising vasculitis. Rickettsial infections vary greatly in severity, depending on the infecting species. Most are febrile infections with a characteristic rash. An 'eschar', a black ulcerated lesion, may develop at the site of inoculation. Severe, often fatal, multisystem involvement occurs with several species.

All rickettsial infections are rare as imported diseases to the UK, with the exception of tick typhus, which occurs occasionally in tourists after rural exposure, e.g. on safari.

Coxiella burnetii and organisms of the genus *Rochalimaea* are currently classified with the rickettsiae, but are biologically distinct. Q fever, the disease caused by systemic infection with *Coxiella burnetii*, occurs in the UK but is rare (see below). *Rochalimaea* spp. have recently been shown to be responsible for most cases of cat-scratch disease (➤24) and a number of syndromes in immunocompromised patients, especially in HIV (➤121).

Clinical features: Summarised on Tables 93–95 below.

Diagnosis: Usually clinical, confirmed by serology. Infection with rickettsiae induces antibodies that react with certain strains of the bacterium *Proteus*. This cross-reaction forms the basis of the Weil–Felix test, which uses different strains of *Proteus* to differentiate between different rickettsial infections. The Weil–Felix test is neither sensitive nor specific and has been replaced by specific serology for all important rickettsial infections. Organisms

may be seen on biopsy of the skin lesions of Rocky Mountain spotted fever.

Management: *Rickettsia* spp.: doxycycline 100 mg 12-hly or tetracycline 500 mg 6-hly for all rickettsial infections. Chloramphenicol 50 mg/kg/day (adult max: 4 g/day, child < 8 years max: 2 g/day) may be used in children under 8 years and in pregnancy.

For diagnosis and management of *Coxiella burnetii* and *Rochalimaea* spp. ➤236, 237.

Organisms related to the genus *Rickettsia* (Table 95)

Coxiella burnetii (Q fever, 'Balkan grippe')

Coxiella burnetii is biologically distinct from other rickettsiae. It grows in phagosomes rather than in the cytoplasm of infected cells and survives in the environment for prolonged periods.

Epidemiology and transmission: Zoonosis acquired by aerosol or direct contact, usually from occupational exposure to cattle or sheep. Person-to-person spread occurs, but not often enough to merit isolation of cases. Exposure to parturient cats or stillborn kittens is an important risk factor. The organism is highly infectious, and is a hazard to staff in the laboratory and post-mortem room. Σ ~150.

In some areas (e.g. Spain and Australia) *Coxiella burnetii* is more common, accounting for a significant proportion of community-acquired atypical pneumonias.

Table 93 *Rickettsia* I: spotted fever group

Species	Disease	Distribution	Ecology	Hosts/route	Incubation (days)	Clinical features
R. rickettsi	Rocky Mountain spotted fever	USA, Canada, Mexico, S America	Typically rural, but may occur in urban areas	Ticks, rodents, dogs, foxes/tick bite	7 (2–14)	Fever, severe headache, myalgia. Eschar in 20%. Widespread maculopapular rash on days 3–5, becoming petechial, purpuric and necrotic. Severe multisystem involvement (pulmonary, renal, GI, neurological, cardiac). Thrombocytopenia, DIC. Mortality 15–20% untreated
R. conori	African tick typhus* ('boutonneuse fever')	Mediterranean, Black Sea, Caspian Sea littorals, Middle East, India, Africa	Usually associated with rural exposure to ticks	Rodents, dogs/ tick bite	5–7	Eschar with tender local lymphadenopathy. Generalised maculopapular rash and conjunctival injection on days 4–5. Systemic features otherwise mild. Mortality very rare
R. australis	Queensland tick typhus	Australia	As for African tick typhus	Marsupials/tick bite	7 10	As for African tick typhus
R. siberica	Siberian tick typhus	Central Europe, Central Asia	As for African tick typhus	Rodents/tick bite	2–7	As for African tick typhus
R. akari	Rickettsialpox	N America, S Africa, CIS, Korea	Urban over-crowding, rodent contact	Rodents/mite bite	5–10	As for African tick typhus. Rash is vesicular, resembling chickenpox

*Also known as Mediterranean tick fever, Mediterranean spotted fever, Marseilles fever, Kenya tick typhus, India tick typhus.

Clinical features: After an incubation period of ~2–5 weeks, sudden onset of fever, rigors, headache, myalgia, arthralgia, chest pain and dry cough. Q fever may present as a respiratory infection, with signs consistent with atypical pneumonia (➤22), as a systemic febrile illness or as an acute hepatitis. Rash occurs rarely. Rarer presentations are reported, including pleuropericarditis, haemolytic anaemia, meningitis, arthritis, nephritis and epididymo-orchitis. Infection is almost always self-limited, even without therapy. **Q fever in pregnancy** is associated with increased risk of miscarriage.

Organisms: *Coxiella burnetii.*

Microbiological investigations: Culture is difficult and hazardous for laboratory staff. Diagnosis is confirmed by serology. *Coxiella burnetii* undergoes antigenic variation during infection. Antibodies to phase II antigens in-

Table 94 *Rickettsia* II: typhus group

Species	Disease	Distribution	Ecology	Hosts/route	Incubation (days)	Clinical features
R. prowazeki	Epidemic louse-borne typhus ('classic typhus')	Worldwide	In colder areas, where people are louse-infested. Typically associated with war and famine	Humans are the reservoir/ transmitted by louse faeces scratched into skin	12 (7–14)	Fever, headache, severe constitutional symptoms. Early neurological (deafness, delirium) and GI symptoms. Generalised maculopapular rash on day 4–7 of illness. Thrombocytopenia. Severe multisystem involvement. Mortality 20–50% untreated
	Brill–Zinsser disease		Recrudescent infection in latently infected persons	B–Z patients may act as reservoir for epidemic typhus		Months to years after recovery from typhus, patients develop a similar but milder illness, lasting ~2 weeks, with no significant mortality
R. typhi (*mooseri*)	Murine typhus ('endemic or flea typhus')	Worldwide	Where rats and humans share buildings	Rodents/flea faeces scratched into skin	12 (7–14)	Clinical features similar to louse-borne typhus, but much milder. Mortality < 1%
R. tsutsugamushi (*orientalis*)	Scrub typhus ('tsutsugamushi fever, mite typhus')	Asia, India, Australia, Oceania	Circumscribed rural foci ('typhus islands') where rats, mites and rickettsiae coexist	Rodents/mite bite	12 (6–21)	Eschar is common. Otherwise similar to louse-borne typhus, but usually less severe. Significant mortality occurs

dicate acute infection. Phase I antibodies are associated with chronic Q fever.

Other investigations: Abnormal liver function is common. CXR often shows diffuse infiltration and rounded opacities, even if auscultation is normal.

Antibiotic management: Treatment is indicated for all cases to reduce risk of developing chronic Q fever. Doxycycline, tetracycline or chloramphenicol for 2 weeks. Ciprofloxacin is active *in vitro* but has not been subjected to clinical trial.

Table 95 Organisms related to the genus *Rickettsia*

Species	Disease	Distribution	Ecology	Hosts/route	Incubation (days)	Clinical features
Q fever group						
Coxiella burnetii	Q fever	Worldwide	See below			
Rochalimaea spp.						
Rochalimaea quintana	Trench fever	Europe, Africa, N America	Associated with overcrowding – typically during war of famine	Humans are the reservoir/ transmitted by louse faeces scratched into skin	7–30	Fever, headache, transient macular rash. Splenomegaly. No significant mortality
Rochalimaea henselae	Cat-scratch disease	Worldwide	See below			
	Bacillary angiomatosis (BA), peliosis hepatis, chronic bacteraemia	Worldwide				Seen in immunocompromised patients, particularly with HIV (≻121). BA occurs rarely in immunocompetent. May also be caused by *R. quintana*

Comments: Chronic Q fever is very rare. It presents as a culture-negative endocarditis, usually affecting the aortic valve. Most patients have pre-existing rheumatic heart disease. Prolonged, even lifelong, treatment with tetracycline and rifampicin or co-trimoxazole is required; valve replacement is often necessary.

Cat-scratch disease (CSD)

Risk factors: Cats, especially flea-infested kittens.

Clinical features: Local suppurative lymphadenopathy developing ~3 weeks after a cat scratch. Often preceded by a papule or pustule at the site of inoculation. Fever, malaise, anorexia, sore throat and arthralgia may occur. Approximately 2% have complications, which include involvement of CNS (encephalopathy and/or fits), granulomatous

hepatitis, infection of spleen, lung, bone and skin.

Organisms: Most cases are due to *Rochalimaea henselae*. *Afipia felis* (≻206) may be responsible for some cases.

Microbiological investigations: Diagnosis is clinical. Histology of lesions is characteristic, with organisms visible on Warthin–Starry silver staining. Organism may be cultured with difficulty. Serological tests are available (↛). A skin test, based on material from cases of CSD, is used in some specialist centres, but is not widely available. Eosinophilia is common.

Supportive management: Spontaneous resolution occurs after 2–4 months. Aspiration of suppurative lymph nodes should be carried out, but open surgery should be avoided if possible as this may leave a non-healing wound.

Antibiotic management: Response to antibiotics is disappointing, in contrast to bacillary angiomatosis and other syndromes due to the same organism in patients with HIV, which respond to erythromycin (➤121). Rifampicin, ciprofloxacin, co-trimoxazole and gentamicin have all been used with some success but antibiotic therapy is generally not indicated for CSD.

27: Virology

This section describes the basic features of the medically important viruses. In many instances clinical features of infection are dealt with in Section I.

Classification of viruses

Viruses are obligate intracellular parasites which require host cells to replicate. They con-

tain either DNA or RNA but not both, and this forms the basis of the fundamental classification into DNA and RNA viruses. Viruses are then grouped into families on the basis of shared biological and structural properties, but members of the same family can cause very different diseases. Similarly, almost identical illnesses may be caused by viruses which are structurally entirely different.

Table 96 Medically important viruses

Group	Important members
DNA viruses	
Adenoviridae	**Adenoviruses**
Herpesviridae	**Herpes simplex types 1 and 2, Epstein–Barr virus, varicella-zoster virus, cytomegalovirus, human herpes virus type 6**
Poxviridae	Vaccinia, variola, molluscum contagiosum, orf, cowpox, paravaccinia
Parvoviridae	**Parvovirus B19**
Papovaviridae	**Human papillomaviruses**, polyomaviruses (JC virus, BK virus)
Hepadnaviridae	**Hepatitis B virus**
RNA viruses	
Orthomyxoviridae	**Influenza types A, B and C**
Paramyxoviridae	**Parainfluenza, mumps, measles, respiratory syncytial virus**
Coronaviridae	**Coronavirus**
Picornaviridae	**Poliovirus, Coxsackievirus types A and B, echovirus, other enteroviruses, hepatitis A virus, rhinovirus**
Reoviridae	**Rotavirus**, reovirus
Retroviridae	HTLV-I, HTLV-II, **HIV types 1 and 2**
Togaviridae	**Rubella**. Arthropod-borne viruses causing encephalitis
Flaviviridae	**Yellow fever, dengue, hepatitis C virus**. Arthropod-borne viruses causing encephalitis
Bunyaviridae	Hantaan virus. Arthropod-borne viruses causing encephalitis. Crimean–Congo haemorrhagic fever
Arenaviridae	Lymphocytic choriomeningitis, Lassa, Machupo, Junin
Filoviridae	Marburg, Ebola

continued on p. 240

Table 96 contd

Group	Important members
Rhabdoviridae	**Rabies**
Small round structured viruses	**Norwalk agent**
Astroviridae	**Astrovirus**
Caliciviridae	**Calicivirus**

Adenoviruses

Icosahedral virion 70–90 nm. dsDNA genome (MW ~23 × 10⁶).

A family of DNA viruses divided into over 40 serotypes, causing a broad range of clinical syndromes, in particular respiratory tract infection and conjunctivitis. Many serotypes have not been associated with human disease. Some adenoviruses cause tumours in animals. Common worldwide.

Key biological features: Virus replication occurs in epithelial cells. Latent infection of lymphoid tissue may occur.

Reservoir: No animal reservoir for serotypes causing human disease.

Transmission: Respiratory, direct contact or faeco-oral, depending on serotype.

Incubation period: Typically 4–5 days; 4–28 days for epidemic keratoconjunctivitis.

Immunisation: Not available.

Diagnosis: Serology, viral culture.

Major clinical associations: Certain serotypes are particularly associated with particular clinical syndromes (Table 97).

Antiviral therapy: None.

Comments: Patients on immunosuppressive therapy or with AIDS may develop severe disseminated adenovirus infection, which may be fatal.

Table 97 Disease associations of adenovirus serotypes

Clinical syndrome	Serotypes	Comments	
Upper respiratory tract infection	1, 2, 4, 5, 6	Primarily in children under 5 years	➤17
Lower respiratory tract infection	3, 4, 7	Primarily young adults	➤20
Pharyngoconjunctival fever	3, 7	'Swimming-pool conjunctivitis'—primarily in children under 10 years	➤82
Epidemic keratoconjunctivitis	8, 19, 37	'Shipyard worker's eye'	➤83
Meningoencephalitis	1, 6, 7, 12	Primarily in children under 10 years	➤77
Haemorrhagic cystitis	11, 21		
Intussusception	1, 2, 3, 5	Primarily in children under 5 years	
Diarrhoea	40, 41		
Encephalitis	7, 12, 32	In AIDS and other immunocompromised	
Pneumonia, urinary tract infection, disseminated infection	5, 34, 35, 39	patients	

Table 98 Human herpesviruses

Subfamily	Important human viruses	
Alphaherpesviruses	Herpes simplex types 1 and 2	HHV-1, HHV-2
	Varicella-zoster virus	HHV-3
Gammaherpesviruses	Epstein–Barr virus	HHV-4
Betaherpesviruses	Cytomegalovirus	HHV-5
	Human herpesvirus type 6	HHV-6

Herpesviruses

Enveloped virion 120–200 nm. (Icosahedral capsid 100–110 nm.) dsDNA genome (MW $\sim$100–150 $\times$ 10^6). Common worldwide (Table 98).

Key biological features: Herpesvirus infections are characterised by primary infection that is often mild or asymptomatic, followed by the establishment of latent infection. Reactivation of the virus occurs months to years later, and may cause asymptomatic shedding of virus or clinical disease, such as cold sores due to HSV or herpes zoster due to VZV, in patients who are immunocompetent. Primary or recurrent infection may be severe in the immunocompromised. EBV has the ability to immortalise B cells *in vitro* and has been associated with malignancies (lymphoma and nasopharyngeal carcinoma).

Reservoir: Humans.

Herpes simplex virus (HSV) infections

(syn. HHV-1 and HHV-2)

HSV-1 and HSV-2 cause a wide range of clinical syndromes. Clinical features depend on the route of infection (e.g. oral, genital, cutaneous) and host factors, particularly previous exposure to HSV, generalised immunodeficiency, intercurrent illness (e.g. eczema). After primary infection, latent infection is established in sensory ganglia (principally the trigeminal ganglion and the dorsal root ganglia of the spinal cord).

Epidemiology: HSV is distributed worldwide. Endemic infection is maintained by asymptomatic shedding of virus from latently infected individuals. In developing countries childhood infection is very common, with seroprevalence typically 90% by age 10 years. In developed countries infection tends to occur later, in adolescence or early adulthood.

Immunisation: Vaccine is not available. Prior exposure to either HSV-1 or HSV-2 gives **partial** immunity to infection by the other virus.

Incubation period: For symptomatic primary infection, 3–6 days. Many primary infections are asymptomatic.

Transmission: HSV-1 is transmitted non-sexually, primarily via saliva, and frequently from asymptomatic shedders. Both HSV-1 and HSV-2 may be transmitted sexually in genital secretions.

Clinical manifestations of HSV infection

Table 99 Clinical manifestations of HSV infection

Clinical syndrome		Relative frequency of HSV-1 and HSV-2	Recommendations for ACV use
Primary infection			
Acute stomatitis	$\succ$102	Usually HSV-1	Systemic ACV may shorten attack
Acute keratoconjunctivitis	$\succ$84	Usually HSV-1. HSV-2 in neonates	Topical ACV

continued on p. 242

Table 99 contd

Clinical syndrome		Relative frequency of HSV-1 and HSV-2	Recommendations for ACV use
Neonatal infection	≻112	HSV-2 in two-thirds of cases	Intravenous ACV (10 mg/kg 8-hly)
Recurrent infection			
Herpes labialis	≻93	HSV-1	Oral ACV may shorten attack. Topical ACV is not effective
Herpes keratitis	≻84	HSV-1	Topical ACV
1° or recurrent infection			
Cutaneous herpes	≻93	HSV-1	Oral ACV (200–400 mg po five times daily) shortens primary attack. Less effective in recurrent disease. Topical ACV is not recommended
Paronychia	≻93	HSV-1 in children, health workers. HSV-2 in adults	As for cutaneous herpes
Genital herpes	≻66	Usually HSV-2	As for cutaneous herpes
Eczema herpeticum	≻93	Usually HSV-1	Intravenous ACV (10 mg/kg 8-hly)
Encephalitis	≻78	Nearly always HSV-1	As for eczema herpeticum
Meningitis	≻77	Usually HSV-2	As for eczema herpeticum
Disseminated disease in immunodeficient		HSV-1 or HSV-2	As for eczema herpeticum

Management: Acyclovir (ACV ≻260) is the drug of choice for all HSV infections. Systemic ACV shortens the duration of primary attacks of cutaneous, oral and genital herpes, but is less effective against recurrent disease, even when started at the onset of prodromal symptoms. For this reason it is generally not indicated for cold sores or recurrent genital herpes, unless particularly frequent or severe. Topical ACV has little effect on the duration of symptoms in recurrent disease and is not recommended. Disseminated or severe HSV infection (e.g. encephalitis) should be treated with intravenous ACV. Ophthalmic HSV infections may be treated topically. In patients with frequent recurrences and in the immunocompromised, prophylactic therapy may be given with ACV 400 mg 12-hly to reduce the frequency and severity of attacks (≻118).

Complications: Disseminated varicelliform infection confined to the skin and due to HSV-1 or HSV-2 occurs occasionally in immunocompetent patients. Severe disseminated visceral infection, which may be fatal, occurs extremely infrequently, most often in women during the third trimester of pregnancy. **Erythema multiforme** (Stevens–Johnson syndrome) is an allergic manifestation, causing target lesions on the skin and mucosal ulceration. Differentiation from HSV infection itself can be difficult, but the vesicular lesions of erythema multiforme have thicker, longer-lived roofs than the vesicles of HSV infection, and virus cannot be isolated from them.

Varicella-zoster virus (VZV) (syn. HHV-3)
Clinical associations: Varicella (➤103), **congenital infection** (➤104), **severe infection in neonates** (➤104), **herpes zoster** (➤105).

Epstein–Barr virus (EBV) (syn. HHV-4)
EBV infects B lymphocytes and epithelial cells. Latent infection is established in B cells. *In vitro* infection of B cells renders them immortal, capable of indefinite *in vitro* propagation ('transformation'). This property of transformation is reflected in the ability of EBV to induce human lymphoma under certain circumstances.

Epidemiology: EBV infection occurs worldwide. Adult seroprevalence rates are typically > 90% in all countries. The age at which infection occurs is lower in developing countries, where infection is typically acquired in childhood.

Transmission: Via oropharyngeal secretions. Asymptomatic shedding of virus is very common.

Clinical associations

Infectious mononucleosis (➤103)

Lymphoma: Burkitt's lymphoma is seen in equatorial Africa and New Guinea. It is associated with a low age of EBV infection and hyperendemic malaria. It presents as a rapidly growing tumour of children, usually affecting the jaw or abdominal organs. **Polyclonal B-cell lymphoma** occurs in immunodeficient patients (e.g. post-transplant or HIV-seropositive). They may sometimes respond to withdrawal of immunosuppression or to acyclovir. Antilymphoma chemotherapy is often required.

Oral hairy leucoplakia: Proliferation of the buccal mucosa on the lateral margins of the tongue seen in patients with HIV infection. It responds to acyclovir, but is associated with a poor prognosis and impending progression to AIDS.

Nasopharyngeal carcinoma: EBV is strongly associated with undifferentiated carcinoma of the nasopharyngeal epithelium, seen primarily in Chinese, Inuit and Greenlanders. A chemical cofactor may be involved.

Chronic fatigue syndrome
The chronic fatigue syndrome (CFS, syn. 'postviral syndrome' and 'myalgic encephalitis') is a chronic condition characterised by intermittent feverishness, fatigue, myalgia and various cognitive disturbances, including poor concentration. A set of diagnostic criteria aimed at establishing a case definition has recently been published. Patients in whom CFS is diagnosed almost certainly represent a heterogeneous group in whom both physical and psychological features are important. Extensive studies have failed to demonstrate any firm link between EBV infection and CFS.

Patients with CFS rarely have a diagnosable underlying infectious illness and at present viral serology, including EBV and enterovirus serology, plays no part in the management of CFS.

Severe persistent illness associated with EBV is extremely rare, but a few patients have been described with immunodeficiency and disseminated viral infection, including hepatitis, pneumonitis, splenomegaly and pancytopenia. Such individuals have an unusual serological profile, with high titres of anti-VCA IgG and anti-EA, and low titres of anti-EBNA antibodies.

Cytomegalovirus (CMV) (syn. HHV-5)
CMV causes only mild disease in the immunocompetent, but can be serious in the immunosuppressed or when infection occurs in pregnancy. Like other herpesviruses, acute primary infection is followed by the establishment of latency. Reactivation and clinical disease may occur if the patient becomes immunodeficient, e.g. post-transplantation.

Epidemiology: Infection occurs worldwide. In developed countries, peaks of seroconversion occur during early childhood, and then during the second and third decades of life, when patients become sexually active. Seroprevalence increases throughout life and is > 80% at age 60 years.

Transmission: Mainly via oropharyngeal secretions or urine, particularly from children.

Asymptomatic shedding of virus and sexual transmission are common. Transmission by blood products or solid organ transplant are important, particularly as transplant recipients will be immunosuppressed.

Incubation period: Variable. Typically 3–8 weeks when the time of transmission is known (e.g. following infection by blood transfusion).

Immunisation: Not available.

Diagnosis: Seroconversion or a rise in antibody titre suggests active CMV infection. Culture of CMV does not always indicate active infection, as healthy seropositive individuals continue to shed virus intermittently in saliva and urine. **CMV viraemia** detected by isolation of virus from buffy coats correlates well with active infection. Conventional culture is slow and a number of methods have been developed in which CMV is demonstrated early in culture by immunofluorescent detection of viral antigens. **Biopsy** of infected tissue may be diagnostic; CMV causes characteristic histological changes, including 'owl's eye' inclusion bodies.

Clinical associations

Acute mononucleosis: Acute primary CMV infection in immunocompetent patients causes a mononucleosis-like illness with fever, malaise and hepatosplenomegaly. Pharyngitis and lymphadenopathy occur in only ~30% of patients, in contrast to EBV-associated mononucleosis. Abnormal liver function tests and atypical mononucleosis are normally seen. Heterophile antibodies do not occur (➤106). Guillain–Barré syndrome and Bell's palsy have been reported as complications.

Congenital infection: Primary maternal infection during pregnancy results in fetal infection in 50% of cases. Congenital infection and structural defects are seen in approximately 10% of these. Infants with cytomegalic inclusion disease present within a few days of birth with hepatosplenomegaly, thrombocytopenia and petechial rash. Intrauterine growth retardation and failure to thrive are common.

Encephalitis, microcephaly and intracranial calcification may occur. Mental and physical retardation affects the majority of patients. Infected infants who do not present with these features have a significant risk of sensorineural deafness (TORCH screening ➤111).

Neonatal infection: Premature infants who acquire CMV (e.g. by transfusion) may develop 'grey baby' syndrome, with pallor, hypotension and respiratory distress.

Infection in the immunocompromised: CMV infection of variable severity may occur post-transplantation of solid organs, causing fever, hepatitis, leucopenia, pneumonitis and graft rejection. In bone marrow transplant patients a severe, frequently fatal, interstitial pneumonitis occurs after CMV infection or reactivation (➤136). Infection in HIV patients causes a number of clinical syndromes, including chorioretinitis, colitis and pneumonitis (➤122, 127).

Antiviral therapy: Infection in immunocompetent patients does not require treatment. In the immunocompromised host, ganciclovir (GCV) and foscarnet are both effective. Interstitial pneumonitis in bone marrow transplant patients responds poorly to GCV, but may respond to GCV given with CMV hyperimmune globulin. Acyclovir is not effective as therapy for established CMV infections, but is useful as prophylaxis in transplant patients.

Human herpesvirus 6 (HHV-6)

Clinical association: exanthem subitum (➤107).

Poxviruses

Brick-shaped virion 300 × 240 × 100 nm. dsDNA genome (MW 85–~140 × 10⁶).

A large family of DNA viruses, members of which infect invertebrate and vertebrate hosts. Nine have been shown to cause disease in humans.

Major clinical associations

Table 100 Major clinical associations of poxviruses

Virus	Group	Major hosts	Disease
Poxviruses restricted to humans			
Variola	Orthopoxvirus	None	Smallpox ⊠ (eradicated)
Molluscum contagiosum	Molluscipoxvirus	None	Molluscum contagiosum (≻94)
Common zoonotic poxviruses			
Orf	Parapoxvirus	Sheep, goats	Orf (≻94)
Vaccinia	Orthopoxvirus	Laboratory virus	Used as smallpox vaccine
Paravaccinia	Parapoxvirus	Cows	'Milker's nodules': small indolent papules on hands
Rare zoonotic poxviruses			
Monkeypox	Orthopoxvirus	Monkeys, squirrels	Smallpox-like systemic illness
Cowpox	Orthopoxvirus	Cows	Localised skin lesions with lymphadenopathy, fever and systemic upset
Tanapox	Yabapoxvirus	Monkeys	Localised skin infection
Yabapox	Yabapoxvirus	Monkeys	Localised skin infection

Reservoir: There is no animal reservoir for molluscum contagiosum and smallpox (a fact which was essential for the eradication of smallpox by vaccination). Other poxviruses are acquired as zoonoses from a variety of animals.

Transmission: Direct contact with an infected person or animal. Orf is the only zoonotic poxvirus common in the UK. Patients always have occupational exposure to sheep or goats, and often the animals are known to have orf.

Antiviral therapy: None.

Parvoviruses

Icosahedral virion 20 nm. ssDNA genome (MW ~1.5–2 × 10⁶).

Parvovirus B19 is the only member of this group pathogenic in humans.

The only known host cell for human parvovirus is the erythrocyte precursor; this site of infection explains the ability of the virus to cause aplastic crises in patients with pre-existing haemolytic anaemia (e.g. sickle-cell disease).

Reservoir: Humans.

Epidemiology: Worldwide. Common in children. Seroprevalence rates ≥ 50% in adults in developed countries.

Transmission: Highly contagious, probably via respiratory route.

Incubation period: Four to 20 days.

Immunisation: Not available.

Diagnosis: By detection of specific IgM or a rise in IgG. Molecular techniques, such as nucleic acid hybridisation, have been used to demonstrate parvovirus antigens in serum, but these techniques are not yet routinely available.

Clinical associations: Erythema infectiosum ('fifth disease') in children (≻107), aplastic crises in patients with sickle-cell disease, viral arthritis in adults (≻107), congenital infection causing hydrops fetalis (≻112).

Persistent infection causing chronic anaemia may occur in the immunodeficient (e.g. AIDS patients, patients with congenital immunodeficiency syndromes and those receiving chemotherapy). Commercial immunoglobulin preparations contain antibodies against parvovirus (reflecting the frequency of infection in the community) and may be helpful in this situation.

Papovaviruses

Icosahedral virion ~50 nm. dsDNA genome (MW ~3–5 × 10^6).

Table 101 Papovaviruses

Subfamily	Important human viruses	Comments
Papillomaviridae	Human papillomaviruses	Cause warts and cervical cancer
Polyomaviridae	JC virus, BK virus	Cause disease in the immuno-compromised host

Papillomaviruses

Very many papillomaviruses have been described. They are each strictly restricted to one host species. Over 60 human papillomaviruses (HPVs) have been isolated.

Key biological features: HPVs grow only in epithelial cells, where they cause benign proliferation of the epithelium. HPVs associated with mucosal infection do not infect skin and vice versa. Certain types of HPV are strongly associated with cervical cancer. Others may cause skin cancers in immunosuppressed individuals and in patients with the rare inherited disorder epidermodysplasia verruciformis.

Reservoir: Humans.

Transmission: By direct contact with an infected person or contaminated object. Swimming-pool transmission occurs. Older children and young adults are most affected; ~10% of the adult population have warts. Genital warts are spread by sexual contact. Infection may be clinically silent.

Incubation period: Warts develop between 1 and 20 months after infection.

Immunisation: None.

Diagnosis: Diagnosis is clinical. Viral culture is not available.

Major clinical associations of human papillomaviruses

Table 102 Major clinical associations of human papillomaviruses

Clinical manifestation	Type
Cutaneous warts	
Plantar warts	1
Common warts	2, 4
Flat warts	3, 10, 28, 41
Mucosal (primarily genital) warts (>69)	
Condylomata acuminata	6, 11
Flat condylomata	6, 11, 16, 18, 31 and others
Cervical cancer	
Strong association	16, 18
Moderate association	31, 33, 35, 45, 51, 52, 56
Weak or no association	6, 11, 42, 43, 44
Association with vulval cancer	16
Respiratory papillomata	6, 11
Conjunctival papillomata	6, 11
Oral mucosal warts	6, 11, 13, 16, 32
Warts on lips	2

Juvenile-onset respiratory papillomata are due to infection with HPVs causing mucosal warts, probably acquired intrapartum from the maternal genital tract.

Antiviral therapy: Specific antiviral therapy is not available. For cutaneous warts topical preparations of salicylic acid are available commercially. For genital warts local caustic agents such as podophyllin or trichloracetic acid may be used. Podophyllin is very irritant and excess topical application can lead rarely to systemic toxicity with nausea, vomiting, lethargy and neuropathy. It is antimitotic and is therefore contraindicated in pregnancy and infancy. Cryotherapy and surgery are necessary in some cases.

Polyomaviruses

Two viruses in this group cause disease in humans. Both JC virus (JCV) and BK virus (BKV) are usually only clinically significant in immunosuppressed patients. In both cases clinical disease is usually due to reactivation of latent viral infection.

Transmission: Probably via the respiratory route. Seroprevalence among children in the developed world is 50% at 3 years for BKV and 10–14 years for JCV.

Immunisation: Not available.

Diagnosis: Serology is not helpful, as latent infection is very common. Detection of virus by electron microscopy of urine or tissue or demonstration of viral antigens or DNA by ELISA or PCR is required to confirm active viral replication.

Major clinical associations: JCV causes **progressive multifocal leucoencephalopathy** (≻124) in patients with AIDS.

BKV causes **haemorrhagic cystitis** in immunosuppressed patients, particularly bone marrow transplant recipients. Viruria is common post-renal transplant, but does not always indicate significant disease. BKV infection has been implicated in the development of post-transplant ureteric stenosis.

Hepadnaviruses

Spherical virion 42 nm. Partially ss/partially dsDNA genome (MW ~1.8 × 10⁶).

This family includes hepatitis B and a variety of related viruses causing hepatitis in animals (e.g. ground squirrel hepatitis virus, duck hepatitis B virus).

Key biological features: As well as causing acute hepatitis, HBV establishes latent infection in a small percentage of patients, causing chronic active hepatitis, cirrhosis and hepatocellular carcinoma. **Hepatitis D virus** is a defective RNA virus that depends on HBV for replication, and is coated in HBV surface antigen. Infection is therefore restricted to those who are previously or simultaneously infected with HBV.

Reservoir: Humans.

Transmission: By blood and blood products, by sexual transmission and vertically before, during and after delivery. Infectivity varies, depending on carrier status (≻50).

Diagnosis: By serology (≻50).

Immunisation: Is now available (≻51).

Major clinical associations: Hepatitis B (≻49), **hepatitis D** (≻51), **chronic active hepatitis, cirrhosis, hepatocellular carcinoma**.

Orthomyxoviruses: influenza virus types A, B and C

Enveloped spherical virion 80–120 nm. ssRNA genome (MW ~5 × 10⁶).

Influenza viruses primarily cause upper respiratory tract infection. Their importance lies in their ability to cause epidemic disease. Most clinical infections are due to types A and B.

Key biological features: Influenza viruses are classified serologically into types A, B and C. The antigens that differentiate the three types are internal nucleoproteins, which are relatively stable and are not accessible to host antibodies. The virus also carries two major surface antigens, haemagglutinin (HA) and neuraminidase (NA), which are variable and are important targets for host antibodies. All three types of virus may alter both HA and NA gradually by mutation, a process known as **antigenic drift**. In addition, for influenza type A (but not types B or C) there exist at least 13 subtypes of HA and at least nine subtypes of NA. The emergence of strains expressing different combinations of surface antigens is called **antigenic shift**. So far only H_{1-3} and N_{1-2} have been found in human influenza viruses. These two processes allow the virus to escape host immune responses.

Epidemiology: Infection occurs worldwide. Endemic cases occur continuously in most communities. Focal epidemics associated with antigenic drift occur every few years. Pandemics due to antigenic shift occur every 10–20 years. For example, the severe pandemic of 1918 followed the replacement of H_1N_1 by H_2N_2 as the predominant strain. Infection is commonest in children but more severe in the elderly, in whom secondary bacterial pneumonia is more common.

Reservoir: It is suggested that animal orthomyxoviruses may serve as a reservoir of antigenic variants. Human influenza viruses may acquire new segments of RNA from them, and thus undergo antigenic shift, during a process known as reassortment, which can occur when cells are infected by two viruses of different strains.

Transmission: Droplet spread by the respiratory route.

Incubation period: One to 5 days.

Infectious period: For 1 week after the development of symptoms.

Immunisation: Vaccine is prepared on an annual basis from recently isolated viruses to take account of antigenic drift. It is usually trivalent, containing two type A strains and one type B strain and typically gives ~70% protection for about 1 year. It is usually given in late October/early November. It is recommended for patients with cardiac, renal and pulmonary disease (including asthma), for patients with diabetes mellitus and other endocrine disorders, for the immuno-compromised, and for residents of old people's homes and nursing homes (➤337). Influenza vaccination is also advocated for patients on long-term aspirin treatment in an attempt to reduce the risk of Reye syndrome.

Diagnosis: Most cases occur in the context of local epidemics. Diagnosis may be confirmed by serology or viral culture from respiratory secretions.

Clinical features: Acute onset of fever, rigors, cough and constitutional symptoms, including headache, malaise and myalgia. Coryza and sore throat are common but less pronounced than with other viral causes of URTI. Fever and constitutional symptoms usually last 3–4 days. Cough and malaise usually resolve by 1 week. Nausea, vomiting and diarrhoea may occur, particularly in children.

Complications: Secondary bacterial pneumonia is common in the elderly and is frequently severe (➤23). Infection by *Staphylococcus aureus* is commoner post-influenza than under other circumstances and cases of toxic shock syndrome have followed flu (➤63). Primary viral pneumonia is rare but frequently severe (➤20). It occurs most often in patients with previous cardiac disease, such as mitral stenosis, and during the third trimester of pregnancy. Myocarditis, polymyositis and neurological sequelae, including encephalo-

pathy and Guillain–Barré syndrome, occur very rarely. Reye syndrome occurs very rarely, usually in association with aspirin use and influenza B.

Antiviral therapy: Amantadine is effective for the treatment and prophylaxis of influenza A, but not B or C. It is not frequently used but is recommended (100 mg 24-hly) for patients in the following categories:

• unimmunised patients in risk groups (as defined above under 'Immunisation') or health workers, for 2 weeks whilst immunisation takes effect;

• patients in risk groups in whom immunisation is contraindicated for the duration of the outbreak.

Side-effects, which occur in 1–5% of patients, include insomnia and agitation.

Paramyxoviruses

Enveloped spherical virion 150–300 nm. ssRNA genome (MW ~5–7 × 10⁶).

Table 103 Paramyxoviruses

Genus	Important human viruses	Comments
Paramyxovirus	Parainfluenza types 1–4	
	Mumps	(➤102)
Morbillivirus	Measles	(➤100)
Pneumovirus	Respiratory syncytial virus (RSV)	

Key biological features: Mumps and measles cause systemic infection, but the clinical manifestations of parainfluenza infection are confined to the respiratory tract (unlike influenza). Parainfluenza does not have the capacity for antigenic shift and drift, and does not therefore cause epidemic disease.

Parainfluenza virus
Reservoir: Humans.
Transmission: Droplet spread by the respiratory route.

Epidemiology: Infection occurs worldwide. Children under 5 years are most often affected.
Incubation period: Two to 6 days.
Immunisation: Not available.
Diagnosis: Viral culture. Serology is unhelpful because infection is widespread, and differentiation between types 1–4 is difficult.
Major clinical associations: Upper respiratory tract infection in children under 5 years (≻17). **Lower respiratory tract infection** which may be severe is seen in infants under 6 months. Parainfluenza type 3 is particularly associated with bronchiolitis in this age group (≻20).
Antiviral therapy: None.

Respiratory syncytial virus
Transmission: Self-inoculation of mucous membranes after contact with infected secretions or contaminated objects.
Epidemiology: In temperate parts of the world, RSV infection has a striking seasonal incidence with peaks occurring in the winter months. These do not occur in tropical areas, and are thought to be due to crowding rather than any climatic effect.
Incubation period: Two to 6 days.
Immunisation: Not available. Repeated infections cause progressively less severe illness due to the development of humoral and cell-mediated immunity.
Diagnosis: Serology is unhelpful. Viral culture and rapid diagnostic tests for viral antigens (including ELISA and direct immunofluorescence) in material obtained by nasopharyngeal aspiration are widely used.
Major clinical associations: Upper respiratory tract infection (≻17), **croup** (≻18), **otitis media** (≻15), **bronchiolitis** in infancy (≻20), **viral pneumonia** (≻20).
Antiviral therapy: Ribavarin administered by aerosol is partially effective, and may be helpful in the management of most severe cases such as infants with bronchiolitis or pneumonia, who may require mechanical ventilation.

Coronaviruses

Enveloped spherical virion 60–220 nm. ssRNA genome (MW ~6 × 10⁶). Two coronaviruses

(strains 229E and OC43) cause disease in humans.
Reservoir: Humans.
Transmission: Respiratory droplet spread.
Epidemiology: Infection occurs worldwide, primarily in children. Seroprevalence is 90–100% in adults in most communities.
Incubation period: Two to 5 days.
Immunisation: Not available.
Diagnosis: Viral culture is difficult. Serology is not routinely available.
Clinical features: Upper respiratory tract infection resembling the common cold, with fever, cough coryza and sore throat. Lower respiratory involvement is extremely rare.
Antiviral therapy: Not available.
Comments: Coronavirus-like particles have been seen by electron microscopy in the stools of some patients with diarrhoea, but these viruses have not been isolated and their identity has yet to be established.

Picornaviruses

Icosahedral virion 25–30 nm. ssRNA genome (MW ~2.3 × 10⁶).

The family picornaviridae contains two large genera of medical importance, the genus enteroviridae and the genus rhinoviridae. The enteroviruses include the polioviruses, hepatitis A virus, echoviruses, Coxsackieviruses and other enteroviruses (Table 104). They were all originally isolated from stools, often as part of efforts to control poliomyelitis. The original classification of non-polio enteroviruses, into Coxsackie A and B, and echoviruses was made on the basis of their pathogenicity for suckling

Table 104 Classification of picornaviruses

Group	Serotypes
Poliovirus	1, 2, 3
Coxsackie A	1–22, 24
Coxsackie B	1–6
Echovirus	1–9, 11–27, 29–33
Enterovirus	68–71
Hepatovirus	Hepatitis A virus (≻49)
Rhinovirus	Over 100 serotypes

mice (Coxsackie A viruses are those that cause flaccid paralysis in mice and type B viruses cause spastic paralysis), and does not reflect the clinical features of infection in humans. Echoviruses (enteric cytopathic human orphan viruses) are those enteroviruses which do not cause disease in mice. Since 1967 this system of classification has been abandoned and newly discovered enterovirus serotypes are now assigned to the group enterovirus and numbered sequentially (e.g. enterovirus 70). Hepatitis A virus has recently been reclassified as the only member of a new genus, hepatovirus.

Polioviruses ✉ ⓘ

Key biological features: Poliovirus types 1, 2 and 3 are distinguished serologically but cause similar disease. The primary site of infection is the epithelium of the intestine and respiratory tract. Neurological involvement with destruction of anterior horn cells and development of paralysis is relatively infrequent.

Reservoir: Humans.

Transmission: Mainly faeco-oral. Spread via the respiratory route occurs and is more important in the developed world, where standards of sanitation are higher.

Epidemiology: Infection occurs worldwide but is now very rare in the developed world as a result of successful mass immunisation. Polio, like smallpox, is a realistic target for global eradication as there is no animal reservoir and the vaccine gives good protection. Most cases occurring in the developed world are now associated with vaccine strains (see below).

Incubation period: Seven to 14 days (range 3–35).

Infectious period: From 36 h after *exposure*. Virus continues to be excreted in the stools for many weeks (typically 2–4 but often longer).

Immunisation: Inactivated (Salk) polio vaccine (IPV) was introduced in 1956 and replaced by live attenuated oral polio vaccine (OPV, the Sabin vaccine) in 1962. Persons born before 1958 may therefore not have been immunised. OPV contains live attenuated strains of all three polio types and provides good mucosal immunity. Vaccine-strain virus may be excreted in the stools for many weeks after ad-

ministration. Because of the very small risk of OPV-associated polio, recently immunised patients and parents of immunised infants should observe careful personal hygiene (particularly washing hands after changing nappies). Paralytic polio following OPV has been estimated to occur in ~1 in 1 200 000 recipients and 1 in 5 000 000 contacts.

OPV is currently recommended for the immunisation of infants from the age of 2 months. Three doses at monthly intervals should be given at the same time as diphtheria/tetanus/pertussis and Hib vaccine (➤337). Adults should also receive three doses at monthly intervals. Travellers to polio-endemic or epidemic areas and health care workers exposed to cases of polio should receive a booster dose. OPV is safe for use in HIV patients but is contraindicated in other immunosuppressed patients, for whom IPV is available.

Diagnosis: Culture of virus from stools, throat swab or CSF is required to confirm the diagnosis. Two stool samples 24–48 h apart should be obtained as soon as possible after the onset of paralysis in suspected cases.

Clinical features: Fever, headache, malaise and mild gastrointestinal symptoms constitute the only signs of illness in the majority of cases. A small number of patients develop neurological involvement with meningism, usually occurring 3–10 days after the onset of illness. In ~1 in 1000 cases in children (1 in 75 in adults) paralytic polio follows with rapid onset of asymmetrical paralysis, usually affecting the legs. The tendon reflexes are reduced or absent, and there is no sensory deficit. Muscle pain is common. Bulbar paralysis or involvement of the muscles of respiration may also occur. Some functional recovery (occasionally complete) may occur. Denervation is followed by atrophy of affected muscle groups. Neuromuscular symptoms may in some cases continue to progress for many years after acute poliomyelitis.

CSF protein and glucose are usually normal. There is a CSF pleocytosis consistent with viral meningitis (➤75). Differentiation from the Guillain–Barré syndrome (GBS) is important since in that condition the prognosis is better. In GBS paralysis and sensory deficit are usually symmetrical and ascending, fever is usually absent, the CSF protein is grossly elevated, and pleocytosis is usually mild or absent.

Antiviral therapy: There is no specific antiviral therapy. Physical exercise may exacerbate paralysis and bedrest is indicated during the acute attack. Supportive therapy, including mechanical ventilation, may be required if the respiratory muscles are involved.

Coxsackieviruses, echoviruses, enteroviruses 68–71

Key biological features: Like poliovirus, these viruses multiply in the epithelium of the respiratory and gastrointestinal tracts. Virus may be isolated from the stools for many weeks after infection.

Reservoir: Humans.

Transmission: Faeco-oral. Person to person, via respiratory or conjunctival secretions.

Incubation period: Typically 2–5 days.

Infectious period: From the onset of symptoms for several weeks as virus persists in stools.

Epidemiology: Infection occurs worldwide. Epidemics due to one serotype occur on the background of endemic cases.

Immunisation: Not available.

Diagnosis: By viral culture from stools, respiratory secretions or CSF. Serology not very useful because of cross-reaction between serotypes and high incidence of previous infection.

Major clinical associations: Infection is often asymptomatic or associated with a mild febrile 'flu-like' illness. Most clinical syndromes are associated with a number of different serotypes. With few exceptions, clinical features are not sufficiently distinctive to allow clinical diagnosis of the serotype involved.

Viral meningitis (➤77).

Rarely **viral encephalitis** (➤78) or a paralytic illness resembling polio but not as severe.

Upper respiratory tract infection (➤17), **herpangina** (➤108), **hand, foot and mouth disease** (➤107).

Myocarditis (➤43), **pericarditis** (➤42).

Acute haemorrhagic conjunctivitis (➤83), usually due to enterovirus 70 or Coxsackie A24.

Disseminated neonatal infection (➤112).

Bornholm's disease (syn. 'devil's grip'):

Sudden onset of severe unilateral pain in the intercostal muscles of the chest, worse on breathing. There may be pain in the muscles of the trunk, neck and limbs. Pleurisy and pericarditis may occur. Resolution takes place over 2–3 weeks.

Antiviral therapy: Not available.

Comments: Persistent enterovirus infection has been proposed as a cause of the chronic fatigue syndrome (CFS, ➤243), but the evidence for this is not conclusive, and the role of enteroviruses in CFS is not widely accepted.

Rhinoviruses

Reservoir: Humans.

Transmission: Via respiratory secretions, by direct contact, droplet spread or fomites.

Incubation period: One to 4 days.

Infectious period: Usually for ~7 days after the onset of symptoms. Viral shedding may occasionally continue for several weeks.

Immunisation: Not available.

Clinical features

Common cold: Fever, malaise, sneezing and coryza lasting 3–7 days. Infection may be asymptomatic. (➤17).

Complications: Sinusitis (➤15), exacerbation of chronic obstructive airways disease (➤21) and secondary pneumonia (➤22). Viral pneumonia does not occur.

Reoviruses

Icosahedral virion 60–80 nm. dsRNA genome (MW ~11–15 × 10^6).

Table 105 Reoviruses

Genus	Important human viruses	Comments
Reoviruses		Human reoviruses have been isolated, but not shown to cause disease
Rotaviruses	Rotavirus groups A and B	An important cause of diarrhoea. Discussed elsewhere (➤44, ➤258)
Orbiviruses	Colorado tick fever virus	

Colorado tick fever
Reservoir: Rodents.
Transmission: By tick vector–*Dermacentor andersoni*.
Epidemiology: Infection is restricted by the geographical distribution of the tick vector to western USA and Canada. Infection is always associated with an occupational or recreational history of tick exposure.
Incubation period: Three to 6 days.
Immunisation: Not available.
Diagnosis: Serology, detection of viral antigens in serum by immunofluorescence. Not routinely available.
Clinical features: Fever, rigors, headache, malaise. Recovery is usually complete by 7–10 days.
Antiviral therapy: Not available.

Retroviruses (Table 106)

Enveloped spherical virion 100 nm. Diploid ssRNA genome (MW ~5 × 10^6).
Key biological features: Retroviruses have a reverse transcriptase enzyme that transcribes their RNA genome into DNA, which may then integrate into the host genome. This is associated with the potential of oncoviruses to cause malignancy and the prolonged 'latency' seen with lentivirus infection. The biology of HIV infection is discussed elsewhere (➤114).

HTLV-I
Reservoir: Humans.
Transmission: Sexual transmission. By blood products (therapeutic or as a result of IVDU).
Vertical transmission, particularly by breast-feeding.
Epidemiology: Infection is common in certain countries, particularly Japan, the Caribbean islands and South America. It is unusual in UK residents.
Immunisation: Not available.
Diagnosis: Serology will indicate infection, but disease is infrequent, affecting only a small percentage of infected individuals.
Major clinical associations: No acute clinical illness has been associated with acquisition of and seroconversion to HTLV-I.

    Adult T-cell leukaemia/lymphoma affects 1–5% of infected individuals. It presents at a mean age of 50 years and the latent period between infection and development of disease is ⩾20 years. It presents as an aggressive leukaemia or lymphoma due to clonal expansion of lymphocytes which can be shown to contain the virus.

    Tropical spastic paraparesis presents as a progressive spastic myelopathy with pyramidal, sensory and sphincteric disturbance. It occurs after a variable latent period, which has been as short as a few months in patients infected by blood transfusion, but is usually many years. The fact that 20–40% of patients are seronegative for HTLV-I suggests that this is a heterogeneous syndrome. Most patients have high-titre antibodies and infectious virus in their CSF.

HTLV-II
This virus appears to be transmitted by blood products, as there is a high prevalence among

Table 106 Human retroviruses

Genus	Important human viruses	Comments
Oncoviruses	Human T-cell lymphotrophic virus (HTLV) I and II	Genus includes many oncogenic animal viruses
Lentiviruses	Human immunodeficiency virus (HIV) 1 and 2 (➤114)	Animal viruses include slow viruses (e.g. visna) and immunodeficiency viruses (e.g. simian immunodeficiency virus (SIV))
Spumaviruses	No human pathogens	

IVDUs. It has not yet been firmly associated with clinical disease, although it has been isolated from patients with a T-cell variant of hairy cell leukaemia.

Togaviruses (Table 107)

Enveloped spherical virion 60–70 nm ssRNA genome (MW ~4 × 10⁶).

Flaviviruses (Table 108)

Enveloped spherical virion 40–50 nm. ssRNA genome (MW ~4 × 10⁶).

Yellow fever (YF) ✉

Organism: Yellow fever virus.

Epidemiology: Found in tropical South America and sub-Saharan Africa, between 15°N and 15°S. In urban YF, which currently occurs only in Africa, human-to-human transmission occurs via mosquito bite (*Aedes aegypti*). In jungle YF, infection is maintained by enzootic infection of monkeys, transmitted by *Hemagogus* and *Aedes* spp. mosquitoes. In this situation, human infection follows jungle exposure.

Incubation period: Three to 6 days.

Infectious period: Blood is infective for mos-

Table 107 Togaviruses

Genus	Important human viruses	Comments
Rubiviridae	Rubella	(➤101)
Alphaviridae	Eastern and western equine encephalitis viruses, Venezuelan equine encephalitis virus	Arthropod-borne viruses causing encephalitis (➤79)
	Chikungunya (SE Asia, Africa) O'nyong-nyong (Africa) Ross River virus (Australia, S Pacific) Sindbis (Africa, Asia, Russia, Australia, Europe)	Arthropod-borne viruses causing febrile illness similar to dengue, often with prominent arthralgia (➤97, ➤254)

Table 108 Flaviviruses

Genus	Important human viruses	Comments
Flaviviridae	Yellow fever virus	(See below)
	Dengue	(See below)
	Kyansur Forest disease Omsk haemorrhagic fever	(See below)
	St Louis encephalitis, Murray Valley encephalitis Japanese B encephalitis (➤79, 143) Tick-borne encephalitis (➤79, 143) Powassan	Arthropod-borne viruses causing encephalitis (➤79)
	West Nile virus (India and East Africa)	Arthropod-borne virus causing febrile illness similar to dengue (➤254)
	Hepatitis C virus	(➤52)

quitoes for the first 3–5 days of illness. YF is not transmissible by contact.

Clinical features: Typically a biphasic illness. Abrupt onset of fever, rigors, headache, backache, myalgia, nausea and vomiting. After 3–4 days symptoms and fever remit for 1–2 days and then recur. Jaundice, hepatic and renal failure, which may progress to acute tubular necrosis, disseminated intravascular coagulopathy, mucosal bleeding, GI haemorrhage and myocarditis may occur. Case fatality rate depends on the quality of supportive management but may be as high as 40%.

Investigations: Leucopenia, thrombocytopenia, abnormal liver function tests and disordered clotting. Diagnosis is confirmed by serology, by the identification of viral antigens in serum by a number of rapid diagnostic methods, or by culture of the virus.

Antiviral therapy: None.

Supportive management: Attention to fluid balance, specific treatment for coagulopathy and management of renal and hepatic failure may all be required. Secondary bacterial sepsis may occur.

Immunisation: Recovery from YF gives complete lifelong protection against further attacks. A live attenuated vaccine is available. Immunisation (➤142), confirmed by a valid certificate, is required for entry to many countries. A single dose of vaccine gives ⩾99% protection. Revaccination is required after 10 years, although protection probably lasts for life. Vaccination is currently recommended in the UK for laboratory workers handling infected material, travellers over the age of 9 months intending to visit infected areas, and persons requiring a valid certificate of immunisation for entry into particular countries. Vaccination is not recommended under the age of 9 months, unless exposure is unavoidable.

Dengue
Organism: Dengue virus, serotypes 1–4.
Epidemiology: Widely distributed in Asia, Africa, northern Australia, Central and South America including the Caribbean. Animal reservoirs, e.g. monkeys, exist in some regions. Transmission occurs by the bite of an infected mosquito, usually *Aedes aegypti*.

Incubation period: Three to 14 days (usually 7–10).

Infectious period: Blood is infective for mosquitoes for the first 5 days of illness. Person-to-person spread does not occur.

Clinical features: Abrupt onset of fever, rigors, severe headache and backache, myalgia, arthralgia, nausea and vomiting. Generalised maculopapular rash and lymphadenopathy develop usually as fever wanes after 3–5 days. A second lower peak of fever is often seen. Leucopenia, thrombocytopenia and abnormal liver function tests are usual.

Antiviral therapy: None.

Complications: Dengue haemorrhagic fever (DHF). This syndrome typically presents with rapid clinical deterioration and shock after 2–5 days of milder febrile illness. DHF is thought to be caused by second infections with a different dengue serotype in individuals with protective immunity against one serotype, a phenomenon known as antibody-dependent enhancement. It is commoner in children and may occur in epidemics following the introduction of a new dengue serotype to susceptible populations. DHF is characterised by abnormal vascular permeability, hypovolaemia and abnormal clotting. Classical clinical signs include hypotension and tachycardia, restlessness and sweating, facial pallor with circumoral cyanosis and hepatomegaly. Spontaneous bruising and GI haemorrhage may occur. Mortality rates may be as high as 40%. Fluid replacement and treatment of coagulopathy are required. After 24–36 h of crisis, recovery is fairly rapid in those that survive.

Kyansur Forest disease/
Omsk haemorrhagic fever ⊠
These two closely related viruses are geographically restricted to the Kyansur Forest in India and the steppes of Siberia respectively.

Transmission: By tick bite. Person-to-person spread does not occur.

Incubation period: Three to 8 days.

Clinical features: Febrile illness with myalgia, GI disturbance and conjunctivitis. There may be a papulovesicular eruption on the soft palate and cervical lymphadenopathy. Encephalitis and haemorrhage may occur. Case fatality rate is estimated at 1–10%.

Bunyaviruses

Enveloped spherical virion 90–100 nm. ssRNA genome (MW ~4–7 × 10⁶).

Over 200 bunyaviruses have been described. They are nearly all arthropod-borne infections causing fever and, occasionally, encephalitis. They are restricted geographically and are often named after the region in which they occur. The more widespread examples are listed in Table 109.

Crimean–Congo haemorrhagic fever (CCHF) ⊠

Epidemiology: Widely distributed throughout tropical Africa, the Middle East, southern CIS and the Balkans.

Reservoir/transmission: Hares, birds and *Hyalomma* spp. ticks, which are also the vector for human infection. Nosocomial person-to-person spread has occurred.

Incubation period: Three to 12 days.

Clinical features: Fever, malaise, headache, severe myalgia. Facial flush and conjunctival in-jection. Palatal petechiae and petechial rash on trunk. GI haemorrhage and haematuria may develop in association with severe hepatitis. Leucopenia, thrombocytopenia, disordered liver function tests and abnormal renal function are common. Reported case fatality rates vary from 5 to 50%.

Diagnosis: By serology or by isolation of virus from blood.

Immunisation: Not available.

Hantavirus infection: haemorrhagic fever with renal syndrome (HFRS) ⊠

Epidemiology: Common throughout Japan, Korea, China. Rarer in Europe although serological evidence suggests subclinical infection, including in the UK. Recently many cases have been described in the USA, particularly in association with severe pulmonary involvement.

Reservoir: Rodents.

Transmission: Direct contact with rodent urine, or fomites contaminated with rodent urine. Person-to-person spread does not occur.

Incubation period: Usually 12–21 days (range 5–42 days).

Immunisation: Not available.

Clinical features: Mild non-specific prodrome followed by abrupt onset of fever, headache, myalgia and GI disturbance. Haemorrhage

Table 109 Important bunyaviruses

Serogroup	Important human viruses	Comments
California	California La Crosse Jamestown Canyon	Arthropod-borne viruses causing encephalitis (>79)
Phlebovirus	Rift Valley fever	Mosquito vector. E Africa
	Sandfly fever	Sandfly vector. Mediterranean area and Middle East
	Toscana virus	Sandfly vector. Italy
Nairovirus	Crimean–Congo haemorrhagic fever virus	
Hantavirus	Haantan virus	

(petechiae and GI) may develop, with severe hypovolaemic shock and acute renal failure. Leucocytosis, thrombocytopenia, abnormal renal function and prolonged bleeding time are commonly seen.

A severe respiratory illness, **Hantavirus pulmonary syndrome,** has recently been described in the USA, associated with a new serotype (Four Corners virus). Severe pulmonary oedema is characteristic and case fatality rates of ~75% have been reported.

Viral haemorrhagic fever (VHF) ✉ ④

Viruses from several families cause febrile infections associated with severe haemorrhage and shock, including bunyaviruses (Crimean–Congo HF, HFRS ➤255), arenaviruses and filoviruses. Dengue may also cause haemorrhagic disease in patients with previous infection by a different dengue serotype (➤254).

Arenaviruses ✉ ④

Enveloped spherical virion 50–300 nm. ssRNA genome (MW ~3–5 × 10^6).
Epidemiology: VHFs are geographically restricted as indicated. Infection is associated with rodent exposure which may be occupational, e.g. in rural areas, or may be due to rodent infestation in dwellings.
Reservoir: Rodents. For LF, the multimammate mouse *Mastomys natalensis.*
Transmission: From rodent to human by contact with urine. Person-to-person transmission has been recorded, but it is not common.

Incubation period: Usually 6–21 days.
Infectious period: Virus may be isolated from the urine of patients with LF for 3–9 weeks post-infection ④.
Immunisation: Not available. See below for use of convalescent serum.
Diagnosis: Serology, viral culture.
Clinical features: Gradual onset of fever, headache, myalgia, vomiting and diarrhoea. Pharyngitis with exudate is common in LF but unusual in AHF and BHF. Bleeding from mucosal surfaces and into skin may occur (15–20% of LF, >50% in AHF and BHF). Petechiae and jaundice are not seen in LF, but a petechial rash is common in AHF and BHF. Death is associated with haemorrhage, shock and pneumonitis. Case fatality rates of 15–30% are reported, but serology suggests that subclinical infection is common.
Antiviral therapy: LF: ribavarin (➤260) improves prognosis significantly. AHF: convalescent serum has been shown to be of benefit. Ribavarin has not been proven to be of benefit in AHF and BHF.

Filoviruses (Table 111) ✉ ④

Filamentous virion with helical nucleocapsid ~800 × 80 nm. ssRNA genome (MW ~4 × 10^6).
Reservoir: Probably monkeys, possibly bats.
Transmission: Person-to-person   transmission occurs by direct contact ④.
Immunisation: Not available.
Diagnosis: Serology, viral culture.
Clinical features: Causes VHF similar to LF.

Table 110 Arenaviruses

Virus	Distribution	Comments
Lymphocytic choriomeningitis virus (LCV)	Worldwide	A pathogen of mice. Human cases are rare. May cause severe meningoencephalitis
Lassa fever (LF)	W Africa	
Argentine HF (AHF, Junin)	Argentina	
Bolivian HF (BHF, Machupo)	Bolivia	

Table 111 Filoviruses

Virus	Incubation period	Comments
Ebola	2–21 days	Has caused outbreaks of HF in Zaïre, Sudan
Marburg	3–9 days	Caused HF in German laboratory workers in contact with African green monkeys

Case fatality rates usually > 50%.
Antiviral therapy: Not available.

Rhabdoviruses

Bullet-shaped virion 180 × 75 nm. ssRNA genome (MW ~4 × 10⁶).

Rabies ≅ ④
Key biological features: Rabiesvirus causes encephalitis and neuronal degeneration. Post-mortem histology of brain shows changes similar to other viral encephalitides. Negri bodies are pathognomonic cytoplasmic inclusion bodies, present in 70–90% of cases. Virus may also be found extracranially, e.g. in salivary glands, corneal epithelium and cutaneous nerves.
Epidemiology: Rabies is now rare in all developed countries, but remains common elsewhere. Rabies-free areas include the UK, most West Indian islands, Finland, Iceland, Sweden, Japan, Taiwan, New Zealand.

Table 112 Rhabdoviruses

Genus	Important human viruses	Comments
Lyssavirus	Rabiesvirus	
Vesiculovirus	Vesicular stomatitis virus	Infrequent cause of fever with oral mucosal vesicles. Sandfly vector. Widespread distribution in tropical and sub-tropical regions

Reservoir: Many different mammalian species, particularly canines, cats, bats. Since 1903 all UK cases have been imported, nearly all after dog bites.
Transmission: Infection occurs by inoculation of virus into peripheral tissues, usually by the bite of an infected animal. Virus ascends along peripheral nerves to the CNS and then descends to skin, cornea and salivary glands. Virus does not penetrate intact skin. Human-to-human transmission via saliva is theoretically possible but has only been recorded after corneal grafting. Isolation procedures are indicated. Infection has occurred by inhalation and inoculation on to mucous membranes.
Incubation period: Usually 3–78 days, > 90 days in 15%. Range 9 days to several years. Heavy contamination and cephalic location of bite are associated with short incubation.
Immunisation: Human diploid cell vaccine (HDCV) is safe and effective. Older vaccines, such as duck embryo vaccine (DEV), are cheaper but are associated with a high incidence of minor local and systemic adverse effects, and very infrequently with encephalitis. DEV is still widely used in developing countries. Rabies-specific immunoglobulin (RIG) is now prepared from serum of hyperimmunised individuals. See below under 'Prevention' for recommendations on vaccine use.
Diagnosis: Serology, viral culture, antigen detection in tissue and histology.
Major clinical associations: Infection is not inevitable after exposure. Risk depends on degree of contamination, post-exposure treatment and vaccination status. Once infection is established, death is inevitable (three cases of recovery have been reported). Following incubation there is a 2–10-day prodrome of fever, headache, GI symptoms, anorexia and fatigue. Mental changes may be present at this stage. Pain and paraesthesiae at the site of the bite may occur. The prodrome is followed by the neurological phase, which lasts 2–7 days. This may be 'furious', with disorientation, hallucinations and hyperactivity. Pharyngeal and laryngeal spasms causing choking or vomiting may be triggered by attempts to eat or

drink, causing the classical symptom of hydro-phobia. Other stimuli such as cold air, loud noises or bright lights may also trigger spasms, which may progress to generalised convulsions. Approximately 20% develop 'dumb' rabies with paralysis, either ascending and symmetrical, or more pronounced on the side of the bite. The neurological phase is followed by coma (usual duration 3–13 days) and death.

Antiviral therapy: No treatment is effective once infection has developed. Full supportive therapy is given but the chance of survival is very slight.

Prevention: Prevention depends on avoiding contact with infected animals, pre-exposure vaccination of those at risk of contact, and post-exposure vaccination of patients who present after being bitten. Fox rabies has been well controlled in Europe by the use of oral vaccine distributed on bait.

Pre-exposure vaccination is currently recommended in the UK for laboratory workers handling virus, those likely to have occupational exposure to imported animals (e.g. zoo workers, customs officials), workers in enzootic areas whose occupation puts them at risk of exposure, and travellers to enzootic areas who are at risk of being infected and who are undertaking long journeys where medical aid may not be immediately available. Three doses of HDCV are given on days 0, 7, 28.

Post-exposure management: Bite wounds should be scrubbed with soap and water for 5 minutes under a running tap as soon as possible. The animal should be captured and observed for 10 days if possible. Local advice should be sought about the risk of rabies associated with the species of animal involved. If preventive treatment is considered necessary, HDCV (six doses on days 0, 3, 7, 14, 30, 90) should be started immediately. Rabies-specific immunoglobulin (20 iu/kg) should be given; half is infiltrated around the bite and half is given im. Previously immunised individuals should receive two doses of HDCV. RIG is not required.

In the UK this situation always involves patients returning from enzootic areas. Advice on the level of risk in different countries may be sought from the PHLS Virus Reference Laboratory, Colindale, the Communicable Diseases (Scotland) Unit and the Department of Health (Northern Ireland).

Viral gastroenteritis

Diarrhoea and vomiting may be caused by viruses from a number of families. (Table 113).

Epidemiology: Infection occurs worldwide. In the developed world rotavirus is responsible for ≥ 50% of diarrhoeal illness in children requiring hospitalisation. In the developing world viral diarrhoea and dehydration account for several million childhood deaths per

Table 113 Viral causes of gastroenteritis

Family/Genus	Structure	Comments
Reovirus: rotavirus	60–80 nm icosahedral virion. dsRNA genome	➢251
Norwalk agent and other small round structured viruses (SRSVs)	20–40 nm round virion. ssRNA genome	
Caliciviruses	35–40 nm round virion. ssRNA genome	Hepatitis E virus has been shown to be a calicivirus (➢52)
Astroviruses	27–32 nm round virion. ssRNA genome	Caliciviruses and astroviruses have characteristic appearances on electron microscopy, but detailed knowledge of their structure is lacking

annum. Rotavirus infections have a seasonal incidence in temperate regions, peaking in winter months. Rotavirus, astrovirus and calicivirus are typically infections of infants and children. Norwalk agent is more often associated with epidemics or family outbreaks and affects individuals of all ages.

Key biological features: Replication occurs in the small intestine, causing malabsorption and osmotic diarrhoea. Colitis is not a feature and faecal pus cells are not seen.

Reservoir: Humans.

Transmission: Faeco-oral, by direct contact, contaminated water or food, particularly cold foods requiring handling such as salads and sandwiches. Inhalation of aerosol from vomit or faeces. The infectious dose is estimated at 10–100 virions, and during acute infection faeces may contain 10^{11} virions/g. Minor contamination of the environment may therefore be highly significant, particularly in nosocomial infection.

Incubation period: One to 2 days.

Immunisation: Not available.

Diagnosis: Electron microscopy of stools. This can be made more sensitive by using specific antisera to concentrate viruses (immuno-electron microscopy). For rotavirus rapid diagnostic methods based on specific monoclonal antibodies, such as latex agglutination or ELISA, are in widespread routine use.

Clinical features: Vomiting, diarrhoea, abdominal cramps, dehydration. Fever and constitutional symptoms such as headache and myalgia are common. Recovery normally occurs in 2–4 days. Infection may be severe or prolonged in immunodeficient or malnourished patients. Asymptomatic infection and faecal shedding are common.

Antiviral therapy: No specific antiviral therapy. Supportive treatment, in particular correction of dehydration, is paramount.

Comments: Rotavirus infection has been tentatively associated with a number of 'non-infectious' syndromes such as haemolytic uraemic syndrome (➤188), Kawasaki's disease (➤154), Reye syndrome and neonatal necrotising enterocolitis (➤113).

Slow virus CNS infections and prions

Several conventional viruses (Table 114), and a number of 'unconventional' agents or 'prions' cause CNS infections that develop over months or years.

Prions ♀

The physical nature of these agents remains uncertain, but it is likely that they are infectious proteins, containing neither DNA nor RNA. Closely related diseases in animals include scrapie in sheep and bovine spongiform encephalopathy.

KURU

Restricted to the Fore people of Papua New Guinea, who practised cannibalism. With the discontinuation of this practice, the disease is disappearing. Sufferers developed ataxia, dysar-

Table 114 Conventional viruses causing slow CNS infection

Family	Virus	Disease	Comments
Polyoma	JC virus	Progressive multifocal leucoencephalopathy	(➤124)
Paramyxovirus	Measles	Subacute sclerosing panencephalitis	(➤101)
Togavirus	Rubella	Rubella panencephalitis	Very rare complication of congenital or early childhood rubella. Presents in teens with intellectual impairment, seizures, myoclonus, spasticity and ataxia

thria and tremor, progressing to chorea, flaccid paralysis and death 3–9 months after onset.

CREUTZFELD–JAKOB DISEASE

Occurs worldwide. Sporadic cases affect about $1/10^6$ persons per year. About 10% of cases are familial with an autosomal dominant pattern of inheritance.

Clinical features: Memory loss, abnormal behaviour and personality change, followed by myoclonus, ataxia and extrapyramidal rigidity. Progression to death over 4–7 months. **Gerstmann–Sträussler syndrome** is a variant, with familial inheritance and extensive spinocerebellar involvement, causing severe gait disturbance, incoordination and dysarthria in addition to dementia.

Investigations: CSF is normal. EEG is abnormal but the changes are not diagnostic. Experimental methods that may be useful in confirming diagnosis include detection of abnormal proteins in CSF and brain tissue. Diagnosis is usually made clinically and confirmed by post-mortem neuropathology.

Prions are resistant to treatments that inactivate conventional viruses, such as boiling, irradiation and disinfectants including alcohol, aldehydes and β-propriolactone. They are an infection hazard to staff handling neurological material *post mortem*. Transmission of Creutzfeld–Jakob disease has occurred after corneal and dura mater transplantation, by purified human growth hormone and by contaminated

Table 115 Summary of antiviral therapy

Agent	Indications	Administration	Adverse effects
Acyclovir	Herpes simplex and herpes zoster virus infections	For doses and indications ➤241. For doses in renal failure ➤319	Rare. Rash, GI upset, CNS toxicity. Renal toxicity due to crystalluria
Idoxuridine	Alternative agent for herpes simplex keratitis	Topical use only. Use 4-hly	
Ganciclovir	Life- or sight-threatening CMV infection in immunocompromised patients. For use in HIV infection ➤128	Parenteral use only. Administer into fast-flowing iv line. Induction dose: 5 mg/kg 12-hly. Maintenance dose: 6 mg/kg daily 5 days/week	Common. Severe myelotoxicity. Contraindicated in pregnancy and lactation. Fever, rash, abnormal liver function. For use in renal failure see manufacturer's data sheet
Foscarnet	Alternative to ganciclovir for CMV retinitis in AIDS (➤128)	Induction dose: 60 mg/kg 8-hly. Maintenance dose: 90 mg/kg daily 5 days/week. Administration with pentamidine may cause severe hypocalcaemia	Nephrotoxicity, hypo/hypercalcaemia, hyper-phosphataemia, anaemia, hepatotoxicity, nausea. Maintain hydration and reduce dose in renal impairment
Amantadine	Prophylaxis of influenza A (➤248)	100 mg 24-hly.	Nausea, insomnia, fits
Ribavarin	Severe RSV bronchiolitis in infants (➤20). Experimental use in Lassa fever (➤256), haemorrhagic fever with renal syndrome (➤255) and Congo–Crimea HF (➤255).	Aerosol inhalation (via small-particle nebuliser) of 20 mg/ml solution for 12–18 h for at least 3 days	No significant adverse effects, but administration to ventilated children is difficult

stereotactic electrodes. Before invasive procedures are performed on patients who have, or may have, these syndromes, always discuss management with a microbiologist ☎.

Summary of antiviral therapy

Viruses use host cellular mechanisms to replicate. Targets for drug action are difficult to identify and therefore antiviral drugs are few and tend to be toxic (Table 115).

28: Protozoa

The taxonomy of protozoan parasites is complex, and includes many non-pathogenic species. For practical purposes, the protozoa of medical importance fall into three groups: flagellates, sporozoa and the amoebae (including the ciliate protozoan *Balantidium coli*, which causes bloody diarrhoea similar to amoebic dysentery).

Pneumocystis carinii (➤119) has been reclassified as a fungus, on the basis of DNA homology.

The following tables given brief details of less important protozoa; page references are given for details of the more important species.

Table 116 Protozoa of medical importance I: flagellates

Species	Epidemiology	Clinical features	Diagnosis	Therapy
Giardia lamblia	See giardiasis (➤266)			
Trichomonas vaginalis	See trichomoniasis (➤70)			
Dientamoeba fragilis	Worldwide. True incidence unknown	Disputed pathogen. May cause mild intermittent diarrhoea and bloating and biliary involvement	Stool microscopy	None proven. Iodoquinol, tetracycline or paromomycin may be effective
Trypanosoma spp.	See trypanosomiasis (➤272)			
Leishmania spp.	See leishmaniasis (➤274)			

Table 117 Protozoa of medical importance II: sporozoa

Species	Epidemiology	Clinical features	Diagnosis	Therapy
Plasmodium spp.	See malaria (➤268)			
Toxoplasma gondii	See toxoplasmosis (➤264)			
Isospora belli	Worldwide. Commoner in subtropics and tropics	Diarrhoea with abdominal cramps and weight loss. Self-limiting in immunocompetent, but may be severe and prolonged in immunodeficient	Stool microscopy	Co-trimoxazole 960 mg 6-hly for 1 week is curative

continued on p. 263

Table 117 contd

Species	Epidemiology	Clinical features	Diagnosis	Therapy
Cryptosporidium parvum (➤122)	Worldwide. Many mammalian hosts. Transmitted human to human and via contaminated water. Σ 5000	Diarrhoea with abdominal cramps and weight loss. Common in children in UK. Self-limiting in normal host, but may be severe and prolonged in immunodeficient. Common in AIDS patients, who may also develop cholangitis, cholecystitis and extraintestinal infection.	Stool microscopy	No reliable therapy. None is required in the normal host. Experimental agents include paromomycin
Sarcocystis hominis, S. suihominis, S. bovihominis	Acquired by eating meat containing tissue cysts	Asymptomatic intestinal infection	Stool microscopy	None required
Babesia microti, B. divergens	Malaria-like illness in cattle, transmitted by ticks. Human infection is very rare	Malaria-like illness with intraerythrocytic parasites. May last several months. Particularly severe in splenectomised patients	Blood film	Quinine and clindamycin

Table 118 Protozoa of medical importance III: amoebae and ciliophora

Group and species	Epidemiology	Clinical features	Diagnosis	Therapy
Amoebae				
Entamoeba histolytica	See amoebiasis (➤267)			
Endolinax nana, Iodamoeba buetschlii, Entamoeba coli	Non-pathogenic protozoa found in stools, which may be confused with *E. histolytica*			
Naegleria fowleri	Free-living amoeba. Acquired by exposure of nasal passages to contaminated fresh water, e.g. swimming	Unusual cause of severe meningo-encephalitis with high mortality. Epidemics may occur related to a common source of contaminated fresh water	Wet preparation of CSF ☛	Amphotericin B, miconazole and rifampicin

continued on p. 264

Table 118 contd

Group and species	Epidemiology	Clinical features	Diagnosis	Therapy
Acanthamoeba spp.	Free-living amoeba. Frequent contaminant of contact lens cases	Keratitis (➤84). Rare cause of meningoencephalitis	Conjunctival scrapings (☎ special stains and culture)	Topical dibromo-propamidine and neomycin
Ciliophora				
Balantidium coli	Intestinal parasite of humans, pigs and rodents. Worldwide, wherever humans and pigs associate	Bloody diarrhoea with colonic ulceration. Perforation may occur. Disputed pathogen	Stool microscopy (thin smear, special stains) ☎	Oxytetracycline **or** metronidazole
Microsporidia				
Encephalitozoon cuniculi, Entero-cytozoon bieneusi, Nosema connori, etc.	Animal parasites	Rare cause of myositis, diarrhoea and CNS infection in immunocompromised patients. Probably also travellers' diarrhoea and keratitis in the immunocompetent	Microscopy ☎. Sometimes confused with cryptosporidia	None known

Toxoplasma gondii

Epidemiology and transmission: Worldwide. Seroprevalence varies with age and between countries (UK ~35%, France ~85%). Σ ~800.

Life cycle: *Toxoplasma gondii* is an intracellular parasite of macrophages infecting a wide range of birds and mammals. Cats are the definitive hosts for the sexual phase of the life cycle. Infected cats excrete oocysts in faeces which become infectious 2–3 days after they are passed and may remain infectious for many months in warm moist soil. Ingestion of oocysts by other cats completes the cycle. Ingestion by non-felines (including humans) causes acute infection, followed by formation of tissue cysts in many tissues. Cysts contain slowly replicating parasites ('bradyzoites') and are asymptomatic, but may reactivate during immunodeficiency, to cause clinical disease, particularly in the CNS.

Human infection is acquired by ingestion of infectious oocysts in cat faeces, by eating poorly cooked meat containing tissue cysts, transplacentally or rarely via blood transfusion.

Clinical features

Incubation time: For acute infectious mononucleosis-like syndrome, 5–20 days.

Symptoms and signs: Infection is rarely symptomatic in the normal population. *Toxoplasma gondii* causes disease in four situations.

Acute infectious mononucleosis-like illness, due to acute primary infection in immunocompetent individuals. Generalised lymphadenopathy, fever, headache, malaise, sore throat, myalgia, hepatosplenomegaly and abnormal liver function tests. Reactive lymphocytosis may occur (➤106).

Chorioretinitis (➤85) presents in older children and adults and is usually due to reactivation of congenital infection. Only ~1% of acquired infections result in eye disease.

Chorioretinitis occurs in AIDS patients, usually in association with CNS disease. It presents with visual loss. On fundoscopy, acute lesions are yellowish patches with surrounding hyperaemia. Older lesions are atrophic white plaques with distinct borders and choroidal pigmentation.

Reactivation during immunodeficiency, particularly AIDS (➤124), typically causing encephalitis.

Congenital infection (➤112).

Investigations: In acute infection, **lymph node histology** is characteristic, with follicular hyperplasia and collections of enlarged epithelioid cells with abundant pale cytoplasm, vesicular nuclei and prominent nucleoli. Organisms are rarely seen on histology. Isolation of *Toxoplasma gondii* is complex and expensive and is rarely performed. Diagnosis is usually confirmed by **serology**. A large number of tests are available for detecting IgG and IgM antibodies, including the Sabin–Feldmann dye test, the indirect fluorescent antibody test and complement fixation and agglutination tests. Since infection is common, interpretation of tests can be difficult. Table 119 is a guide only, and liaison with local and reference labs is essential ☎.

Table 119 Interpretation of toxoplasma serology

Situation	Comments
Suspected acute toxoplasmosis in immunocompetent patient	Negative serology excludes toxoplasmosis. Seroconversion, a fourfold rise in titre at 3-week interval or positive IgM supports diagnosis. IgM may persist for several years
Ocular disease	Seropositivity is common in most populations. Titres do not correlate with active chorioretinitis, and serology is therefore not usually helpful
Suspected toxoplasmosis in immunodeficient patients	Titres do not usually rise during reactivation, and serology is therefore not usually helpful. Only ~3% of AIDS patients with toxoplasma encephalitis are seronegative for *Toxoplasma gondii*
Infection during pregnancy	Documented seroconversion confirms infection. The interpretation of positive serology discovered during pregnancy requires consultation with reference laboratory. Fetal blood sampling may be used to confirm foetal infection
Congenital infection	Confirmed by rising titres or positive IgM

Table 120 Management of toxoplasmosis

Situation	Comments
Acute toxoplasmosis in immunocompetent patient	No therapy required
Ocular disease	Pyrimethamine, folinic acid and sulphadiazine for 1 month.* Steroids and laser may also be used to limit lesion size.
Toxoplasmosis in immunodeficient patients	Pyrimethamine, folinic acid and sulphadiazine or clindamycin for 6 weeks followed by indefinite prophylaxis*
Infection during pregnancy	Treatment reduces fetal infection rate. Pyrimethamine is contraindicated in first trimester. Ideal treatment regimens not established. Spiramycin 1.5 g 12-hly or

continued on p. 266

Table 120 contd

Situation	Comments
	sulphadiazine* alone are commonly used for first trimester, followed by pyrimethamine/ sulphadiazine* continuously or alternating with spiramycin. Consultation with reference lab essential
Congenital infection	Pyrimethamine, folinic acid and sulphadiazine, alternating with spiramycin, plus steroids. Consultation with reference lab essential

* For doses and precautions ➤125.

Giardia lamblia

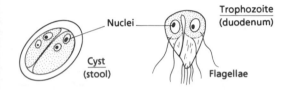

Epidemiology and transmission: Worldwide, but commoner in developing countries. Transmission occurs by contaminated water and food, and by direct person-to-person contact. Mammalian reservoirs are often important in local epidemiology, e.g. by contaminating water supplies. Σ > 6000.

Life cycle: *Giardia lamblia* has two stages. The flagellated motile trophozoite is fragile and cannot survive outside the host; the chitin-walled cyst is the infective stage, and can survive in the environment, particularly in moist cool conditions. Cysts are highly infectious—the infectious dose is estimated at between 10 and 100 cysts. After ingestion cysts develop into trophozoites in the duodenum and small intestine, where they adhere to gut epithelial cells and multiply by binary fission. Tissue invasion does not occur.

Clinical features

Incubation time: One to 3 weeks.

Symptoms and signs: Infection is often asymptomatic. Diarrhoea is the primary symptom, with bulky, pale, offensive stools, but no blood. Anorexia, nausea, abdominal bloating and low-grade fever may occur. Tiredness may be a prominent feature. Arthralgia, myalgia, urticaria and eosinophilia are rare. In 30–50% there is progress to chronic diarrhoea, of whom ~50% develop malabsorption, sometimes severe, particularly in malnourished or immunodeficient patients, especially those with hypogammaglobulinaemia.

Investigations: Stool microscopy for cysts is positive in ~80% of patients if three samples are examined. Trophozoites may be seen in duodenal juice or biopsy material obtained at endoscopy. In the 'hairy string test' the patient swallows the end of a string which passes into the duodenum, before being pulled back and examined for parasites. Immunological tests for the detection of *Giardia lamblia* antigens in stools are being developed.

Management: Metronidazole 2 g 24-hly for 3 days or 400 mg 8-hly for 5 days. Treatment failure is common (~10%). The course should be repeated, and reinfection from family members excluded.

Entamoeba histolytica ✉ ②

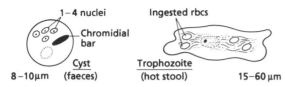

1–4 nuclei

Chromidial bar

Cyst (faeces)

8–10µm

Ingested rbcs

Trophozoite (hot stool)

15–60 µm

Epidemiology and transmission: Worldwide: ~10% of the world's population are chronically infected, mainly in underdeveloped countries. Infection is unusual in the UK except in returning travellers, homosexuals and residents of institutions. Σ ~1000.

Life cycle: *Entamoeba histolytica* exists in two forms. The motile trophozoite is responsible for clinical disease, but is incapable of surviving outside the host. Trophozoites develop into cysts in the colon. The cyst form may survive in the environment for weeks and is responsible for transmission. Asymptomatic carriage of non-pathogenic strains of *Entamoeba histolytica* is common. Clinical disease is caused by distinct pathogenic strains. *Entamoeba histolytica* adheres to colonic epithelium and invades it directly, causing lysis of mucosal cells.

Clinical features

Incubation time: Variable, from a few days to months. Commonly 2–4 weeks.

Symptoms and signs: Infection may be **asymptomatic** or cause only mild diarrhoea and colicky abdominal pain ('non-invasive disease'). Epithelial invasion causes **amoebic dysentery**, an acute rectocolitis with abdominal pain, tenderness and bloody diarrhoea. Constitutional symptoms are few; fever occurs in ~30%. Immunosuppressed patients, children or pregnant women are at risk of developing **fulminant amoebic colitis**, which may cause perforation or toxic megacolon. Chronic localised invasive disease, usually in the right colon, causes an inflammatory mass, an **amoeboma**, which resembles colonic carcinoma on barium enema, but responds rapidly to amoebicidal therapy. **Amoebic liver abscess** (ALA) presents with weight loss, fever, right upper-quadrant pain and tenderness. In

returning travellers to the UK it usually develops 2–5 months after exposure and there is often no history of dysentery. Symptoms and signs may be minimal and jaundice is rare. Untreated, ALA grows until it ruptures, either through skin, diaphragm, pericardium (rarely) or into peritoneal cavity, causing acute abdominal pain. Metastasis to brain and lung may occur rarely. **Cutaneous amoebiasis** is a rare complication that develops from sites of skin exposure to amoebae, such as ALA ruptures sites or perianal region, causing progressive destructive and sometimes extensive ulceration.

Investigations: Stool microscopy for cysts and trophozoites. In amoebic dysentery stools contain blood but few pus cells. Motile trophozoites containing red blood cells are usually seen. Diarrhoea from other causes (e.g. bacterial dysentery) may accelerate gut transit time, resulting in the presence of amoebae in stools of patients who were previously asymptomatically passing cysts, but the characteristic sign of invasive amoebiasis is ingestion of red blood cells by amoebae. In asymptomatic infection, cysts are seen in ~30%; at least three samples should be examined to exclude carriage. Examination of stools for cysts is only relevant in patients who have left the endemic area or who are pregnant. In ALA, stools are positive for cysts or trophozoites in ~20%. *Entamoeba histolytica* cysts are differentiated from commensal *Entamoeba coli* cysts by size, number of nuclei and chromatidal bar.

Serology: Many methods exist for demonstrating antibodies; currently in the UK sera are screened using IFAT, and positive tests confirmed by a cellulose acetate precipitin test (CAP). These are positive in acute dysentery

(~75%), amoeboma and ALA (~95–100%, often to high titre), and asymptomatic carriage (~40%).

Diagnosis of ALA: Leucocytosis, anaemia and raised ESR are usual. Liver function tests are usually normal. CXR may show raised hemidiaphragm, right basal shadowing and pleural effusion, even in the absence of diaphragmatic rupture. Diagnosis may be confirmed by USS or CT scanning. Abscesses may be multiple (less commonly than pyogenic liver abscess ➤56) and are most frequently located in the right lobe. Aspiration may be carried out to exclude pyogenic liver abscess, or to prevent rupture. Indications for aspiration are bulging of the rib cage or abdominal wall, a very raised hemidiaphragm, marked local tenderness or oedema or failure to respond to medical therapy. Abscess contents resemble 'anchovy sauce'. Amoebae are found in ~80% of cases. Pus cells are not seen as the abscess contains only the liquid remains of digested liver cells and amoebic products are leucotoxic. Aspiration to dryness is essential.

Management: Dysentery and asymptomatic carriage: metronidazole 800 mg 8-hly **followed by** the luminal amoebicide diloxanide furoate, 500 mg 8-hly for 5 days to prevent relapse. In severe cases, tetracycline 500 mg 8-hly should be added. ALA: metronidazole 800 mg 8-hly **followed by** diloxanide furoate, 500 mg 8-hly for 10 days. If ALA fails to respond to treatment (see above for indications), diagnostic/therapeutic aspiration should be performed.

Malaria ⊠

There are ~1900 imported cases of malaria p.a. in the UK and deaths still occur. Factors contributing to this are failure to consider the diagnosis, delay in starting therapy, failure to recognise the onset of severe complications and misplaced trust in the efficacy of prophylaxis and 'negative' blood films.

Epidemiology and transmission: Malaria occurs throughout the tropics and subtropics, although some areas have achieved eradication. WHO estimates $>10^8$ cases/year worldwide and $>10^6$ child deaths/year in Africa alone. Four species of *Plasmodium* cause malaria in humans (Table 121).

Transmission occurs by bite of the female *Anopheles* mosquito. Control programmes are aimed principally at eradication of the mosquito vector. Vertical, transfusion and organ transplant transmission may occur.

Life cycle: The mosquito injects *sporozoites*, which rapidly attach to and enter liver cells.

Table 121 Species of malaria parasite

Species	Disease	Areas of greatest prevalence	Key biological/clinical features
P. falciparum Σ ~1050	Malignant tertian malaria	Worldwide. Predominant species in Africa. Common in SE Asia, S America	Potentially fatal. Chloroquine resistance common
P. vivax Σ ~700	Benign tertian malaria	Predominant species in Indian subcontinent. Common in Central/South America, SE Asia	Rarely severe. Late relapses can occur due to persistence in liver ('hypnozoites'). Chloroquine resistance very rare.
P. ovale Σ ~130	Ovale tertian malaria	Least common species. Mainly African	As for *P. vivax*
P. malariae Σ ~20	Quartan malaria	Widely distributed in Africa	Rarely severe. Causes nephrotic syndrome in children

An asymptomatic period of 1–2 weeks follows, during which parasites mature and multiply within liver cells, forming *hepatic schizonts* ('exoerythrocytic' forms). These rupture, releasing *merozoites*, which enter RBCs and mature and multiply through *ring* and *trophozoite* forms to become *schizonts*. This process takes 48 h (72 h for *P. malariae*), following which the schizonts rupture, releasing between six and 24 merozoites, depending on the species, which may then infect further RBCs. This cycle repeats causing the well-recognised pattern of cyclical fevers. Some merozoites develop in RBCs into sexual forms, *gametocytes*, which may be taken up by a biting mosquito. Sexual reproduction takes place in the mosquito and the cycle is completed. Each stage in the life cycle for each species has a characteristic morphology, which allows diagnosis and speciation.

P. vivax and *P. ovale* have hepatic schizonts which lie dormant in the liver and cause late relapse (*hypnozoites*).

Pathogenesis: Febrile episodes are related to schizont rupture. Only *P. falciparum* causes severe complications, such as cerebral malaria. *P. falciparum* may infect RBCs of all ages (other species are restricted to RBCs at particular stages of development) and can therefore cause very high rates of parasitaemia (> 1% of all RBCs). It also causes sequestration of infected RBCs in vascular beds, leading to severe disturbance of microcirculation. Anaemia is due to haemolysis, splenic sequestration and depressed erythropoiesis.

Partial immunity develops with repeated attacks but wanes in emigrants from endemic areas. Infection is usually only severe in children, non-immune travellers and pregnant women.

Clinical features

Incubation time: Primary attack: 7–30 days. Relapse of *P. vivax* or *P. ovale*: up to 1 year, typically 38 weeks.

> **Practice point:** *P. falciparum* infection causes life-threatening complications in returning travellers. *P. falciparum* **infection is a medical emergency.**

Symptoms and signs: There may be a short prodrome mimicking viral infection with malaise and fatigue. Paroxysmal fever is the cardinal symptom. Patients typically notice three stages: shivering with rigors; then flushed and pyrexial for several hours; finally drenched in sweat as the fever resolves. The typical pattern of cyclical fever takes ≥ 1 week to develop and is unusual in patients in the UK. Hyperpyrexia may occur, and occasionally patients with severe falciparum malaria may be apyrexial. On examination, anaemia and jaundice due to haemolysis may be detectable clinically. Tachycardia with flow murmur, hepatosplenomegaly and abdominal tenderness are common.

Complications: These occur almost exclusively with *P. falciparum* and are common and severe only in non-immune patients, i.e. children, travellers and pregnant women. **Cerebral malaria** presents with disturbed level of consciousness, fits and, less often, focal neurological deficits, progressing to coma and death. Mortality is ~20–50%. It is usually, but not always, associated with heavy parasitaemia. Patients who survive usually

Table 122 Natural history of untreated malaria

Species	Natural history of **untreated** infection
P. falciparum	If the patient survives the primary attack, there may be recrudescences at increasing intervals due to persistence of blood forms between attacks. These die out after ~1 year unless reinfection occurs
P. vivax, P. ovale	Relapses due to dormant liver forms ('hypnozoites') occur for up to 5 years
P. malariae	Recurrent fevers for many years (≤ 50 years). Anaemia and hepatosplenomegaly are common

have full recovery of neurological function. Pathogenesis is related to sequestration of parasitised RBCs in cerebral circulation, but exact mechanism remains controversial. Cerebral oedema is not a feature and steroids are **not** indicated. **Renal failure** occurs due to acute tubular necrosis secondary to hypovolaemia and shock and occasionally massive haemolysis and haemoglobinuria ('blackwater fever'). **Hypoglycaemia** is common, due to glucose use by parasites, impaired hepatic gluconeogenesis and stimulation of insulin secretion by quinine. It is particularly severe in patients with cerebral malaria or receiving intravenous quinine. **Adult respiratory distress syndrome** presents with tachypnoea and bilateral interstitial shadowing on CXR. Similar appearances may be due to fluid overload and diagnosis and management depend on haemodynamic monitoring of fluid status. **Algid malaria** describes septic shock due to Gram-negative bacteraemia complicating severe malaria. **Thrombocytopenia** is very common, but significant bleeding and disseminated intravascular coagulation occur only rarely.

P. malariae causes severe nephrotic syndrome in children, which rarely resolves after antimalarial treatment.

Malaria in pregnancy is often more severe, even in patients who would otherwise have partial immunity. Severe haemolytic anaemia may occur and hypoglycaemia is more frequent. There is increased risk of fetal death, small birth weight and prematurity, attributable to placental microcirculatory damage. Mefloquine and halofantrine are relatively contraindicated in pregnancy, but chloroquine and quinine may be given safely. **Congenital malaria** occurs rarely, more often due to *P. vivax* than to *P. falciparum*. It presents as progressive haemolytic anaemia, and should be treated as appropriate for the species involved, with the exception that primaquine is not required, because the fetus is infected by blood forms which cannot re-enter the liver.

Investigations: Anaemia, thrombocytopenia and leucopenia are common. Prolonged coagulation tests and positive fibrin degra-

dation products suggest DIC, which is often due to secondary Gram-negative septicaemia, probably secondary to gut microvascular damage. Diagnosis of malaria is made by examination of **thick and thin blood films** processed using special stains (Field's, Leishman's, Giemsa). Thin films comprise a single layer of RBCs; parasite morphology is preserved, so it is possible to determine species reliably, but many high-power fields may have to be examined. Thick films are made by allowing a thick smear of blood to dry. RBCs are then lysed, leaving parasites concentrated in a small area. This allows more rapid diagnosis of malaria, but parasite morphology is damaged and it may not be possible to determine species. If in doubt, *P. falciparum* infection should be assumed. At least three negative films taken at intervals are required to exclude malaria, particularly as levels of parasitaemia fall between febrile paroxysms. New methods of detecting parasites based on immunological and molecular technology are becoming available, but at present examination of films remains the gold standard and the only method in widespread use. **Serology** is not used for the diagnosis of acute illness, but is sometimes helpful in excluding malaria as a cause of recurrent fever, e.g. in old soldiers or retrospectively.

Management: Chloroquine resistance in *P. falciparum* has been reported from almost all areas except the Middle East and N Africa, and all patients returning to the UK with *P. falciparum* should be assumed to have chloroquine-resistant malaria. Serial blood films are recommended to follow response to therapy. The other species remain susceptible, although there have been reports of chloroquine-resistant *P. vivax* in Papua New Guinea. Fansidar resistance has been reported from many areas, and is sufficiently prevalent in Thailand, Burma and Kampuchea for patients with *P. falciparum* returning from those countries to receive alternative therapy.

Antimalarial drugs
Specific recommendations for treatment
Non-falciparum malaria: Choroquine 600 mg po initially, 300 mg after 6 h, then 300 mg 24-

Table 123 Antimalarial drugs

Drug	Important side-effects	Comments
Chloroquine	GI upset, headache, retinal damage and cataracts, rarely myelotoxicity, psychosis. Contraindicated in epilepsy.* Reduce dose in renal failure	Resistance is widespread, but confined to *P. falciparum*. Not active against dormant hepatic forms ('hypnozoites') of *P. vivax* and *P. ovale*
Proguanil	GI upset, rarely mouth ulcers. Reduce dose in renal failure	Prophylaxis only
Fansidar (pyrimethamine and sulfadoxine)	Skin rash, myelotoxicity	For eradication of *P. falciparum* infection
Maloprim (pyrimethamine and dapsone)	Skin rash, myelotoxicity	Prophylaxis only
Halofantrine	Contraindicated in pregnancy. GI upset, pruritus, transient elevation of serum transaminases, cardiotoxicity	Treatment of uncomplicated *P. falciparum* infection
Primaquine	GI upset, haemolysis, particularly in G6PD deficiency	Eradication of dormant hepatic forms ('hypnozoites') of *P. vivax* and *P. ovale*
Mefloquine	Contraindicated in first trimester, breast-feeding, neurological disease, epilepsy* (including family history), liver disease, concurrent β-blocker therapy. Causes neuropsychiatric effects and GI upset. Avoid pregnancy for 3 months after stopping treatment. Treatment duration should not exceed 1 year	Prophylaxis and treatment of chloroquine-resistant *P. falciparum* malaria
Quinine	Tinnitus, hypoglycaemia, headaches, flushing, GI upset, rash, myelotoxicity	Agent of choice for treatment of chloroquine-resistant or severe *P. falciparum* malaria

* Doxycycline is an alternative in epileptic patients.

hly for 6 days (children 10 mg/kg, then 3 doses of 5 mg/kg). If patient unable to swallow, slow iv infusion of 10 mg/kg over 8 h may be given, followed by oral therapy if possible or a further 15 mg/kg iv over 24 h. Failure to clear parasitaemia should raise the question of mixed infection with *P. falciparum* or chloroquine resistance, and quinine should be substituted—see below. After chloroquine treatment for *P. vivax* and *P. ovale*, give primaquine 15 mg 24-hly for 15 days (21 days for travellers from SE Asia) to destroy hypnozoites. Check glucose-6-phosphate dehydrogenase (G6PD) levels, as primaquine causes haemolysis in G6PD deficiency. Primaquine is also contraindicated in pregnancy. In pregnancy or G6PD deficiency, give chloroquine 300 mg weekly for 6 months instead.

Uncomplicated falciparum malaria (see below for definition of 'complicated'): quinine (sulphate, hydrochloride or dihydrochloride) 600 mg 8-hly for 7 days (child 10 mg/kg 8-hly) **plus** Fansidar (pyrimethamine/sulfadoxine) three tablets stat (see BNF for child doses). Dose of quinine may be reduced to 12-hly if side-effects (esp. tinnitus) are severe. Doxycycline (200 mg loading dose, then

100 mg 24-hly for 6 days) may be substituted for Fansidar, particularly if Fansidar resistance is likely, as in patients returning from Thailand, Burma and Kampuchea.

Alternative regimens: Mefloquine 10 mg/kg (max. 700 mg) two doses 6 h apart (child > 15 kg and < 45 kg, 12.5 mg/kg two doses 6 h apart). Contraindicated in pregnancy, in patients on β-blockers, in neurological disease including epilepsy. **Or** halofantrine, 500 mg (child 8 mg/kg) three doses at 6-h intervals repeated after 1 week. Contraindicated in pregnancy.

Complicated falciparum malaria: This is defined by the presence of one of the following complications: impaired conscious level, renal failure, respiratory distress syndrome, haemorrhage, severe anaemia, shock, haemoglobinuria, hypoglycaemia, fits, prostration, parasitaemia > 2%, jaundice, hyperpyrexia or continued vomiting. Quinine dihydrochloride 20 mg/kg (max. 1.4 g) loading dose, infused over 4 h; then, after 8–12 h, maintenance dose of 10 mg/kg (max. 700 mg) infused over 4 h every 8 h until patient can swallow oral quinine **plus** Fansidar or doxycycline as above under uncomplicated falciparum malaria. Omit loading dose if patient has received quinine or mefloquine in preceding 24 h. **Exchange transfusion** has been advocated for patients with very heavy parasitaemia (≥ 10%) but there has been no controlled trial and indications for its use are not yet defined. Urgent specialist consultation is strongly recommended.

Antimalarial prophylaxis (➤139)

Table 124 Stand by treatment for malaria

Chloroquine resistance	
No	Chloroquine (Fansidar for those taking chloroquine prophylaxis)
Yes	Fansidar, mefloquine, or quinine (followed by Fansidar or tetracycline)

Standby treatment: Travellers to particularly remote areas where medical help is unavailable may be given **standby treatment** to take in the event of fever.

The choices in Table 124 are appropriate.

Trypanosomiasis

Four species of *Trypanosoma* infect humans (Table 125).

African trypanosomiasis (sleeping sickness)

Epidemiology and transmission: Occurs in focal areas of tropical Africa. There are 10 000–20 000 cases reported p.a. *T. b. rhodesiense*, found mainly in E Africa, causes a more severe and rapid illness than *T.b. gambiense*, which is commoner in W and Central Africa. Transmission is via the bite of the tsetse fly. Σ ~1.

Pathogenesis: In mammals the parasite is a flagellated organism that circulates extracellularly in blood, lymph and extracellular fluid, replicating by binary fission. Trypanosomes have a glycoprotein surface coat that

Table 125 *Trypsanoma* species

Species	Disease	Vector	Reservoir
Trypanosoma brucei rhodesiense	African trypanosomiasis ('Rhodesiense sleeping sickness')	Tsetse fly	Wild mammals, e.g. bushbuck, hartebeest
Trypanosoma brucei gambiense	African trypanosomiasis ('Gambiense sleeping sickness')	Tsetse fly	Mainly other humans, but also domestic animals, e.g. pigs
Trypanosoma cruzi	South American trypanosomiasis (Chagas' disease)	Reduviid bug	Many wild and domestic mammals
Trypanosoma rangeli	Non-pathogenic		

undergoes spontaneous antigenic variation during infection, thus avoiding host antibodies; each change in antigenic structure is followed by a surge in parasite replication. This mechanism allows the organism to persist for years, eventually entering the CNS.

Clinical features

Incubation time: The bite may be inconspicuous or may develop after ~5 days into a painful inflamed nodule (trypanosomal chancre).

Symptoms and signs: This is followed by fever, headache, myalgia and lymphadenopathy. Splenomegaly, transient painful cutaneous oedema and generalised pruritus occur and a circinate erythematous rash is commonly seen in Caucasians. In *T. b. gambienese* infection CNS invasion occurs after months to years, causing a chronic meningoencephalitis with dementia and behavioural changes, including sleep reversal. Focal signs, tremor and ataxia follow, progressing to coma and death. *T. b. rhodesiense* causes a more rapid and severe infection, which is often fatal within weeks. Myocarditis, causing congestive heart failure and arrhythmia, and disseminated intravascular coagulation commonly cause death before CNS invasion takes place. Features of CNS disease are similar to *T. b. gambienese* infection, but develop more rapidly.

Investigations: Anaemia, lymphocytosis and a marked elevation of total serum IgM are characteristic. Trypanosomes may be seen on blood films processed as for malaria. Concentration methods are used to detect scanty parasitaemia. Lymph node puncture or bone marrow material can also be examined for parasites. CSF is abnormal after CNS invasion has occurred, with raised opening pressure, raised protein and IgM and a lymphocytic pleocytosis. Mott cells ('morula cells') are characteristic plasma cells with intracellular aggregations of IgM, seen in CSF. Organisms are sometimes seen in centrifuged deposit of CSF. Serology (IFAT) is also widely used.

Management: Treatment with suramin and pentamidine is most effective before CNS invasion has occurred. After CNS invasion, the trivalent arsenical melarsoprol (Mel B) or eflornithine is given. These agents are all toxic; 1–5% of patients treated with Mel B

die of side-effects, including encephalopathy ☞.

South American trypanosomiasis (Chagas' disease)

Chagas' disease, due to infection by *Trypanosoma cruzi*, is a major cause of cardiovascular death and GI disease in S America.

Epidemiology and transmission: Most prevalent in Brazil, Bolivia, Argentina and Chile. *T. cruzi* infection is associated with poverty. The reduviid bug vector lives in roofs and walls of rural/slum housing and emerges at night to bite the occupants. Bug faeces containing trypanosomes is then rubbed into the bite wound or conjunctiva. Congenital and transfusion-related infections also occur. Σ ~1.

Pathogenesis: Parasites replicate intracellularly in many cells, especially muscle, macrophages and central/peripheral nervous tissue, causing progressive inflammation and destruction.

Clinical features: Asymptomatic acute infection is common.

Incubation time: About 1–2 weeks after inoculation, unilateral orbital oedema (Romaña's sign) or an area of cutaneous oedema (chagoma) may develop

Symptoms and signs: This is associated with fever, malaise and generalised lymphadenopathy. This usually resolves after 4–8 weeks, although ~10% (usually children) die due to acute myocarditis or meningoencephalitis. After resolution of acute infection there is an asymptomatic period lasting many years, following which ~10–30% develop evidence of chronic sequelae. These present in early adulthood or middle age and include dilated cardiomyopathy, arrhythmias, heart block and denervation of the gastrointestinal tract presenting as megaoesophagus or megacolon.

Investigations: Diagnosis is made by finding *T. cruzi* in blood films, by special blood culture for trypanosomes, or by xenodiagnosis (feeding laboratory-reared 'clean' bugs on the patient and examining the bugs for infection 3–4 weeks later). Serology is also used.

Management: Nifurtimox and benznidazole are used for acute infection; they terminate parasitaemia but do not eradicate intra-cellular parasites. They are not helpful once chronic sequelae have developed ☙.

Leishmaniasis

Visceral and cutaneous leishmaniasis are different diseases best considered separately.

Visceral leishmaniasis (kala-azar)

Caused by *Leishmania donovani* in both Old and New Worlds.

Epidemiology and transmission: Widely distributed around Mediterranean, in tropical Africa, S America, E and Central Asia. Wild mammals, especially rodents and canines, are reservoirs. Transmitted by bite of sandfly. In the sandfly, parasites are flagellated *promastigotes*; in mammals they become small non-flagellate intracellular *amastigotes*. Transfusion and person-to-person sexual transmission have been reported rarely. Infection is more likely to progress in the malnourished. Σ ~5.

Pathogenesis: A local inflammatory reaction occurs at the site of the bite and infection can be eradicated at this stage. Dissemination is followed by replication within cells of the reticuloendothelial system.

Clinical features:

Incubation time: Three to 18 months.

Symptoms and signs: Reaction at the site of the bite produces a nodule ('leishmanioma'). Dissemination is associated with recurrent fever, night sweats and weight loss. On examination, cachexia, lymphadenopathy and moderate to massive hepatosplenomegaly with anaemia, hypoalbuminaemia and oedema. Patients are immunocompromised and secondary bacterial infections and tuberculosis account for ~95% of deaths. Untreated visceral leishmaniasis is fatal usually within 2 years, although spontaneous recovery is reported. Cirrhosis, glomerulonephritis and amyloidosis are rare complications.

Investigations: Normocytic, normochromic anaemia, leucopenia and thrombocytopenia (frequently with haemorrhagic complications, e.g. epistaxis) are usual. Marked polyclonal increase in IgG occurs and underlies the outdated and non-specific formol gel test for leishmaniasis, in which a drop of formalin is added to patient's serum, which then coagulates due to hyperglobulinaemia. Hypoalbuminaemia is common. Diagnosis is made by demonstrating amastigotes by microscopy, culture or animal inoculation. If the spleen is enlarged, splenic puncture is safe in experienced hands and gives the best yield. Bone marrow, liver biopsy and buffy coat may also be examined. Serology (IFAT) is available although false positives may occur, particularly in autoimmune disease. DNA probes are under assessment.

Management: Pentavalent antimony (sodium stibogluconate, Pentostam™) is the drug of choice. Important side-effects include malaise and arthralgia, disordered liver function tests and cardiotoxicity. Treatment failures and relapses occur and pentamidine and amphotericin are used as second-line drugs. TB should be excluded in patients who fail to respond to therapy ☙.

Post-kala-azar dermal leishmaniasis: Following apparent cure of visceral leishmaniasis, relapse may occur in the skin, causing disseminated erythematous and hypopigmented nodules and papules, which are rich in parasites and act as a reservoir of infection, particularly in India where there is no animal reservoir.

Cutaneous leishmaniasis (CL)

CL is caused by many *Leishmania* species. Each is geographically restricted by the distribution of its specific sandfly vector and animal reservoir, and they produce different clinical patterns. CL occurs in travellers returning to the UK, particularly from S and Central America. Knowledge of *Leishmania* species prevalent in the areas visited is essential to guide management (Table 126).

Epidemiology and transmission: Life cycle is essentially as for *L. dononvani* (see above).

Clinical features: CL typically presents with a persistent erythematous skin ulcer at the site of the bite, which heals over a number of months. Lesions are solitary and dry or multiple and exudative ('wet CL'). Relapses occur after apparent healing and occasionally lesions become chronic ('recidivans CL'). Disseminated or 'diffuse CL' is associated with

Table 126

Species	Distribution	Diseases	Reservoir
Old World cutaneous leishmaniasis			
L. tropica	North-west India, west Asia, Pakistan, Afghanistan, Mediterranean area	Old World CL, recidivans CL	Humans
L. major	Afghanistan, Iran, Israel, North Africa, Sudan, Senegal, Niger, CIS (E of Caspian Sea)	Old World CL; multiple sores are frequent	Various desert rodents
L. aethiopica	Ethiopia	Old World CL; small number develop disseminated CL (DCL)	Hyrax
New World cutaneous leishmaniasis			
*L. viannia braziliensis	S America, esp. Amazon basin. As far north as Belize	S American CL, mucocutaneous leishmaniasis ('espundia')	Forest rodents
*L. viannia guyanensis	Guyanas, and adjacent parts of Venezuela and Brazil	S American CL ('forest sore' or 'pian bois')	Various sloths
*L. viannia panamensis	Panama, probably elsewhere in S America	S American CL, very rarely mucocutaneous leishmaniasis	Sloths and other forest mammals
L. mexicana mexicana	Central America esp. Belize	S American CL ('chiclero's ear')	Forest rodents
L. mexicana amazonensis	Brazil	S American CL, DCL	Forest rodents
L. mexicana pifanoi	Venezuela	S American CL, DCL	Unknown
L. peruviana	Peruvian Andes, Argentina	Uta	?Dog

* L. viannia group was previously called L. braziliensis (e.g. L. braziliensis braziliensis).

impaired host immunity and causes diffuse or nodular infiltration of skin with depigmentation but little ulceration.

Mucocutaneous disease ('espundia') is a serious destructive complication, usually involving the mucocutaneous junction of the nose and spreading inwards to destroy adjacent tissue over a number of years. It is only seen with L. viannia group infections (principally L. viannia braziliensis, complicating ≤5% of cases). Secondary bacterial infection may be important and there is significant mortality.

Investigations: Diagnosis is by biopsy of the lesions. Biopsy is taken from the edge of the ulcer and impression smears made before it is fixed. Liaison with histology is essential. Serology is available but is usually negative in returning UK travellers with early disease. Culture of organisms from lesions is possible and allows typing by isoenzyme studies. Polymerase chain reaction is under assessment at some research centres and may allow typing directly from biopsy material.

Management: It is essential to treat infection by L. viannia group to prevent mucocutaneous disease. Old World CL and L. mexicana group infections do not cause mucosal disease and are usually self-limiting. The decision to treat is made on an individual basis. Speciation of Leishmania is not usually possible clinically, and information about species prevalent in the area of travel is usually lacking. Thus many patients suspected to have L. mexicana group infections are treated in case they have L. viannia infection. Pentavalent antimony is used, the dose depending on the species. Second-line drugs include pentamidine, amphotericin B and the imidazoles ☎.

29: Helminths

Guide to helminth infections (Table 127)

Table 127

Helminths are divided into three groups:
- nematodes (roundworms);
- trematodes (flatworms or flukes);
- cestodes (tapeworms).

Although they may produce innumerable larvae or eggs, which may themselves cause disease, adult worms cannot usually reproduce without a period of development outside the body, often involving specific environmental conditions, animal hosts and/or vectors. Therefore the total 'worm burden' cannot increase without constant re-exposure to infection. For this reason clinically significant helminth infections are very rare in the UK, even in travellers returning from the tropics. Figures given below (Σ) to indicate relative frequency usually represent imported infections. The exception is *Enterobius vermicularis*, which is common in the UK because it produces eggs which are directly infective for humans.

Soil-transmitted intestinal nematodes

These are all nematode infections that are transmitted from human to human. The egg or larva is not usually infectious when first passed, but must undergo development in the soil. Transmission depends on contamination of soil with faeces, and appropriate environmental conditions. Diagnosis is usually made by identifying characteristic eggs of each species in faeces. The **prepatent period** is the interval between infection and the appearance of eggs in the stool.

Ascaris lumbricoides – the large roundworm

Egg in faeces

Adults: cream-coloured, 15–30 cm, resident in small intestine.
Epidemiology: Common worldwide, mainly in tropics. Most prevalent in children. Σ ~600.
Transmission and life cycle: Eggs are swallowed and develop into larvae in the intestine. Larvae then migrate through tissues, penetrating

gut wall and travelling via circulation to lungs. After penetrating the alveolus they travel up the trachea and are swallowed. Arriving in the gut a second time, they develop into adult worms, mate and produce eggs, which are passed in faeces.

Clinical features
Prepatent period: Sixty to 75 days.
Life expectancy of adult worm: Approximately 1 year.
Symptoms and signs:
Larval migration is associated with cough, fever, wheeze, dyspnoea, CXR infiltrates and eosinophilia, occurring 10–14 days after infection and lasting a few days.
Adult worms are usually asymptomatic or may cause only abdominal discomfort, but may rarely cause intestinal obstruction. They may contribute to malnutrition or cause mechanical damage/inflammation by entering biliary tree, pancreatic duct, appendix. If bowel is opened at surgery, *Ascaris lumbricoides* will disrupt the suture line and enter peritoneum. Prevent this by prophylactic or intraoperative antihelminthics.
Diagnosis: Stool microscopy for eggs. Adults passed in stools are distinguished from earthworms by their lack of segmentation.
Management: Piperazine 75 mg/kg (max 4 g) on 2 successive days **or** pyrantel 10 mg/kg (max 1 g) single dose **or** mebendazole 100 mg 12-hly for 3 days (contraindicated in pregnancy) **or** levasimole (not on UK market) 150 mg single dose.

Ancylostoma duodenale,
Necator americanus – the hookworms
Adults: 1 cm, attached to jejunal mucosa.
Epidemiology: Widespread in tropics and subtropics. Σ ~500.
Transmission and life cycle: Eggs passed in faeces develop into infectious larvae in the soil. These penetrate intact skin, e.g. on the feet, and travel via the circulation to the lungs and thence to the gut. Adult worms attach to jejunal mucosa and suck blood, each worm causing the loss of about 0.1 ml/day.
Clinical features
Prepatent period: Forty to 100 days.
Life expectancy of adult worm: One to 5 years.

Symptoms and signs: Itchy papules may develop at the site of larval penetration ('ground itch'). Mild pulmonary symptoms associated with lung migration (compared with severe manifestations associated with *Ascaris lumbricoides*). Hookworm infection is an important cause of **iron-deficiency anaemia**, which may be severe, particularly if dietary iron intake is poor.

Diagnosis: Stool microscopy for eggs.

Egg in faeces

Management: Iron supplements. Pyrantel (course extended to 3 days in heavy infections) or mebendazole: doses as for *Ascaris lumbricoides*.

Trichuris trichiura – whipworm

Adults: 2–5 cm long, reside partly buried in the mucosa of the large bowel.

Epidemiology: Worldwide, commonest in tropics. Σ ~1000.

Transmission and life cycle: Eggs are ingested and develop into adults in the gut. There is no tissue migratory phase.

Clinical features

Prepatent period: Seventy to 90 days.

Life expectancy of adult worm: One year.

Symptoms and signs: Usually asymptomatic. Heavy infection may cause bloody diarrhoea, rectal prolapse, anaemia, wasting and eosinophilia. Worms may be seen on sigmoidoscopy.

Diagnosis: Stool microscopy for eggs. Often co-exists with *Ascaris*.

Egg in faeces

Management: Mebendazole 100 mg 12-hly for 3 days (contraindicated in pregnancy and under 2 years), **or** albendazole 400 mg stat.

Enterobius vermicularis – pinworm, threadworm

Adult worms: 5–10 mm long, resident in large bowel. May emerge from anus.

Epidemiology: Worldwide, commoner in temperate regions than tropics. The only common helminth infection in the UK. Infection is commonest in children; other members of the same household are often also infected.

Transmission and life cycle: Female emerges from anus at night to lay eggs on perianal skin. These become infectious after ~4 h. After ingestion they develop into adults with no tissue migratory phase.

Clinical features

Prepatent period: Approximately 40 days.

Life expectancy of adult worm: Eight weeks.

Symptoms and signs: Pruritis ani. Very rarely worms migrate into vagina and uterus causing endometritis and salpingitis. Appendicitis is a rare complication.

Diagnosis: Microscopy of sellotape swab from perianal region.

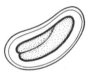

Egg in sellotape slide

Management: Mebendazole 100 mg stat repeated after 2 weeks **or** pyrantel 10 mg/kg (max 1 g) repeated after 2 weeks **or** piperazine citrate elixir (750 mg/5 ml) 15 ml 24-hly for 7 days (daily doses for children: < 2 years, 0.5 ml/kg; 2–3 years, 5 ml; 4–6 years, 7.5 ml; 7–12 years, 10 ml). Other family members usually need to be treated at the same time.

Strongyloides stercoralis

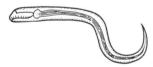

Larva in faeces

Adults: 2 mm long, live burrowed into mucosa of small intestine.

Epidemiology: Worldwide in tropics and sub-tropics. Σ ~60.

Transmission and life cycle: *Strongyloides stercoralis* is unusual because adult worms can reproduce within one host. Adult females lay eggs, which develop into larvae within the gut. These are normally non-infectious and must undergo development in the soil before penetrating intact skin and travelling via the lungs to the gut, as for hookworm (➤277). Sometimes larvae develop into the infective form before they leave the host, and are then able to penetrate perianal skin or intestinal wall, travelling from there to the lungs. This 'autoinfective cycle' maintains infection for many years in patients who have left the tropics and is responsible for hyperinfection in patients who become immunocompromised. This can occur 50 or more years after infection (e.g. Far East prisoners of war). Larvae may also enter a free-living cycle, when they can survive in the soil in appropriate tropical conditions.

Clinical features
Prepatent period: Seventeen to 28 days.
Life expectancy of adult worm: Not known.
Symptoms and signs: Occasional pruritus at the site of larval entry, or pulmonary symptoms related to larval migration. Development of adult worms in the gut may cause malabsorption with eosinophilia. Most patients become asymptomatic after a few weeks. If infection is maintained by autoinfection, signs of established infection occur. These include intermittent diarrhoea and **larva currens**, a raised serpiginous wheal due to larval migration that appears on the skin, usually of the trunk. It is very itchy, migrates at several centimetres/hour and usually resolves within 24 h.

  Hyperinfection occurs when patients become immunocompromised. Penetration of gut wall by filariform larvae causes diarrhoea and malabsorption, paralytic ileus, peritonitis, secondary Gram-negative bacteraemia, meningitis and pulmonary symptoms. Diagnosis is made by finding larvae in clinical material, particularly stools and sputum. Eosinophilia is rare in hyperinfection.

Diagnosis: Stool microscopy for larvae. Microscopy of duodenal string test, duodenal aspirate or jejunal biopsy. Stools may be cultured for larvae – this takes 3 weeks (🦠). Filaria ELISA cross-reacts in ~90% of cases – a specific serological test for strongyloides is also available.

Management: Thiabendazole 25 mg/kg 12-hly for 3 days **or** mebendazole 100 mg 8-hly for 7 days. Often ineffective in hyperinfection. Repeated courses of suppressive treatment may be needed. Consider prophylaxis for patients from endemic areas prior to transplantation, etc.

Larva migrans
Visceral larva migrans (VLM) is due to *Toxocara canis* and *T. cati*, the dog and cat roundworms. Σ ~20. Eggs (from animal faeces) ingested by humans develop into larvae and migrate through tissues for 1–2 years. Heavy infections in children may cause fever, hepatomegaly, eosinophilia and asthma. Severe VLM may be treated with mebendazole 200 mg 12-hly for 5 days **or** albendazole 5 mg/kg/day for 5 days. **Ocular disease** is more important. Larvae trapped in the retina cause a granulomatous reaction which presents as a solid retinal mass and may cause blindness in the affected eye. Eosinophilia is not usually seen in ocular toxocariasis. Serology is

Table 128 Rarer zoonotic intestinal nematodes

Species	Natural host	Most prevalent in	Comments
Trichostrongylus spp.*	Various mammals	Japan, Indonesia, Egypt	Usually asymptomatic
Capillaria phillipensis†	Birds	Philippines, Thailand	Severe fatal diarrhoea may occur with heavy infection. Autoinfection occurs
Anisakis spp.†	Sea mammals	Japan	Eosinophilic gastritis

* Acquired by eating vegetables contaminated with larvae. † Acquired by eating undercooked, infected fish.

available, but false positives are common due to previous asymptomatic VLM. High-titre antibodies in aqueous humour are strongly predictive of infection. Antigen detection is also available: ✚. Steroids (systemic and intraocular) and thiabendazole are used, although antihelminthics have not been shown to influence outcome. Differential diagnosis includes retinoblastoma and other retinal tumours.

Cutaneous larva migrans is due to the dog hookworms *Ancylostoma caninum* and *Ancylostoma braziliense*, which are common in North, Central and South America, including the Caribbean. Larvae penetrate the skin, usually on the buttocks or feet of humans exposed to warm sandy soil contaminated with dog faeces. Migration of larvae causes **creeping eruption**—a very itchy serpiginous track advancing about 1 mm/day and persisting for several weeks before resolving spontaneously (in contrast to 'larva currens' due to *Strongyloides stercoralis* ➤279). *Ancylostoma caninum* larvae may occasionally reach the bowel, causing eosinophilic enteritis. Topical or systemic thiabendazole (25 mg/kg po daily in divided doses for 5 days repeated after 1 week, or 10% thiabendazole in petroleum jelly applied daily for 5 days) may speed resolution. Individual larvae may be killed by freezing the skin with ethyl chloride spray.

Tapeworms

Taenia saginata—beef tapeworm

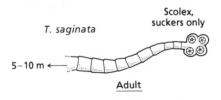

T. saginata

Scolex, suckers only

5–10 m ←

Adult

Adult worms: 5–10 m long, resident in small intestine.
Epidemiology: Worldwide. Σ ~50.
Transmission and life cycle: Humans acquire infection by eating undercooked beef containing encysted larvae. Cysts mature into adult segmented worm in the small intestine, attached to the mucosa by the head. Segments

(*proglottids*) full of eggs are shed from the tail end of the worm. Proglottids, and eggs from proglottids that rupture in the gut, are shed in faeces and contaminate pastureland, where they infect cattle.

Clinical features
Prepatent period: Twelve weeks.
Life expectancy of adult worm: Up to 30 years.
Symptoms and signs: Patients may notice white motile proglottids in stools or emerging from the anus. Otherwise usually asymptomatic.
Diagnosis: Stool microscopy for eggs and proglottids.

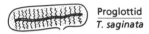

Proglottid
T. saginata

Management: Niclosamide, two doses of 1 g, 1 h apart **or** praziquantel (not on UK market, but available on named-patient basis) 10 mg/kg stat.

Taenia solium—pork tapeworm and cysticercosis

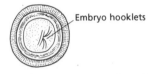

Embryo hooklets

Egg of *solium* or *saginata* (faeces)

Adult worms: 3–5 m long in small intestine.
Epidemiology: Worldwide; very rare in UK. Σ ~20.
Transmission and life cycle: As for *Taenia saginata* (pigs substituting for cattle), with the very important difference that **eggs are infectious for humans,** who may unwittingly act as secondary hosts. Eggs consumed by humans hatch in the gut and develop into *onchospheres*, which enter the circulation and are carried to muscles, CNS and other organs, where they develop into larval cysts—this is called **cysticercosis**.
Clinical features
Prepatent period: Three to 6 months.

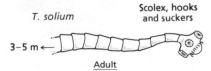

T. solium

Scolex, hooks and suckers

3–5 m ←

Adult

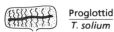 Proglottid
T. solium

Life expectancy of adult worm: Up to 25 years.

Symptoms and signs: Infection by adult worms is usually asymptomatic, except for passage of proglottids. Manifestations of cysticercosis depend on magnitude of infection and location of cysts. Infection is often asymptomatic and diagnosed coincidentally by discovery of spindle-shaped calcified tissue cysts on X-ray. Epilepsy developing 3–5 years after infection is the most common presentation; other neurological defects include raised intracranial pressure without focal signs, due to chronic basal meningitis.

Diagnosis: Adult *T. solium*: stool microscopy for eggs and proglottids. **Cysticercosis:** serology (IFAT), demonstration of cysts in muscle by X-ray or in CNS by CT/MRI. CSF shows lymphocytic pleocytosis, raised protein, eosinophilia (50% of cases) and reduced glucose (25% of cases).

Management: Adult *T. solium*: niclosamide, as for *T. saginata*. It is usual to give an antiemetic 1 h before and a purgative 1 h after treatment to avoid the risk of autoinfection by eggs released from the dying worm. **Cysticercosis:** praziquantel and aldendazole have both been used effectively. Anticonvulsants may be required ☞.

Echinococcus granulosus and *Echinococcus multilocularis*

Dog tapeworms, causing **hydatid disease** in sheep, cattle and humans.

Epidemiology: Worldwide, associated with sheep and cattle rearing and contact with dogs. Incidence varies widely depending on degree of human contact with dogs and degree to which dogs feed on herbivore car-

casses. *Echinococcus granulosus* accounts for most human infections. Σ ~25.

Transmission and life cycle: Dogs are the definitive host for the small adult tapeworms. Eggs passed in dog faeces infect secondary host—usually sheep or cattle—where they develop in the intestine, enter the circulation and form cysts in the viscera. Cysts are encapsulated by host fibrous tissue and may continue to grow for many years. Dogs are infected by eating herbivore carcasses containing cysts. Humans are infected from dog faeces and act as a secondary host, developing visceral cysts.

E. multilocularis is associated with wild canines and rodents, and human infection is rare. Unlike *E. granulosus*, cysts are multiloculated, not contained within a capsule and may spread through surrounding tissue like a malignant tumour.

Clinical features: Cysts are found in the liver (70%), lungs (25%) and other organs. Hepatic cysts may be very large (e.g. 15 l capacity). Symptoms may occur months to years after infection and are due to mechanical pressure or the release of allergenic cyst contents, causing urticaria or anaphylaxis. Ruptured cysts may seed multiple secondary cysts or cause death by anaphylaxis. Cysts may become secondarily bacterially infected.

Diagnosis: USS and CT are used to delineate cysts but aspiration is **absolutely contraindicated** because of the risks described above. Serology (ELISA) is helpful but false negatives occur. Eosinophilia occurs (25% of cases).

Management: Surgical removal is most effective but requires extreme care and use of specialised techniques to avoid rupture. Prolonged treatment with albendazole is used before and

Table 129 Minor tapeworms

Species	Definitive host	Secondary host	Clinical features
Diphyllobothrium latum	Humans	Freshwater fish	Usually asymptomatic. Rare cause of B_{12} deficiency
Hymenolepis nana	Humans	None	Occasional GI upset

after surgery and in patients with multiple cysts or who are unfit for surgery (e.g. albendazole 400 mg 12-hly for 28 days, followed by 14 days' rest; the cycle may be repeated up to three times). *E. multilocularis* is usually fatal untreated. Surgical removal is often impossible, and very prolonged albendazole treatment is used.

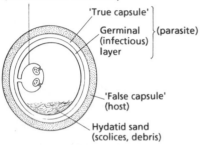

Brood capsule containing scolices
(not infectious to humans)

'True capsule'
Germinal (infectious) layer ⎫⎬ (parasite)

'False capsule' (host)

Hydatid sand (scolices, debris)

Hydatid cyst in intermediate host (sheep, man)

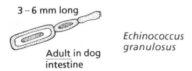

3–6 mm long

Echinococcus granulosus

Adult in dog intestine

Tissue nematodes

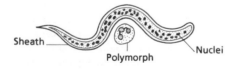

Sheath

Polymorph

Nuclei

W. bancrofti in thick blood smear

Wuchereria bancrofti, Brugia malayi and *Brugia timori*

Thread-like adult worms, 4–10 mm long, living in lymphatics and causing **lymphatic filariasis.**

Epidemiology: *Wuchereria bancrofti* is endemic throughout the tropics. *Brugia malayi* is found is SE Asia and the Indian subcontinent and *Brugia timori* is found in Indonesia. Σ ~5.

Transmission and life cycle: Adult worms mate and produce large numbers of larvae (*microfilariae*) which are present in blood and are taken up by biting mosquitoes. Human infection is acquired by mosquito bite.

Clinical features

Life expectancy of adult worm: Approximately 30 years.

Symptoms and signs: Symptoms usually develop at least 6 months after infection. Microfilaraemia may be asymptomatic or cause recurrent fever, malaise and headache. Recurrent attacks of lymphangitis occur at irregular intervals due to adult worms in lymphatics draining limbs and external genitalia, causing fever, tenderness and redness over lymphatics with temporary lymphoedema, resolving over 2–3 weeks. After repeated attacks there is irreversible damage to lymph drainage, with hydrocoele, chronic peripheral oedema, overgrowth of soft tissue and ultimately elephantiasis of limbs, scrotum, breast or vulva. Secondary bacterial infection is frequent. Chyluria—the presence of chylous lymph in the urine—is due to rupture of dilated lymphatics in the renal pelvis.

Diagnosis: Demonstration of microfilariae in blood. Species are distinguished by morphology. Concentration methods (e.g. membrane filtration) are used to demonstrate scanty parasitaemia. Microfilariae show marked nocturnal periodicity, being present in large numbers only during the night (except in Pacific strains, which show 'diurnal periodicity'). These patterns are determined by host sleep patterns and synchronise with vector biting behaviour; blood for microfilariae should be taken at midnight (microfilaraemia adapts to changed time zones in returning travellers within one week). Serology is also available.

Management: Diethylcarbamazine (DEC) has been the drug of choice until recently. It kills microfilariae and adult worms if given for long enough, but is associated with adverse effects due to release of worm antigens. Ivermectin is a newer less toxic agent that effectively abolishes microfilaraemia for months after a single dose. It is used in mass chemoprophylaxis regimens; its full effect on adult worms is under investigation.

TROPICAL PULMONARY EOSINOPHILIA (TPE)
An immune-mediated response to infection by *Wuchereria bancrofti* or *Brugia malayi*, which

affects children and young adults, especially in the Indian subcontinent. Gradual onset of low fever, lassitude, cough and wheeze are associated with marked eosinophilia ($\leqslant 20 \times 10^9/1$), high IgE and high-titre antifilarial antibodies. CXR may be normal or show patchy shadows. DEC (2 mg/kg 8-hly for 10 days) causes rapid and complete recovery.

Dracunculus medinensis – Guinea worm

Adult worm up to 1 m long, living subcutaneously and emerging through the skin of the leg.

Epidemiology: Widespread patchy distribution throughout Middle East, Africa, Asia and S America. $\sum \sim 1$.

Transmission and life cycle: Humans acquire infection by swallowing a small crustacean (*Cyclops*) in contaminated fresh water. *Dracunculus medinensis* eggs hatch in the human gut and larvae penetrate the intestinal mucosa. They develop into adults in the subcutaneous tissues. After ~1 year the female worm, which may be up to 1 m long, approaches the skin and a blister forms. On contact of skin with water, blister bursts and larvae are discharged, escaping to infect *Cyclops* and complete the cycle. Prevention depends on establishment of clean water supplies. Infected persons should avoid contaminating supplies. Sieving of water through two layers of ordinary shirting is sufficient to remove *Cyclops* and prevent transmission.

Clinical features

Incubation period: Approximately 1 year.

Life expectancy of adult worm: Approximately 1 year.

Symptoms and signs: Localised pain, swelling and itching. Fever and urticaria. The appearance of the ulcer is characteristic with a central pearly loop formed by the worm's uterus. A drop of water placed on the ulcer causes reflex contraction of the uterus and expulsion of larvae. Secondary bacterial infection, localised responses to dead worms and arthritis, (either immune-mediated or due to worms migrating through joint spaces), may all occur.

Management: The ulcer should be bathed for several days to deplete larvae, then the end of the worm is attached to a small stick and re-moved by carefully winding it out, over the course of 10–14 days. Metronidazole (400 mg 8-hly for 10 days) reduces inflammation and eases extraction.

Onchocerca volvulus – onchocerciasis, 'river blindness'

Adult worms (males 4 cm, females 50 cm) live free in subcutaneous tissues or in fibrous subcutaneous nodules.

Epidemiology: Focally distributed across equatorial Africa. Also found in some areas of C America and Yemen. Foci of infection are located near fast-flowing rivers, which are breeding areas of the blackfly vector. $\sum \sim 10$.

Transmission and life cycle: Infection is acquired by the bite of the blackfly (*Simulium* spp.). Adult worms live free in subcutaneous tissues unless they are contained by fibrous nodules. Large numbers of motile larvae (*microfilariae*) are produced; it is the inflammatory response to the microfilariae which is responsible for most clinical features.

Clinical features

Incubation period: Approximately 1 year.

Life expectancy of adult worm: Approximately 20 years.

Symptoms and signs: Nodules (2–5 cm) tend to occur over bony prominences and it is postulated that the worms become trapped between bone and skin, allowing host defence mechanisms to attack them. Symptoms due to microfilariae include a papular rash and severe pruritus (which may affect normal-looking skin) and excoriation, which is often secondarily infected by bacteria. These eventually progress to depigmentation, loss of elasticity and severe premature ageing of the skin. These changes and inguinal lymphadenopathy give rise to the 'hanging groin' appearance. There may be minor elephantiasis of the legs or scrotum. Migration of microfilariae into the eye causes severe keratitis, iritis and retinitis, eventually leading to blindness.

Diagnosis: By finding microfilariae in skin snips taken from pruritic areas.

Management: A vigorous effort has been made to eradicate onchocerciasis, initially with vector control programmes and lately with mass chemoprophylaxis with ivermectin, which kills microfilariae, thus preventing transmission and removing the cause of the symptoms. Ivermectin is also used for treatment of individual cases. Global eradication is a real possibility. Palpable nodules represent only some of the adult worms, so removal is not logical, except for nodules on the head, which should be removed because of the increased risk of ocular damage. (Microfilariae density is highest close to nodules.)

Loa loa–loiasis, Calabar swelling
Adults 3–7 cm long live free in subcutaneous tissues.

Epidemiology: Forest areas of West and Central Africa. Σ ~10.

Transmission and life cycle: Transmitted by the biting fly, *Chrysops*. Adult worms take about 1 year to develop before mating to produce microfilariae; these are found in the circulation (showing diurnal periodicity) and are taken up by the fly.

Clinical features
Incubation period: One year.

Life expectancy of adult worm: Twenty years or more.

Symptoms and signs: Usually asymptomatic. Sudden painful itchy subcutaneous swellings ('Calabar swellings') occur, often related to minor trauma. Occasionally worms may be seen crossing the conjunctiva—this is associated with intense irritation and periorbital swelling. Eosinophilia is common.

Diagnosis: By detection of microfilariae in the blood, or by seeing the worm under the conjunctiva.

Management: DEC kills microfilariae and adult worms, but reactions to treatment are common, including fever, headache, tender subcutaneous swellings around dead worms, very high eosinophilia and encephalitis. Reactions are less severe if DEC is introduced gradually (e.g. day 1, 50 mg; day 2, 50 mg 8-hly; day 3, 100 mg 8-hly; days 4–21, 2 mg/kg 8-hly). Ivermectin kills microfilariae without adverse effects, and will be an important agent in the control of this disease.

Prevention: ➤138

Trichinella spiralis

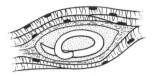

Cyst within skeletal muscle

Epidemiology: Worldwide, particularly in Europe and the USA (Table 130). Σ ~5.

Transmission and life cycle: Infection is acquired by eating undercooked meat containing encysted larvae. These hatch in the gut and mature in the small intestine. After mating, larvae are produced which migrate to striated muscle, where they encyst. Transmission continues when the new host is eaten.

Clinical features: Usually asymptomatic. Approximately 1 week after ingestion, GI disturbance associated with intestinal development of worms may occur. After 2–8 weeks, there may be fever, headache and cough, with muscle tenderness and swelling. Periorbital oedema and conjunctivitis are common. Splinter haemorrhages may occur. Neurological signs (deafness, encephalitis, fits, focal signs), myocarditis and pneumonitis occur rarely. Severe cases may be fatal.

Diagnosis: Suspected in any patient with fever, eosinophilia, myositis and periorbital oedema who has recently eaten pork. Leucocytosis

Table 130 *Trichinella spiralis* species

Species	Source of human infection	Distribution
Trichinella spiralis spiralis	Domestic pigs	USA, Europe
Trichinella spiralis nelsoni	Wild pigs	Africa, S Europe
Trichinella spiralis nativa	Wild mammals (bear, walrus, seal)	Arctic

and raised creatine phosphokinase are common. Serology (IFAT) becomes positive 3–4 weeks into illness, at which time larvae may be demonstrated on muscle biopsy.

Management: During the GI phase, mebendazole 7.5 mg/kg 12-hly for 3 days. During muscle migration phase, mebendazole 5 mg/kg 12-hly for 10–13 days (no proof of therapeutic efficacy). Steroids and aspirin are also given in severe cases (prednisolone 40–60 mg 24-hly).

Minor tissue helminths (Tables 131 & 132)

Blood flukes

Schistosomiasis–bilharzia

Terminal spine

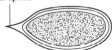

Ovum *S. haematobium* (urine, occasionally faeces, rectal biopsy)

Adult worms 1–2 cm long live in veins draining the bowel or bladder; the female lives in a groove on the ventral surface of the male. Most disease is due to inflammatory response to eggs. Five species of schistosome cause disease in humans (Table 133), although only the first three are common.

Epidemiology: Children are most heavily infected. Infection is acquired by contact with contaminated fresh water containing infected snails, and efforts have in the past been directed at control of snails. Mass chemoprophylaxis with praziquantel (see below) is now used. Σ ~150.

Transmission and life cycle: Female worm lays eggs in terminal venules. Eggs penetrate the vein wall and traverse the wall of the bowel or bladder to be excreted in urine or faeces. Eggs hatch in water and infect particular species of snail. After 2–3 weeks, minute motile *cercariae* are released. These penetrate human skin and migrate via the lungs and liver to become adults in the vesical or mesenteric veins.

Table 131 Mansonella spp. (formerly *Dipetalonema* spp.)

Species	Distribution	Vector	Site of adult worms	Clinical features
Mansonella perstans	Tropical Africa. S America	Midges	Peritoneum	Serositis. Usually asymptomatic
M. streptocerca	W Africa	Midges	Dermis	Pruritus, hypopigmented macules
M. ozzardi	S and C America	Midges, blackflies	Peritoneum	Usually asymptomatic

Table 132 Nematodes causing eosinophilic meningitis

Species	Distribution	Host	Acquired from	Clinical features
Angiostrongylus cantonensis	SE Asia, Japan, India, Oceania	Rat	Ingestion of infected molluscs (on vegetables or undercooked)	Eosinophilic meningitis
Angiostrongylus costaricensis	Costa Rica	Rats		Abdominal pain, eosinophilia
Gnathostoma spinigerum	SE Asia	Cats and dogs	Fish	Larva migrans with cutaneous swellings, creeping eruption. Eosinophilic meningitis

Table 133

Species	Distribution	Location of adult worms	Eggs excreted in	Complications
Schistosoma haematobium	Africa, Middle East	Vesical plexus	Urine	Obstructive uropathy
S. mansoni	Africa, Middle East, S America	Lower mesenteric veins	Faeces	Portal hypertension
S. japonicum	Asia, Philippines	Lower mesenteric veins	Faeces	Portal hypertension, fits
S. mekongi	SE Asia	Lower mesenteric veins	Faeces	Portal hypertension
S. intercalatum	Africa	Lower mesenteric veins	Faeces	Portal hypertension

Clinical features: Skin penetration may be associated with an itchy papular rash ('swimmer's itch'). Initial illness ('Katayama fever') is usually only recognised in travellers: 2–8 weeks after exposure they may develop fever, urticaria, eosinophilia, hepatosplenomegaly, diarrhoea, cough and wheeze. These symptoms resolve spontaneously. Most important sequelae of infection are due to granulomatous reaction to eggs:

S. haematobium: Terminal haematuria, dysuria, fibrosis and calcification of the bladder and obstructive uropathy (hydronephrosis, renal failure). Kidney stones and squamous-cell carcinoma of the bladder are late complications. In heavy infections eggs may reach the lungs via the inferior vena cava, causing pulmonary hypertension and cor pulmonale.

S. mansoni and *S. japonicum*: Bloody diarrhoea may occur. Long-standing infection causes periportal fibrosis with portal hypertension, hepatosplenomegaly and oesophageal varices. Hepatocellular function is characteristically well preserved. Eggs may reach lungs via portocaval anastamoses to cause cor pulmonale.

Adult worms of all species (particularly *S. japonicum*) occasionally migrate into other tissues, such as the spinal cord and brain.

Schistosomiasis is also associated with increased prevalence of *Salmonella typhi* urinary carriage (➤190) and recurrent salmonella septicaemia.

Diagnosis: Demonstration of eggs in stool or urine, or on rectal biopsy. Eosinophilia is common. ELISA is available but is not ideally sensitive and is only useful in travellers and visitors to endemic regions. In long-standing cases AXR may show pathognomonic ring calcification of the bladder.

Management: Praziquantel is the drug of choice for all species. It is free of serious adverse effects. Dose for *S. japonicum, S. mekongi*, 60 mg/kg in three divided doses; other species, 40 mg/kg as a single dose.

Practice point: Differential diagnosis of a returning traveller with eosinophilia and diarrhoea includes schistosomiasis, strongyloidiasis (➤278), capillariasis (➤279) and trichuriasis (➤278). To exclude schistosomiasis in the returning traveller with compatible symptoms, check for eosinophilia and send serum for ELISA at 6 and 12 weeks after return. If negative and schistosomiasis is still suspected, send three terminal urine specimens collected at midday and three stool samples for ova, cysts and parasites at least 3 months after exposure.

Other trematode infections: the flukes

Diagnosis: Stool microscopy for eggs (sputum microscopy for lung flukes). Serology is also available.

Management: Praziquantel, 25 mg/kg 8-hly for 3 days.

Comments: A large number of flukes normally parasitic on other mammals may rarely infect humans.

Table 134

Species	Acquired from	2° host	Distribution	Size (mm)	Clinical features
Liver flukes—adults resident in human biliary tree					
Clonorchis sinensis	Freshwater fish	Snail	China, SE Asia	15 × 3	Abdominal pain, pancreatitis,
Opisthorchis fileneus			Eastern Europe	10 × 2	cholangitis, cholangiocarcinoma;
Opisthorchis viverrini			Thailand	10 × 2	often asymptomatic
Fasciola hepatica	Freshwater plants	Snail	Worldwide	25 × 18	Eosinophilia, hepatitis, biliary colic, obstructive jaundice
Lung fluke—adults resident in human lung					
Paragonimus westermani	Freshwater crabs, crayfish	Snail	Far East, SE Asia	10 × 5	Cough, haemoptysis, chest pain, fever. CXR shadowing with cavitation. Flukes may rarely migrate to many other organs, including CNS
Intestinal flukes—adults resident in human intestine					
Fasciolopsis buski	Edible water plants	Snail	SE Asia	30 × 12	Usually asymptomatic. Heavy infection may cause abdominal pain and diarrhoea
Heterophyes heterophyes	Fish	Snail	China, Japan, Egypt	1.5 × 0.5	
Metagonimus yokogawai	Fish	Snail	Far East	1 × 0.5	

Antihelminthic drugs

Table 135

Drug	Common indications	Important adverse effects
Mebendazole	Threadworm, roundworm, whipworm, hookworm	Diarrhoea, rash. Contraindicated in pregnancy and children <2 years
Piperazine	Threadworm, roundworm	GI disturbance, rash, bronchospasm. Rarely, dizziness, ataxia, drowsiness, convulsions. Contraindicated in first trimester, epilepsy
Pyrantel	Threadworm, roundworm, hookworm	GI disturbance, rash, headache
Levamisole	Roundworm, whipworm	GI disturbance
Niclosamide	Intestinal tapeworms	GI disturbance, pruritus

continued on p. 288

Table 135 Contd

Drug	Common indications	Important adverse effects
Albendazole	Threadworm, roundworm, whipworm, hookworm, strongyloidiasis, hydatid disease, cysticercosis	GI disturbance, rash, fever, headache. Abnormal liver function tests. Myelotoxicity
Praziquantel	Trematodes	Mild dizziness. Contraindicated in ocular cysticercosis
Diethylcarbamazine	Filariasis, *Loa loa*	Headache, dizziness, nausea, fever, allergic reactions to death of worms
Ivermectin	Onchocerciasis	Fever, pruritus, rash (all mild)
Thiabendazole	Strongyloidiasis, larva migrans, trichinosis	GI disturbance, headache, rash; rarely, tinnitus, collapse, hepatitis

30: Fungi

Primitive eukaryotes, the vast majority of which are saprophytic and do not cause disease in humans. Many of the remainder are frequent human commensals. Most pathogenic fungi are **dimorphic** (capable of existing in two forms, depending upon environmental conditions). Each pathogenic fungus causes infection within the human body in one or other of these two forms:
• **hyphal** or mould-like (e.g. *Aspergillus* spp.): branching filaments, interweaving to form a mycelium, often (outside the body) forming specialised reproductive bodies carrying asexual or sexual spores (Table 136);

• **yeast-like** (e.g. *Candida* spp.): single spherical or oval cells, reproducing by asexual budding. Yeast forms often produce unbranched chains of elongated cells known as a pseudomycelium (Table 137).

Provisional identification of fungi is performed in most diagnostic laboratories by a combination of microscopical and colonial morphology, and some biochemical tests. All stain Gram-positive. Atypical or unfamiliar isolates ⇒ ✈. Antimicrobial sensitivity testing of fungi requires experience (✈).

Table 136 Moulds

Genus	Species	Notes
Aspergillus	***fumigatus, flavus,*** *niger, terreus, nidulans,* etc.	Cause allergic, localised and invasive aspergillosis (➤290)

(*Mucor* spp., *Rhizopus* spp. and *Absidia* spp. cause rare, invasive infections in the immunocompromised and diabetic host, especially of the paranasal sinuses: 'zygomycosis', 'mucormycosis' or 'phycomycosis')

(*Trichosporon beigelii, Pseudallescheria boydii, Fusarium* spp. and *Penicillium* spp. are a miscellaneous group of filamentous fungi, occasionally causing invasive infections in the immunocompromised host)

Epidermophyton spp., *Microsporum* spp. and *Trichophyton* spp. are the ringworm fungi, infecting stratum corneum of skin, hair and nails (➤92)

(*Madurella* spp., *Acremonium* spp., *Actinomadura* spp., *Exophiala* spp., *Fonsecaea* spp., *Phialophora* spp., *Cladosporium* spp., etc. are causes of mycetoma (eumycetoma – involving fungi) and chromoblastomycosis, superficial skin infections in the tropics)

(*Rhinosporidium seeberi* causes rhinosporidiosis, a granulomatous disease of nasal and conjunctival mucosae, especially in India)

Table 137 Yeasts

Genus	Species	Notes
Candida (➤291)	**albicans**, tropicalis, parapsilosis, lusitaniae, glabrata, guilliermondii, krusei	Candida glabrata is also known as Torulopsis glabrata
Cryptococcus	**neoformans**	Capsulate yeast (➤292)
Histoplasma	capsulatum (duboisii)	Widespread environmental distribution, especially in eastern USA and the tropics (➤293)
(Coccidioides immitis, Blastomyces dermatididis, Paracoccidioides brasiliensis)		Restricted environmental distribution, especially in the Americas (➤293)
(Sporothrix	schenkii)	Skin sepsis and lymphangitis following local trauma associated with moist vegetation
Malassezia	furfur	Causes pityriasis versicolor and iv catheter infection and fungaemia in infants receiving parenteral lipid therapy. Also called Pityriasis versicolor and ovale

Aspergillus fumigatus

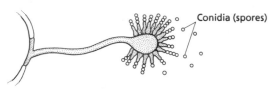

Conidia (spores)

Conidiophore ('fruiting body')

Pathogenesis: Virulence factors largely unknown. Macrophages kill spores ('conidia'), and principally neutrophils kill hyphae.

Epidemiology: Airborne spores ubiquitous from decaying vegetation. Inhalational route, spores germinate within airways; *Aspergillus* spp. can be isolated from nose swabs of ~1% normal individuals (usually transient colonisation), but nasal colonisation does not always precede invasive lung disease. Risk of invasive disease up to 40% in patients after BMT with neutropenia (<0.5 × 10⁹/l) for >20 days.

Higher rate of recurrence in subsequent episodes of chemotherapy in those with previous *Aspergillus* infection (➤133). Occasional outbreaks of invasive disease in the immunocompromised associated with disturbance of fungal growth in hospital buildings (e.g. damp organic insulation material) in construction work, ventilation systems. Strain typing is in its infancy.

Spectrum of disease: Allergic aspergillosis — includes: (i) allergy to inhaled aspergillus antigens, common in atopic patients (raised

IgE levels); (ii) colonisation of airways causing asthma, eosinophilia, plugging of airways; and (iii) inhalation of high spore concentrations ⇒ fever, breathlessness (allergic alveolitis) ⇒ progressive lung damage if repeated (e.g. Maltster's lung from *Aspergillus clavatus*). **Local infection (aspergilloma)** – colonisation of pre-existing pulmonary cavities (esp. posttuberculous) usually asymptomatic, with no local invasion (eventual erosion of pulmonary arteriole ⇒ haemorrhage in up to 50%, but usually minor). **Invasive aspergillosis** (IA) in immunocompromised patients only (➤133). Usual site of invasion is lung, later spread haematogenously to many organs ⇒ arterial thrombosis or infarction with local invasion. Occasional primary invasion of nasal sinuses, and iv catheter infection. Cerebral involvement carries grave prognosis. Rare endocarditis (most commonly PVE, acquired at time of valve insertion) with large, friable vegetations.

Laboratory diagnosis: Allergic aspergillosis – plugs of mycelium visible in sputum, serum precipitins positive. **Aspergilloma** best visualised radiologically; sputum usually microscopy- and culture-negative. Hyphae in **IA** best seen in biopsies; various serological tests under assessment, but none currently reliably sensitive. Growth on Sabouraud's agar visible in 1–7 days (occasionally up to 10 days). Will grow on blood agar, and frequently contaminates plates incubated for long periods. Quantitation and repeated isolation helpful to assess significance. Growth frequently scanty from biopsies in IA, and blood cultures rarely positive even in IE. IA still often diagnosed *post mortem*.

Treatment: Symptomatic aspergilloma usually requires surgical excision; possible role for local instillation of amphotericin B. For IA use amphotericin B; itraconazole under assessment, but seems useful as continuation treatment after initial control with amphotericin. Therapy should begin as soon as diagnosis of invasive aspergillosis seriously entertained – failure is associated with treatment delay.

Prevention: Dust screening of hospital building works. HEPA filtration of air supply to bone marrow transplant units. Antifungal prophylaxis of immunosuppression episodes is under assessment, but nebulised and iv amphotericin B and oral itraconazole have been used with apparent success.

Aspergillus flavus causes similar infections to *fumigatus*, but is less commonly isolated from invasive disease. *Aspergillus niger* forms black colonies on solid media, and is most frequently isolated from chronic otitis externa. It is occasionally isolated from invasive disease.

Many other moulds (e.g. *Penicillium* spp., *Thermoactinomyces* spp.) are associated with extrinsic allergic alveolitis.

Candida albicans

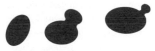

Responsible for ~90% *Candida* spp. infections and ~50% cases of fungaemia.

Pathogenesis: Adhesion to epithelia, phospholipase and proteinase production, and formation of hyphae are major virulence factors.

Epidemiology: Usually causes endogenous infections: *Candida albicans* is a normal oropharyngeal, vaginal and gut commensal. Overgrowth on mucosae follows destruction of normal bacterial flora (yeast takes over epithelial binding sites) – commonly with antibiotic therapy, diabetes, persistently moist skin. Other factors include pregnancy, infancy, old age, steroids, neutropenia, organ transplants, iron deficiency. Bladder catheter ⇒ colonisation, may ⇒ infection. Systemic candidiasis may follow contamination of lemon juice used to dissolve heroin by IVDUs. Epidemiology often difficult to elucidate because recurrent episodes in single patients may involve strains with variation in typing markers. Nosocomial outbreaks occasionally proven.

Spectrum of disease: Thrush – superficial infection of mucous membranes (➤61); may progress to local invasion (e.g. oesophagitis in AIDS ➤121, 122). Moist skin areas, nappy rash, paronychia, otitis externa (➤16). Development of **invasive candidiasis** usually requires several predisposing factors, and haematogenous spread is uncommon without iv access (iv catheter infection, IVDUs). Intraperitoneal infection common following treatment of serious peritoneal bacterial sepsis—especially after pancreatitis. **Endophthalmitis** has been reported in up to 60% cases of candidaemia—hence perform ophthalmoscopy and ask patient about blurred vision. Endocarditis (from candidaemic infection of previously abnormal valves) and PVE (usually acquired at time of implantation). Neonatal candidaemia and meningitis encouraged by iv catheters and prolonged antibiotics.

Laboratory diagnosis: Round or oval budding yeasts; pseudomycelium and mycelium commonly seen in superficial and invasive disease. Strict aerobes, growing on many solid media in 24–72 h ⇒ alcoholic-smelling, heaped colonies. Modern blood culture systems usually positive in most bottles in 48–96 h in cases of candidaemia. Although speciation is slow (commercial biochemical kits or ✢), formation of 'germ tubes' on incubation in serum (3 h) is virtually diagnostic of *C. albicans*, hence implies isolate is likely to be sensitive to azoles. Positive cultures from normal carriage sites need careful clinical interpretation, and quantitation may be helpful. Superficial infections often diagnosed clinically. Consider possibility of invasive disease in ICU patients with superficial candidiasis, iv catheters and fever. Serology rarely useful diagnostically; rapid antigen and cell component detection systems under development (e.g. ELISA for cell-wall mannans or enolase).

Treatment: Topical therapy used for superficial infections (➤306). Virtually all strains sensitive to amphotericin, which remains drug of choice for invasive disease (➤306). Combination with flucytosine possibly of value in systemic neonatal infection, but otherwise avoid because of risk of toxicity. Oral azole therapy usually successful in AIDS oesophagitis (➤122). *C. albicans* rarely resistant to azoles (except after prolonged prophylactic use in, for example, AIDS), which are useful continuation therapy after initial control with amphotericin. IE usually requires

valve replacement for control of infection. Changing urethral catheter may resolve urinary colonisation, and is a prerequisite for successful treatment of catheter-associated infection.

Prevention: Multiple recurrent superficial episodes may respond to intermittent antifungal prophylaxis, at the risk of encouraging resistance. Diabetic control. Oral azole prophylaxis in AIDS. Fluconazole and non-absorbed antifungals reduce incidence of clinical candidiasis during immunosuppressive episodes. Hand hygiene with alcoholic antiseptics between each patient contact.

Candida parapsilosis and *tropicalis* are skin commensals isolated from a higher proportion of iv catheter infections and endocarditis than *C. albicans*; *Candida parapsilosis* multiplies rapidly in glucose-containing solutions and has a propensity to adhere to synthetic materials. *Candida glabrata* (syn. *Torulopsis globrata*) is most commonly isolated from the urine. *Candida krusei* forms elongated yeast cells looking like grains of rice, and is resistant to fluconazole. It is occasionally found in a variety of environmental sites, but only rarely from human mucosae. It is increasingly seen colonising patients receiving fluconazole prophylaxis, and may cause significant infection in this group. It appears to be less virulent than *Candida albicans*.

Cryptococcus neoformans

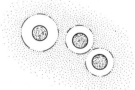

India ink preparation of CSF, showing capsules

Capsulate, spherical yeast.

Pathogenesis: Antiphagocytic mucopolysaccharide capsule; capsule production increased by host immune response.

Epidemiology: Present worldwide in bird droppings and elsewhere in environment. Frequently inhaled to cause asymptomatic or mild infection (lung granuloma), which resolves with intact CMI. Rare chronic cryptococcoma formation, with surrounding fibrosis. Progression (recrudescence or reinfection), especially in AIDS and others with CMI deficits. Typing available (✈).

Spectrum of disease: Commonest cause of fungal **meningitis**; occasionally also chronic skin and pulmonary sepsis, osteomyelitis. Recurrent infections, particularly meningitis, in AIDS (➤125).

Laboratory diagnosis: Seen in CSF wet preparation and Gram stain in up to 50% of cases–differentiated from host lymphocytes by demonstration of capsule by Indian ink negative stain. Sometimes little capsule seen, especially in AIDS. Budding visible, but forms no mycelium or pseudomycelium. Demonstrated by tissue fungal stains in biopsy material. Most rapid, sensitive and specific diagnostic method is capsule detection by latex agglutination or ELISA (many laboratories send to ✈) in CSF and serum. CSF and serum are positive by antigen tests in >90% of cases of meningitis; serum alone positive in 10%. Repeat if initially negative and diagnosis strongly suspected clinically. Usually readily cultured on Sabouraud's agar (~90% cases; also grows on blood agar) to cream, opaque, waxy colonies in 48–96 h, but can take up to 3 weeks. (Confirm in ✈.)

Treatment: Amphotericin B ± flucytosine until stable, then fluconazole (➤126). Antigen detection and serology useful to follow progress of treatment.

Histoplasma capsulatum

Found in soil contaminated with bat and bird droppings, especially in eastern USA, but it is also widespread in tropical and some temperate areas. It normally causes subclinical or self-limited lung infection, but occasionally causes chronic or acutely progressive pneumonia and disseminated infection in the immunocompromised (including AIDS). Diagnosed by microscopy of sputum, pus, tissue biopsies for yeast cells within macrophages. Can be cultured on Sabouraud's agar at low temperature for up to 6 weeks (☠). Serology and antigen detection available (✈). Amphotericin B and azoles have been used in treatment (discuss with ✈).

Histoplasma duboisii mainly causes skin and subcutaneous histoplasmosis in Africa.

Coccidioides immitis

A soil saprophyte, found only in dry regions of the south-western USA and north Mexico. Serological evidence of exposure is common in the indigenous population (over 90% in some areas) following self-limited lung infections. Progressive pulmonary and generalised infection seen in ~1% of those infected, especially with immunosuppression. Diagnosed by seeing 'spherules' in sputum, pus and tissue biopsies. Grows within 3 weeks on Sabouraud's agar (☠). Serology available (✈). Amphotericin B and azoles have been used in treatment (discuss with ✈).

Other fungi

Blastomyces dermatitidis ☠ causes chronic pulmonary, skin and bone infections in patients from parts of the USA and Canada. ***Paracoccidioides brasiliensis*** ☠ causes chronic pulmonary, skin and mucosal infections in patients from tropical forest regions of South and Central America. Both usually diagnosed by microscopy of sputum, pus or tissue biopsies, and grow slowly on Sabouraud's agar. Serology is useful for paracoccidioidomycosis (✈). Amphotericin B and azoles have been used in treatment of both (discuss with ✈).

Section 3:
Antibiotic Therapy

31: Classification of Important Antibiotics

A pharmacological grouping, further divided by spectrum of activity. Many variants of each group exist, often differing only slightly in spectrum of activity or pharmacological properties. In the tables that follow, CSF✓ indicates that the drug in question penetrates CSF sufficiently well to be useful clinically. CSF✗ or urine✗ indicate the converse.

β-Lactams

All excreted via the kidney; excretion of many reduced (hence serum levels increased and prolonged) by probenecid.

Penicillins

'ORDINARY' PENICILLINS

Table 138 'Ordinary' penicillins

	Benzylpenicillin (Pen-G)	Phenoxymethyl penicillin (Pen-V)
Administration, pharmacology	Parenteral only (acid labile). CSF✓ (in high dose, penetration best with inflamed meninges), urine✓	Oral. Variable absorption in adults. CSF✗, urine✓
Sensitive; often useful	Streptococci (*Enterococcus* spp. not killed), *Clostridium* spp., *Neisseria gonorrhoeae* (resistance increasing) and *meningitidis*, *Actinomyces* spp., treponemes, leptospires, Lyme disease, *Listeria monocytogenes*	
Variable; occasionally useful	Staphylococci (but >80% resistant in and out of hospital nowadays), non-sporing anaerobes (resistance increasing)	
Resistant; unreliable	Coliforms, *Pseudomonas* spp., *Haemophilus influenzae*; MRSA	
Side-effects	Hypersensitivity rash, fever (rare anaphylaxis); rare interstitial nephritis, cerebral toxicity with very high doses	

Long-acting depot preparations (e.g. procaine, benethamine and benzathine penicillins) similar activity and side-effects to benzylpenicillin.

BROADER-SPECTRUM PENICILLINS

Table 139 Broader-spectrum penicillins

	Ampicillin	Amoxycillin	Co-amoxiclav (Augmentin)
Administration, pharmacology	Best used iv. CSF✓ (in high dose, penetration best with inflamed meninges), urine✓	Best used orally. More reliably absorbed than Pen-V in adults. Urine✓	Amoxycillin + clavulanic acid (blocks many β-lactamases). Oral and iv. CSF✗, urine✓
Sensitive; often useful	As 'ordinary penicillins', with better activity against *Enterococcus* spp.		As amoxycillin, plus staphylococci, non-sporing anaerobes, most *Haemophilus* spp. and most 'easy' coliforms (➤184)

continued on p. 298

Table 139 contd

	Ampicillin	Amoxycillin	Co-amoxiclav (Augmentin)
Variable; occasionally useful	*Haemophilus* spp. (15% resistant), *Escherichia coli* (35% resistant), *Proteus mirabilis*, staphylococci (80% resistant), non-sporing anaerobes		
Resistant; unreliable	Most coliforms other than *Escherichia coli* and *Proteus mirabilis*; *Moraxella catarrhalis*, *Pseudomonas* spp.; MRSA		'Hard' coliforms (>184), *Pseudomonas* spp.; MRSA
Side-effects	Hypersensitivity, especially 'ampicillin rash' in acute EBV infection, rare anaphylaxis. Nausea. Diarrhoea (5–10%), *Clostridium difficile*		As ampicillin/amoxycillin, but diarrhoea 10–12%

Oral esters of ampicillin (bacampicillin, talampicillin, pivampicillin) converted to ampicillin in gut or on absorption through gut mucosa, giving better oral availability, but are more expensive.

FLUCLOXACILLIN (and other isoxazolyl penicillins—cloxacillin, dicloxacillin, oxacillin—and nafcillin)
Uses: Resistant to staphylococcal β-lactamase. Use for staphylococci and mixed infections with streptococci; combine with gentamicin, fusidic acid or rifampicin for severe staphylococcal infection. Inactive against MRSA and *Enterococcus* spp.
Administration: Parenteral or oral. CSF✓ (in high dose, penetration best with inflamed meninges), urine✓.
Adverse effects: Rare neutropenia, and reversible renal and hepatic dysfunction (cholestasis) with courses over 2 weeks, commoner in the elderly.

ANTI-PSEUDOMONAL/GRAM-NEGATIVE β-LACTAMASE-RESISTANT PENICILLINS (Table 140)

Table 140 Anti-pseudomonal/Gram-negative β-lactamase-resistant penicillins

	Azlocillin and relatives*	Timentin (ticarcillin + clavulanate) and Tazocin (piperacillin + tazobactam)	Temocillin
Administration, pharmacology	Parenteral only. CSF✓ (in high dose, penetration best with inflamed meninges), urine✓	Parenteral only. CSF✗, urine✓	Parenteral only. Urine✓. CSF unknown.
Sensitive; often useful	Mostly like ampicillin + useful activity against many *Pseudomonas* spp. Less active against Gram-positive cocci	Like co-amoxiclav + useful activity against many *Pseudomonas* spp.	Almost all coliforms (including many resistant to other agents by β-lactamase production), haemophili and neisseria
Variable; occasionally useful	More active than ampicillin against some 'hard' coliforms (>184)		
Resistant; unreliable	Most 'hard' coliforms (>184), anaerobes, staphylococci	Most 'hard' coliforms (>184)	Most *Pseudomonas* spp., *Acinetobacter* spp., *Serratia* spp., anaerobes and Gram-positive bacteria

continued on p. 299

Table 140 contd

		Timentin (ticarcillin + clavulanate) and Tazocin (piperacillin +	
	Azlocillin and relatives*	tazobactam)	Temocillin

Side-effects	Overall similar to benzylpenicillin. Sodium load. Occasional reversible platelet dysfunction, liver function abnormalities. Rare convulsions, commoner in renal failure, previous CNS disease and old age

* **Including acylureido penicillins**–azlocillin, piperacillin, mezlocillin–and **carboxy penicillins**–ticarcillin, carbenicillin. Antibacterial differences between these agents of little clinical significance, but acylureido penicillins contain less sodium. All have synergistic interactions with aminoglycosides against *Pseudomonas aeruginosa* (do not mix in same syringe).

OTHER PENICILLINS AND THEIR RELATIVES

Table 141 Other penicillins and their relatives

	Carbapenems (imipenem-cilastatin,* meropenem)	Monobactams (aztreonam; **mono**cyclic beta-**lactams**)
Administration, pharmacology	Parenteral only. CSF✓ (in high dose, penetration best with inflamed meninges), urine✓	
Sensitive; often useful	Moderate to good activity against virtually all groups of bacteria; highly β-lactamase-stable. Meropenem has better antipseudomonal and weaker anti-Gram-positive activity	Good to excellent activity against virtually all coliforms, *Pseudomonas* spp., haemophili, neisseria and other Gram-negative aerobes, highly β-lactamase-stable
Resistant; unreliable	Only MRSA, most *Enterococcus faecium*, and *Stenotrophomonas maltophilia* predictably resistant; rare coliforms/*Pseudomonas* spp. resistant by impermeability of outer membrane	All Gram-positive bacteria and anaerobes. *Stenotrophomonas maltophilia*
Side-effects	Overall similar to benzylpenicillin. Imipenem: nausea reduced by slowing infusion. Occasional reversible liver function abnormalities, convulsions with previous history of epilepsy	Nausea, vomiting, diarrhoea. Occasional reversible neutropenia, thrombocytopenia, liver function abnormalities. Probably usable in patients with benzylpenicillin and other β-lactam allergies

* **Imipenem-cilastatin** combines imipenem with inhibitor of the renal tubular dehydropeptidase that degrades it; thus plasma half-life extended, and renal tubular damage prevented.

Cephalosporins

Best classified in five groups: oral, parenteral, broad-spectrum, long half-life, and broad-spectrum oral. Clinicians need to be familiar with (and most hospitals need to keep in stock) only one example of each of the first three groups. In domiciliary practice, 'oral' cephalosporins will regularly be useful, but 'broad-spectrum oral' agents should be reserved for special indications because of cost, encouragement of resistance and side-effects. Classification in 'generations 1–4' is popular with the pharmaceutical industry, but is a better guide to cost than to usage.

Table 142 lists properties of the oral, parenteral and broad-spectrum cephalosporins. The two remaining groups have special properties, and may be useful for 'niche' indications.

Table 142 Major cephalosporins

Group	Oral (cephalexin, cephradine, cefaclor, cefadroxil)*	Parenteral (cefotaxime, cefuroxime, ceftizoxime, cefamandole, cefoxitin, cefodizime)	Broad-spectrum (ceftazidime, cefpirome)
Administration, pharmacology	High urine levels; often borderline levels elsewhere (**cefadroxil** usable 12-hly)	Good penetration to most sites at high dose. CSF√ (in high dose, penetration best with inflamed meninges), urine√	
Sensitive; often useful	'Easy' coliforms (**cefaclor**: better activity against *Haemophilus* spp.)	As oral group + *Neisseria* spp., staphylococci, strepto-cocci and *Haemophilus* spp. (**cefoxitin**: active against many anerobes)	As parenteral group (**ceftazidime**: many *Pseudomonas* spp. but less Gram-positive activity; **cefpirome**: many 'hard' coliforms (≻184) and enterococci)
Variable; occasionally useful	Staphylococci, streptococci, some 'hard' coliforms (≻184), *Haemophilus* spp.	Some 'hard' coliforms (≻184)	
Resistant; unreliable	Enterococci, many 'hard' coliforms (≻184), clostridia, *Listeria monocytogenes*, *Pseudomonas* spp., many anaerobes		As left, but see individually above
Side-effects	Diarrhoea (*Clostridium difficile*, especially with parenteral agents), β-lactam allergy. Fever, rashes, rare erythema multiforme. Arthralgia. Reversible hepatitis or cholestasis. Neutropenia with high dose in renal failure		

*Cefazolin, cephalothin have similar spectra, but only available im and iv. Cephradine also available im and iv. Cefsulodin is a parenteral agent with good activity against *Pseudomonas aeruginosa* only.

Long half-life cephalosporin: Ceftriaxone — similar spectrum to cefotaxime, but once-daily dosage. Pseudolithiasis common (precipitation of calcium salt in bile), hence avoid in biliary disease.

Broad-spectrum oral cephalosporins: Cefixime — similar spectrum to cefotaxime, but no antistaphylococcal or anaerobic activity. **Ceftibuten** — similar to cefixime but less antipneumococcal activity. **Cefuroxime axetil** — hydrolysed in intestinal mucosa to cefuroxime. Diarrhoea in 15% (including some *Clostridium difficile*). **Cefpodoxime proxetil** — similar spectrum to cefotaxime; promoted for respiratory tract infection.

β-Lactam allergy
Many patients claim to be 'penicillin-allergic', but 90% show no reaction when given penicillins again, and they should not be denied the advantages of β-lactam therapy when it is clearly the treatment of choice. Cross-allergenicity with

Table 143 β-Lactam allergy

Reaction	Frequency	Notes
Immediate (IgE-mediated vs. penicillamine and penicilloic acid breakdown products): anaphylaxis, angio-oedema, urticaria, some maculopapular rashes	1–10% overall; anaphylaxis 1–5% per 10000 courses	Anaphylaxis most commonly with iv benzylpenicillin. Avoid **all** β-lactams in patients after anaphylaxis or angio-oedema

continued on p. 301

Table 143 contd

Reaction	Frequency	Notes
Delayed (some IgG-mediated vs. penicilloyl group): 'serum sickness', haemolytic anaemia, acute interstitial nephritis, neutropenia, rashes, fever		Appear related to dose and duration of therapy. Can present 3 weeks after course finished. Frequent causes of diagnostic confusion during treatment of endocarditis, etc.
Ampicillin/amoxycillin reactions	5–10% overall: approaching 100% with glandular fever, CMV or HIV infection, chronic lymphocytic leukaemia	Maculopapular rashes of uncertain aetiology. These patients can safely be given other penicillins in future, unless the reaction was urticarial

Skin testing in expert hands can identify a patient's current allergic state, but can itself cause anaphylaxis. Desensitisation rarely helpful in practice.

cephalosporins said to be seen in up to 10% with penicillin allergy, but probably under 1% react in practice (Table 143).

Aminoglycosides

Aminosugars glycosidically linked to amino-cyclitols. All have narrow therapeutic indices, but good bactericidal activity against coliforms and many *Pseudomonas* spp. All carry risks of nephro- and ototoxicity, hence serum assay is mandatory for courses over 48 h (➤314). Often best used for less than 5–7 days. Especially valuable in single-dose/short-course prophylaxis,

and in combination with other antibiotics (e.g. a penicillin plus metronidazole) for empirical therapy of serious infection while culture results awaited.

Haemodialysis removes aminoglycosides (➤331).

High-level gentamicin-resistant (HLGR) enterococci (➤175) are defined as strains not killed by gentamicin combined with penicillin or vancomycin.

Neomycin: Used topically (ear drops, nasal cream) for *Staphylococcus aureus* (naseptin ➤305). Oral (non-absorbed) alleged effective for hepatic failure.

Table 144 Aminoglycosides

	Gentamicin, netilmicin	Tobramycin	Amikacin
Administration, pharmacology	Iv or im. Do not mix in same syringe with β-lactams. Major modification of dose by body weight and renal function. Serum assay essential for courses longer than 48h; repeat at least 2x weekly (➤314). CSF✗, urine✓		
Sensitive; often useful	Coliforms, many *Pseudomonas* spp., streptococcal endocarditis (with penicillin); severe *Staphylococcus aureus* infection (with flucloxacillin)	A little more active against *Pseudomonas* spp.	More stable to common aminoglycoside-modifying enzymes; best reserved for resistant organisms
Resistant; unreliable	Streptococci and staphylococci (if used alone), haemophili, anaerobes		
Side-effects	**Nephrotoxicity** (often largely reversible: synergy with vancomycin, amphotericin and other nephrotoxic drugs), **VIIIth nerve** (often irreversible: especially vestibular branch). Effects partially correlate with peak and trough levels and duration of therapy		

Streptomycin: Second-line (in combination) therapy for *Mycobacterium tuberculosis* (➤32). Active against some HLGR enterococci (➤175).

Spectinomycin: Single-dose therapy for *Neisseria gonorrhoeae* (especially with penicillin allergy or resistance). Active against *Ureaplasma urealyticum*, but not *Chlamydia* spp.

Paromomycin: Possibly effective against *Cryptosporidium* in AIDS (➤122).

Trimethoprim and sulphonamides

Co-trimoxazole consists of trimethoprim and sulphamethoxazole; the antibacterial 'synergy' of this combination is of dubious significance *in vivo*, hence trimethoprim is preferred as a single agent, with co-trimoxazole best reserved for special indications (Table 145).

Quinolones

4-Quinolones

Uses: Oral agents with activity against coliforms and *Neisseria* spp. Largely urinary excretion, tissue levels poor. **Nalidixic acid** and **cinoxacin** are oral urinary tract agents. They are inactive against Gram-positive bacteria and *Pseudomonas* spp. **Acrosoxacin** is an antigonococcal agent. A single oral dose is given for urethral and anorectal infection; ineffective against *Chlamydia trachomatis*.

Adverse effects: May cause convulsions (enhanced by NSAIDs); headache, sleep disturbance. Avoid in pregnancy; damage developing cartilage in animals, hence avoid in childhood unless no adequate alternative. Diarrhoea, occasionally *Clostridium difficile*-associated. Photosensitivity.

Table 145 Trimethoprim and sulphonamides

	Trimethoprim	Co-trimoxazole	Sulphonamides*
Administration, pharmacology	Oral, iv formulations	CSF✓, urine✓	
Sensitive; often useful	Coliforms in lower UTI and travellers' diarrhoea; *Haemophilus influenzae* and *Streptococcus pneumoniae* in acute bronchitis and sinusitis. *Staphylococcus saprophyticus. Vibrio cholerae. Listeria monocytogenes*	As trimethoprim + *Nocardia* spp., *Brucella* spp., *Haemophilus ducreyi*. Only current major indication is high-dose therapy for *Pneumocystis carinii* (➤119)	Combined with pyrimethamine for toxoplasmosis and drug-resistant malaria
Variable	*Staphylococcus aureus*		
Resistant; unreliable	*Streptococcus pneumoniae* pneumonia; many streptococcal infections; *Enterococcus* spp.; coliform resistance rate approaching 20%. *Pseudomonas* spp.		Resistance rates in most bacteria now too high for use alone
Side-effects	Nausea, vomiting. Rashes. Exacerbation of haematological abnormalities in patients with folate deficiency	As trimethoprim + sulphonamides. Rashes,† fever, leucopenia, thrombocytopenia common in AIDS	Nausea, vomiting. Fever, rash, eosinophilia, Stevens–Johnson syndrome, epidermal necrolysis. Granulocytopenia, thrombocytopenia. Interference with fetal bilirubin transport (kernicterus)

* Including sulphadiazine and sulphadimidine. Sulfametopyrazine has longer half-life because of high serum protein binding; given as 2 g dose once weekly for UTI.
† Diphenhydramine iv may resolve mild reactions.

Fluoroquinolones: ciprofloxacin, ofloxacin, norfloxacin

Uses: Compared with 4-quinolones the fluoroquinolones have enhanced antibacterial activity against Gram-negative bacteria and improved tissue/blood levels. Little reliable activity against staphylococci (including MRSA—resistance emerges) and streptococci (including *Streptococcus pneumoniae*). Inactive against anaerobes. **Ciprofloxacin** is useful against Gram-negative bacteria resistant to other agents (e.g. UTI, sepsis in ICU); also for gut decontamination (neutropenia), travellers' diarrhoea, neisseria (gonorrhoea; meningococcal prophylaxis), and oral therapy of chronic Gram-negative infection (cystic fibrosis, osteomyelitis). It is the only oral antibiotic with useful antipseudomonal activity, and is also active against *Chlamydia* spp., *Legionella* spp. and some mycobacteria. CSF✓ in high dose. **Ofloxacin** has minor differences. **Norfloxacin** is used for UTI.

Administration: Ciprofloxacin and ofloxacin: oral, iv; norfloxacin: oral.

Adverse effects: Similar side-effects to 4-quinolones (also potentiate warfarin, theophylline; increased nephrotoxicity with cyclosporin).

Macrolides

Erythromycin has been the drug of first choice for many infections in patients allergic to penicillin. Newer macrolides offer pharmacological, antimicrobial and toxicity advantages. Bacteria resistant to one macrolide are considered resistant to all (Table 146).

Tetracyclines

Uses: All tetracyclines have similarly broad spectra of activity, but resistance now common in many bacteria. Still drugs of choice for *Chlamydia* spp., *Coxiella burnetii*, *Mycoplasma* spp., *Brucella* spp., rickettsial infections and granuloma inguinale. Useful in exacerbations of chronic obstructive airways disease. Also used for *Borrelia burgdorferi*, acne, and as second-line agents in chronic prostatitis, sinusitis, acute exacerbations of

Table 146 Macrolides

	Erythromycin	Clarythromycin	Azithromycin
Administration, pharmacology	Oral, iv formulations. CSF ✗, urine ✗	Oral, iv formulations	Oral only; long half-life, hence 3-day courses. High intracellular but low serum levels
Sensitive; often useful	Staphylococci, streptococci (local resistance problems). *Legionella* spp., *Chlamydia* spp., syphilis, mycoplasma, *Campylobacter* spp., *Bordetella* spp., *Moraxella* spp.	As erythromycin + haemophilus	As clarythromycin + *Haemophilus ducreyi*; more activity against *Chlamydia* spp. and some mycobacteria
Variable; occasionally useful	Anaerobes, *Neisseria* spp.		
Resistant; unreliable	Coliforms, *Pseudomonas* spp., haemophili	Coliforms, *Pseudomonas* spp.	
Side-effects	Gastric upset, phlebitis. Ototoxicity at high dose in renal failure. Rare cholestasis with long courses; avoid estolate salt in liver disease*	Much less gastric upset*	

*Potentiate astemizole, terfenadine, midazolam, carbamazepine, cyclosporin.

Spiramycin is a macrolide sometimes used for treatment of toxoplasmosis in pregnancy (➤264).

bronchitis, malaria, *Neisseria gonorrhoeae*. Frequently used for *Vibrio cholerae*, but resistance increasing.

Administration: There are iv and oral preparations. **Tetracycline, oxytetracycline** and **demeclocycline** are given four times and **lymecycline** twice daily. Oral absorption reduced by milk, antacids and salts of calcium, iron and magnesium. **Doxycycline** (once daily) and **minocycline** (twice daily) are not affected by milk and may be used in renal impairment, but are much more expensive.

Adverse effects: Avoid in children <12 years (bone and tooth deposition). Gastrointestinal disturbance common. Avoid in renal failure. Minocycline commonly causes vestibular side-effects.

Glycopeptides: vancomycin and teicoplanin

Uses: Expensive parenteral glycopeptides, active against Gram-positive bacteria only. Resistance currently only seen in rarely pathogenic Gram-positive bacteria (including *Leuconostoc* spp., some *Lactobacillus* spp. and *Enterococcus* spp.). Used for Gram-positive bacteria resistant to other agents (e.g. MRSA, *Staphylococcus epidermidis* infection of prostheses, ampicillin-resistant *Enterococcus* spp.); severe infection in penicillin-allergic patients; CAPD peritonitis treatment (➤54); endocarditis prophylaxis (➤40); oral for *Clostridium difficile* diarrhoea (not absorbed).

Administration: **Vancomycin**: two to four times daily iv dosage, modified by serum assay △, with special care in renal impairment. Serum levels reduced by haemofiltration and CAPD, but not by haemodialysis. CSF ✗, urine ✓. Can be given intrathecally.

Adverse effects: Rapid infusion of **vancomycin** (less than 1 h) causes 'red man syndrome', perhaps from histamine release. Renal and VIIIth nerve (especially auditory branch) toxicity, occasional neutropenia; latest preparations less toxic.

Teicoplanin given iv or im has minor differences in spectrum. Once-daily dosage; said not to require assay except in prolonged

therapy in impaired renal function or in the elderly. No 'red man syndrome', but cross-allergy with vancomycin reported.

Miscellaneous antibiotics

Fusidic acid
Uses: Good clinical activity against staphylococci only. Resistance develops rapidly; use systemically in combination with flucloxacillin, erythromycin or vancomycin. Used in severe staphylococcal infection; topical eye preparation (high concentration, therefore active against most ophthalmic pathogens).

Administration: Oral preparation well absorbed and widely distributed throughout the body: CSF ✗ but penetrates cerebral abscess, urine ✓.

Adverse effects: Liver dysfunction likely to be caused by iv formulation, hence use orally. Check hepatic function.

Metronidazole, tinidazole (imidazoles)
Uses: Only active against obligate anaerobic bacteria (only *Propionibacterium* spp. and *Actinomyces* spp. are commonly resistant) and protozoa, including *Trichomonas vaginalis*, *Giardia lamblia*, *Entamoeba histolytica* and *Balantidium coli*. Major uses are anaerobic infection (including surgical prophylaxis ➤312, *Clostridium difficile* diarrhoea ➤47), protozoal infection. **Nimorazole** used for trichomoniasis and ulcerative gingivitis.

Administration: Oral and iv preparations (and metronidazole suppositories). Widely distributed around the body: CSF✓, urine✓.

Adverse effects: Side-effects include antabuse effect, nausea, metallic taste; peripheral neuropathy after prolonged use, therefore keep courses shorter than 6 weeks.

Mupirocin (pseudomonic acid)
Uses: Active against *Streptococcus* spp. and *Staphylococcus* spp.; resistance rare, but found in some MRSA strains circulating in UK. Useful for treatment of superficial staphylococcal and streptococcal infections, and clearance of nasal carriage of *Staphylococcus aureus*.

Administration: Topical use only (unstable within body), two to three times daily.

Naseptin (chlorhexidine + neomycin cream)

Topical to anterior nares four times daily. Less effective than mupirocin for eradication of *Staphylococcus aureus*.

Chloramphenicol

Uses: Broad spectrum, only *Pseudomonas* spp. and *Nocardia* spp. innately resistant, but acquired resistance common in many bacteria. Newer antibiotics have supplanted systemic chloramphenicol usage in developed countries; used commonly only as topical eye preparation. Occasionally used second-line for typhoid, invasive *Haemophilus influenzae*, meningitis, neonatal sepsis, rickettsial infections.

Administration: Oral, im and iv preparations; CSF✓, urine✓.

Adverse effects: Avoid in pregnancy, breast-feeding. Serum assay required in neonates △ ('grey baby' syndrome, especially in prematurity). Dose-related, reversible marrow suppression (if serum levels > 25 mg/l), plus rare idiosyncratic, irreversible aplastic anaemia.

Urinary tract agents

Oral antimicrobial agents used for the treatment of cystitis or long-term suppression of UTI. Usage decreasing. Most have no useful activity outside the urinary tract. Prevention of recurrent UTI: ➤60.

NALIDIXIC ACID (➤302)

HEXAMINE

Liberates formaldehyde when excreted to acid urine; weakly antibacterial, so only used for suppression of UTI. Commonest side-effect is GI upset. (NB Antacids prevent acidification of urine.) Most bacteria sensitive except powerful urease-producers, e.g. *Proteus* spp.

NITROFURANTOIN

Active in acid solution against many bacteria causing UTI, but not against most *Pseudomonas* spp., and some *Proteus* spp. and *Klebsiella* spp. Useful for treating resistant *Staphylococcus* spp., *Streptococcus* spp. and *Enterococcus* spp. UTI in β-lactam-allergic patients. Safe in preg-nancy but not currently recommended because of adverse effects, which include rare pulmonary fibrosis, and reversible peripheral neuropathy, especially in renal failure. New macrocrystalline preparation causes less nausea and vomiting; rash, fever, eosinophilia and cough also seen.

FOSFOMYCIN

Broad spectrum, with little cross-resistance to other classes of antibiotic. Single dose at bedtime for treatment of UTI. Dose 3 h before and 24 h after for prophylaxis of transurethral procedures. Avoid in pregnancy and renal failure. Occasional nausea, rash.

Clindamycin

Uses: Long-established; active against most obligate anaerobes and many Gram-positive bacteria (of these, *Clostridium* spp. and *Enterococcus* spp. are the least likely to respond). Macrolide (erythromycin)-resistant bacteria best considered resistant to clindamycin also. Widely used in the USA with gentamicin for abdominal surgical prophylaxis. Useful in mixed aerobic/anaerobic soft-tissue infection (➤89), especially in patients allergic to β-lactams; also worth trying in such infections in patients with arterial insufficiency. Endocarditis prophylaxis (➤40). Topical preparation in acne (➤92). **Lincomycin** similar.

Administration: Oral, im or iv preparations, with good tissue distribution and intracellular concentration – CSF ✗, urine ✓.

Adverse effects: Diarrhoea (10–30%), *Clostridium difficile* colitis (1–2%) limits usefulness (commoner >60 years, and with doses > 300 mg qds). Stop treatment if diarrhoea occurs. Also rash, fever, eosinophilia.

Colistin (polymyxin E)

Uses: Active against most Gram-negative bacteria including *Pseudomonas* spp., but excluding *Proteus* spp. and *Serratia* spp. Occasional use for multiply resistant organisms. Oral (not absorbed) for gut decontamination (➤134). Inhalational (not absorbed) for *Pseudomonas aeruginosa* infection in cystic fibrosis.

Administration: Colistin, and the related

polymyxin B, also used in topical preparations (can be absorbed from large burns).

Adverse effects: Systemically toxic (central and peripheral neuro- and nephrotoxicity).

Antituberculous drugs

Including rifampicin (➤32)

Antifungal agents

Antifungal agents have no cross-activity against bacteria, and are frequently prescribed to treat *Candida* spp. superinfections resulting from antibacterial use. Only five different classes of antifungal agent are available. Many can be used topically (including oral usage of non-absorbable antifungals) or systemically. The systemic agents available until recently have been toxic.

Polyenes: amphotericin B

Uses: Active against most yeasts and systemically infecting fungi (including *Aspergillus* spp. and the dimorphic fungi), and the amoebae *Naegleria* spp. and *Hartmanella* spp. Dermatophytes, *Pseudallescheria boydii* and some moulds are less sensitive or resistant. Occasional acquired resistance in *Candida* spp. (*tropicalis, krusei, guilliermondii, parapsilosis* and *lusitaniae*; very rare in the clinically commoner *Candida albicans* and *glabrata*). Sensitivity testing useful if treatment failure, unusual species or endocarditis. Despite toxicity, remains **agent of choice** for most serious fungal infections, including systemic candidiasis, aspergillosis and cryptococcosis. Oral prophylaxis and treatment of GI tract yeast infection. Combination with flucytosine allows lower doses of both in cryptococcal meningitis, but little evidence of benefit for combinations with azoles (theoretical risk of antagonism).

Administration: There are iv and oral preparations; occasionally instilled into abscesses, joints, CSF; not absorbed from gut. CSF ✗, urine ✗. Slow build-up to full dosage reduces unwanted effects, but may risk inadequate early therapy in immunocompromised patients (hence 'accelerated regimen' ➤319). Monitor renal function: creatinine >200 mmol/l an indication to give same daily dose

on alternate days. 'Low-dose' regimen for 10–14 days often used for moderately serious *Candida* spp. infection (e.g. oesophagitis, iv line infection). Serum levels do not correlate with side-effects, so assay not helpful.

Adverse effects: Fever, rigors, vomiting, thrombophlebitis after iv administration; minimised by analgesics, antihistamines, iv pethidine, adding hydrocortisone to infusion. Hypokalaemia, hypomagnesaemia, nephrotoxicity, cardiac arrythmias, hepatic dysfunction, cerebral irritation, peripheral neuropathy.

Liposomal amphotericin: first of several expensive, lipid-complexed preparations with lower toxicity (especially nephrotoxicity). Best reserved for when nephrotoxicity seen with conventional preparation. Efficacy currently unproven, but initial agent of choice in hepatosplenic candidiasis (➤291) and rhinocerebral zygomycosis (➤289).

Nystatin

Oral and topical treatment of mucosal candidiasis; oropharyngeal and gastrointestinal prophylaxis. Resistance rare, but no systemic absorption, so use as treatment only for minor infections. Inactive against other fungi.

Azoles

In vitro sensitivity testing not always predictive of response. For itraconazole, fluconazole, miconazole and ketoconazole *in vitro* and *in vivo* cross-resistance is rare, but well recognised in some *Candida albicans* strains. Use in combination with amphotericin B is controversial (theoretical antagonism).

CLOTRIMAZOLE, ECONAZOLE

Topical treatment of mucosal candidiasis and dermatophyte infection.

FLUCONAZOLE

Uses: Broad spectrum including yeasts (some non-*albicans Candida* spp. show acquired or primary resistance, especially *Candida krusei*) and some dermatophytes. Used single-dose for vaginal candidiasis; prophylaxis, prevention of relapse, and treatment of yeast infections in immunocompromised patients,

especially *Cryptococcus neoformans* meningitis in AIDS (➤125). Ineffective in aspergillosis.
Administration: There are iv and (well-absorbed) oral preparations; CSF✓ (especially with meningitis), urine✓.

ITRACONAZOLE
Uses: Broadly active against many yeasts, dimorphic fungi and *Aspergillus* spp.
Administration: Oral administration; absorption unpredictable especially in AIDS △. CSF ✗, urine ✗.
Adverse effects: Nausea, headache, dizziness, rashes, pruritus; occasional hepatotoxicity, Stevens–Johnson syndrome.

KETOCONAZOLE
Uses: Broad spectrum, including systemic mycoses (not *Aspergillus* spp.), candidosis and dermatophytosis.
Administration: Oral, topical formulations; minimal CSF and urinary penetration, improved with very large doses.
Adverse effects: Gastrointestinal disturbance, pruritus, rashes; rare hepatotoxicity (monitor liver function); occasional painful gynaecomastia, loss of libido (interference with testosterone synthesis).

MICONAZOLE
Uses: Largely superseded by newer azoles; broad spectrum *in vitro* including *Aspergillus* spp., yeasts and dermatophytes, but clinical response in serious infection often poor.

Administration: Oral (little systemic absorption), iv preparations; little CSF or urinary penetration. Can be given intrathecally.
Adverse effects: Phlebitis, pruritus, rashes, fever; nausea, vomiting; cardiac dysrhythmia.

Flucytosine
Uses: Combine with amphotericin B in cryptococcosis (➤292) and severe *Candida* spp. infection. May enable lower dosing of amphotericin. Primary resistance *c.* 10%. Acquired resistance common if flucytosine used alone (except short courses for lower UTI).
Administration: Well absorbed orally (iv available); CSF✓, urine✓. △.
Adverse effects: Marrow aplasia (especially with serum level >100 mg/l), nausea, vomiting, diarrhoea, rashes, CNS effects; rare hepatotoxicity.

Griseofulvin and terbinafine
Griseofulvin is used for the oral treatment of dermatophyte infections when topical therapy inappropriate; skin, scalp, hair and nails. Prolonged therapy needed for nail infections; ineffective for toe web infections. Adverse effects include headache, gastrointestinal disturbance, rashes and occasional disturbance of motor coordination.

Terbinafine is a new alternative to griseofulvin in dermatophyte infections of skin, scalp, hair and nails. More effective in nail infections. Occasional gastrointestinal disturbance, rashes. Rare hepatotoxicity.

32: Antibiotics: Theory, Use and Abuse

An **antibiotic**, strictly, is a substance produced by a micro-organism that kills or inhibits the growth of another micro-organism in high dilution. Most 'antibiotics' today are at least partly synthetic, so **antimicrobial agent** is a better term.

In any community the results of widespread antibiotic usage are reflected in the prevalence and distribution of antibiotic resistance in common pathogens. Antibiotic usage is the only form of medical treatment where the choice of therapy for one patient can affect diseases suffered in the future by another, by selection of resistant organisms followed by cross-infection to the new host.

Mechanisms of action

Rely upon **selective toxicity** versus microbial rather than human structures and metabolism. Common examples are given in Table 147.

Table 147 Mechanisms of antibiotic action

Target	Antibiotic class
Cell wall	Penicillins, cephalosporins, glycopeptides
Protein synthesis	Chloramphenicol, macrolides, fucidin, tetracyclines, aminoglycosides, lincosamides
DNA/RNA synthesis	Quinolones, rifampicin, 5-nitroimidazoles, nitrofurans
Intermediary metabolism	Sulphonamides, diaminopyrimidines

Antibiotic sensitivity, resistance and 'activity'

Sensitivity testing

Results of susceptibility testing of bacteria are reported by most laboratories as 'sensitive' or 'resistant', with some using an 'intermediate' category. These results are based upon *in vitro* tests, which may include the following.

Disc diffusion: zone of inhibition around antibiotic-containing disc after overnight incubation of bacterial lawn on solid agar. If zone diameter of test organism is ≥3 mm less than that of control sensitive organism, result is 'resistant'.

Breakpoint test: growth of a spot inoculum of bacteria on solid medium containing a known concentration of antibiotic, the 'breakpoint concentration', chosen to allow the growth of 'sensitive' micro-organisms and inhibit the growth of 'resistant' ones.

Direct detection of resistance mechanism: e.g. extracellular β-lactamase activity of *Neisseria gonorrhoeae* by rubbing a colony on a paper strip containing chromogenic cephalosporin—colour change = β-lactamase-positive.

More detailed tests, which attempt to quantify the specific 'activity' of antibiotics include the following.

Minimum inhibitory concentration (MIC): lowest concentration of an antibiotic to inhibit multiplication of an organism in broth culture or on solid agar.

Minimum bactericidal concentration (MBC): lowest concentration of an antibiotic to kill an organism—usually shown by subculture of MIC broth on antibiotic-free medium to demonstrate death or viability of bacteria within it.

Laboratory reports of sensitivity or resistance are educated guesses about what may happen in a real patient: disc contents, zone diameters and breakpoint concentrations are chosen based upon past experience, and on likely concentrations of antibiotic achieved at the site of infection. Many factors will modify activity *in vivo*, including protein binding, penetration to abscesses and privileged sites (CSF, eye, inside cells), immune and phagocytic activity, and presence of foreign bodies. Some antibiotics (e.g. β-lactams) reach high concentrations in the urine, so greater zone diameters and breakpoints are used for these agents to denote resistance in urine isolates.

To limit antibiotics tested to practicable numbers, laboratories usually test one example of a particular group and assume results for other members of the group—e.g. methicillin for *Staphylococcus aureus* (assume results for all β-lactams), cephalexin for *Escherichia coli* (assume results for all oral cephalosporins).

Some antibiotics kill organisms *in vitro* (**bactericidal**), others only inhibit their multiplication (**bacteriostatic**); clinical relevance of this is dubious.

Serum bactericidal titre (SBC, back titrations): highest dilution titre of patient's serum that inhibits multiplication of the patient's infecting organism. Serum taken immediately before and usually 1 h after antibiotic infusion. Therapy adjusted and test repeated to give SBC ≥ 1:8. Often requested during treatment of IE (occasionally also osteomyelitis, meningitis), but never proven to be predictive of response, so many laboratories do not perform this test.

Antibiotic resistance

Common resistance mechanisms include: **inactivation** by bacterial enzymes (β lactamases, aminoglycoside-modifying enzymes); **alteration of target molecules** (penicillin-binding proteins); **restriction of entry** to the cell (imipenem in *E coli*); **bypassing of metabolic pathway** (trimethoprim in enterococci).

Use of virtually any antibiotic results in an increased prevalence of resistance in the bacterial flora of an individual patient, and in the population of which he or she is a member—by **selection** and overgrowth of resistant mutants (e.g. rifampicin resistance in *Neisseria meningitidis*), or by **induction** of innate resistance mechanisms latent within initially apparently sensitive subpopulations (e.g. cefotaxime resistance in *Enterobacter cloacae*). Multiple determinants of resistance may be linked on plasmids or other mobile genetic elements, so exposure to one antimicrobial agent may increase the prevalence of all linked resistances in the population.

Selection and induction during antibiotic treatment is most likely with undrained 'sumps' of infected material (e.g. empyema, abdominal abscess). Resistant bacteria may also appear *de novo* at an infected site by **cross-infection** and **superinfection**—most likely with infections that communicate with the mucous membranes or skin (e.g. abdominal abscess treated with open drainage).

Current important examples of resistance: Four bacteria are causing particular resistance problems in the UK and USA at the moment: methicillin-resistant *Staphylococcus aureus* (MRSA) (➤167); high-level gentamicin-resistant (HLGR) and vancomycin-resistant enterococci (➤175); cefotaxime/ceftazidime-resistant *Klebsiella* spp. (➤189); and multiply resistant *Mycobacterium tuberculosis* (➤128, 229).

Counting the costs

At any one time, about 25% hospital in-patients are receiving antibiotics, and about 15% of a large hospital's drug budget is spent on antibiotics. When audited, about 15% of this usage is inappropriate. Antibiotic expenditure rises annually above inflation in all units, with the largest proportional increases seen recently in antiviral and antifungal agents. Considerable savings can be made by agreement of an **antibiotic policy**, allowing bulk purchase of few agents, reduced chance of confusion, and offering treatment guidelines based on local resistance patterns, at the expense of restricted clinical freedom.

The best methods of ensuring cost-effective antibiotic therapy involve: (i) **agreement of treatment guidelines** between microbiologists and clinicians; (ii) **selective sensitivity reporting** by laboratories; (iii) **regular feedback of usage** to prescribers; and (iv) **budgetary inducements** to reduce expenditure.

Principles of antibiotic use

Figure 7 illustrates a rational approach to antibiotic prescribing.

Take specimens for culture before starting antibiotics: Specimens taken after antibiotics have been given (even only a few hours after) may be grossly misleading.

Antibiotic choice: Once it has been decided to

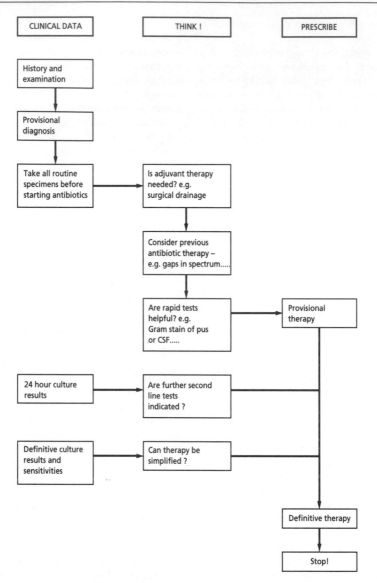

Fig. 7 Principles of antibiotic usage. Antibiotic choice for the individual patient should follow the algorithm given.

treat a patient with antibiotics, there are usually numerous agents that could be **rational therapy**. Few clinical syndromes are so characteristic and their causative organisms so reliably antibiotic-sensitive that a single antimicrobial agent of first choice is always indicated. Rapid tests can sometimes confirm a microbial cause and allow definitive therapy to be started immediately—e.g. Gram stain of CSF confirming *Neisseria meningitidis*, allowing benzylpenicillin monotherapy. Alternatives are always necessary to cater for hypersensitivity in the patient and unusual resistance in the pathogen. Most hospital or practice antibiotic policies give guidelines for antibiotic choice in different clinical situations.

Table 148 Factors influencing antibiotic choice

Factor	Notes
Antibiotic activity	*In vitro* and *in vivo* vs. likely or known pathogens
Concentrations achieved at site of infection	Predictably poor for many in CSF, eye, intracellularly and in abscesses. Some have poor urinary penetration (e.g. macrolides)
Bacterial resistance	Local knowledge of resistance patterns; previous antibiotic therapy; likelihood of inducing resistance in the infecting flora
Pharmacokinetics	Absorption, excretion, metabolism, penetration. Some give poor tissue levels (e.g. nalidixic acid)
Side-effects	Adverse drug reactions and interactions; some patients predisposed (e.g. age, renal or hepatic failure). E.g. toxicity (aminoglycosides and VIIIth nerve), allergy (ampicillin rash), superinfection (thrush, *Clostridium difficile*), administration problems (iv line infection)
Cost . . .	. . . of drug, administration, and monitoring

Factors to be considered when choosing which to use include those listed in Table 148.

Route of administration: Intravenous recommended for severe infection. Bolus doses better than continuous infusion for most indications, but risks of iv access and high costs of administration. **Intramuscular** allows use of depot preparations (e.g. procaine penicillin), but painful (some agents locally toxic), ineffective if patient shocked, and contraindicated with haemorrhagic diathesis. **Oral** best for minor infections and follow-on after initial iv therapy; requires a conscious patient without diarrhoea or vomiting; administration costs low; possibly greater effects on commensal flora of colon. Some antibiotics especially well absorbed orally (e.g. ciprofloxacin, fusidic acid). **Rectal** cheap and often convenient, but not with diarrhoea, and only limited range of agents available for this route (e.g. metronidazole). **Topical** cheap, but hypersensitivity reactions and encouragement of bacterial resistance are problems. Mupirocin (➤304) and antiseptics are preferred.

Combinations of antibiotics: Most commonly to **broaden spectrum** (e.g. benzylpenicillin/gentamicin/metronidazole for mixed infection with faecal flora after colonic perforation); a few specific indications for **synergistic action** (penicillin/gentamicin for streptococcal infective endocarditis) and **to slow development of resistance** (e.g. isoniazid, rifampicin, pyrazinamide + ethambutol for *Mycobacterium tuberculosis*) and **overcome resistance** (e.g. amoxycillin + clavulanate (co-amoxiclav) for many β-lactamase-producing bacteria); rarely enables use of **lower doses of toxic agents** (amphotericin + flucytosine in cryptococcal meningitis).

Guidelines for stopping: 'Measures of response' to antibiotic treatment include: fever, pulse, respiratory rate, CRP, ESR, WBC, culture results. Antibiotic course lengths have been defined by clinical trial for only a few infectious syndromes (including tuberculosis and gonorrhoea). Inferences can be made for others, including lower urinary tract infection, streptococcal infective endocarditis, *Staphylococcus aureus* bacteraemia, meningitis, but length of treatment needed for many common infections, including pneumonias, wound infections, abdominal abscess, osteomyelitis and most severe systemic sepsis, is based upon scant evidence and antibiotics are probably often given for too long. When individual guidelines not available, patients are best treated iv until a clear clinical response is seen, then orally until signs and symptoms have resolved and, for severe, chronic infections such as osteomyelitis, abdominal abscess, 'measures of response' have returned to normal range.

Reaction to apparent treatment failure

• Ask for microbiology or infectious diseases opinion ☎.

- Review diagnosis, results of culture, and therapy:
  Is the provisional diagnosis of infection still likely?
  Was the original culture representative?
  Are further, second-line investigations now indicated?
  Is more time needed for response (serious infections often take 48–72 h to respond clinically)?
- Then consider the following:
  Is drainage or foreign body removal indicated?
  Stop antibiotics and reculture?
  Is this a drug (antibiotic) allergy?
  Is there a superinfection or additional pathogen (original site, or different – e.g. iv line sepsis)?
  Has the original pathogen developed resistance?
  Is there an intracellular-persisting pathogen?

Prophylactic antibiotics

Antibiotics given just before, during and just after the period of exposure to an infectious agent to reduce the risks of establishment of infection. Audit shows that prophylaxis comprises ~25% antibiotic usage in hospitals and up to 50% of these courses are given for too long.

Principles of use: Consider **incidence** of infection to be prevented, **likely organisms**, their **probable sensitivities**, and **period of risk**. Infections deserving prophylaxis should be **common** (e.g. all large-bowel surgery), and/or **catastrophic** (e.g. prosthetic heart valve insertion), and/or **proven** to be reduced by prophylaxis (Table 149).

Disadvantages of prophylaxis: To be weighed against potential advantages: antibiotic costs; encouragement of antibiotic resistance in individual and community; hypersensitivity and adverse drug reactions; false sense of security (prophylaxis is never a substitute for good surgical, aseptic and antiseptic techniques); sometimes delayed presentation rather than prevention of infections.

Choice of prophylactic regimen: Use high doses of antibiotics that reach high levels at the risk site (e.g. rifampicin rather than penicillin to clear nasopharyngeal meningococci); maintain effective levels throughout risk period (e.g. consider repeating doses during long operations).

Surgical prophylaxis

First dose given at time of induction of anaesthesia to ensure adequate tissue levels perioperatively. 'Cover' for > 48 h **never** shown superior to shorter periods, and **single-dose** prophylaxis increasingly proven to be as effective. Prophylaxis proven ineffective for indwelling urinary catheters, CSF leaks, insertion of iv and CAPD catheters.

Protocols are usually decided at individual hospitals, based on local antibiotic resistance patterns and purchasing arrangements. The regimens in Table 150 are suitable if local protocols are unavailable.

Table 149 Note important differences between medical and surgical indications

	Medical indications	Surgical indications
Risk period	Often long and ill-defined	Usually short
Magnitude of risks	Often low with many confounding variables (hence value of prophylaxis hard to prove)	Often high, or many patients at risk under standardised conditions (hence easier to prove)
Routes of antibiotics	Oral usually essential	Parenteral regimen assures high, timely concentrations at sites of risk
Infecting organisms	Often a single organism	More usually a range of possibilities
Repeated risk?	Often yes	Usually single event only

Table 150 Surgical antibiotic prophylaxis

Operation	Normal regimen	Minor[1] penicillin allergy	Major[2] penicillin allergy
Orthopaedics			
Primary insertion of prosthesis	Flucoxacillin 1 g 6-hly × 3 doses	Cefotaxime 2 g 8-hly × 2 doses	Vancomycin 1 g × 1 dose[3]
Urinary catheter insertion during post-op. period[4]	Benzylpenicillin 1.2 g + gentamicin 120 mg × 1 dose	Gentamicin 120 mg × 1 dose	Gentamicin 120 mg × 1 dose
Neurosurgery			
Clean craniotomy, shunts, flaps and external drains	Flucoxacillin 1 g, repeated if op. time >4 h	Cefotaxime 1 g, repeated if op. time >6 h	Vancomycin 500 mg, repeated if op. time >6 h
Acoustic neuroma and transmucosal operations	Cefotaxime 1 g 8-hly for 24 h	Cefotaxime 1 g 8-hly for 24 h	Cefotaxime 1 g 8-hly for 24 h
Abdominal surgery			
Uncomplicated biliary surgery or oesophagectomy	Cefotaxime 1 g, repeated if op. time >6 h	Cefotaxime 1 g, repeated if op. time >6 h	Ciprofloxacin 200 mg
Complicated biliary surgery (e.g. acute infection)	Cefotaxime 1 g 8-hly for 48 h	Cefotaxime 1 g 8-hly for 48 h	Ciprofloxacin 200 mg 12-hly for 48 h
Complicated oesophagectomy (e.g. perforation, spillage)	Cefotaxime 2 g + metronidazole 500 mg 8-hly for 48 h	Cefotaxime 2 g + metronidazole 500 mg 8-hly for 48 h	Ciprofloxacin 200 mg 12-hly + metronidazole 500 mg 8-hly for 48 h
Uncomplicated gastrectomy or colonic surgery	Benzylpenicillin 1.2 g + gentamicin 120 mg + metronidazole 500 mg × 1 dose	Cefotaxime 1 g + metronidazole 500 mg × 1 dose	Ciprofloxacin 200 mg + metronidazole 500 mg × 1 dose
Complicated gastrectomy (e.g. gastric stasis, spillage at operation) or complicated colonic surgery[5] (e.g. AP resection, spillage of gut contents)	Benzylpenicillin 1.2 g 6-hly + gentamicin 120 mg 12-hly + metronidazole 500 mg 8-hly for 48 h	Cefotaxime 1 g + metronidazole 500 mg 8-hly for 48 h	Ciprofloxacin 200 mg 12-hly + metronidazole 500 mg 8-hly for 48 h
Appendicectomy (uncomplicated)	Metronidazole 500 mg pr x 2 doses		
Complicated appendicectomy	As for complicated colonic surgery above		
Aortic/lower limb vascular graft surgery (uncomplicated)	Flucloxacillin 500 mg + gentamicin 120 mg x 2 doses of each 8 h apart	Cefotaxime 1 g x 2 doses 8 h apart	Vancomycin 1 g single dose[3]
Aortic and lower limb vascular graft surgery – bowel ischaemia suspected	Flucloxacillin 500 mg 6-hly + gentamicin 120 mg 12-hly + metronidazole 500 mg 8-hly for 48 h	Cefotaxime 1 g + metronidazole 500 mg 8-hly for 48 h	Ciprofloxacin 200 mg 12-hly + metronidazole 500 mg 8-hly for 48 h

[1] Skin rash only. [2] Anaphylaxis or angioneurotic oedema. [3] Vancomycin infusion is given over 1 h, so start it with premed. [4] Give 1 hour before catheterisation. [5] ⚠ If therapy is prolonged beyond 48 h, gentamicin assays should be performed.

Table 151 Medical prophylaxis

Short-term risks	
Infective endocarditis	(≻40)
Contacts of invasive meningococcal and *Haemophilus influenzae* infection	(≻77)
Syphilis	(≻69)
Gonorrhoea	(≻65)
Diphtheria	(≻181)
Neonatal Lancefield group B streptococcal infection	(≻173)
Medium-term risks	
Neutropenia	(≻133)
Patients in ITU (selective gut decontamination)	
Travellers' diarrhoea	(≻48)
Leptospirosis	(≻226)
Lyme disease	(≻224)
Malaria	(≻140)
Tuberculosis contacts	(≻34)
Long-term risks	
Pneumocystis carinii, toxoplasmosis, candidiasis, HSV in AIDS, transplantation, etc.	(≻118)
Asplenia	(≻132)
Sickle-cell disease: penicillin V 250 mg 12-hly, and see asplenia	
Rheumatic fever	(≻171)
Recurrent UTI	(≻60)

Antibiotic assays ⚠ (Table 152)

- Serum assay is needed when an antibiotic has a narrow 'therapeutic index' (range of serum concentrations between adequate therapy and toxicity), or when absorption, excretion or metabolism is highly variable.
- Timing of assay samples in relation to administration of doses is important for interpretation; write both times on the request card.
- Perform assays around doses given early in the day to avoid delays or the need to do tests 'on call'. Many laboratories have standardised on samples taken immediately before a dose ('pre-sample' or 'trough' level) and 60 minutes after the same dose ('post-sample' or 'peak' level).

Table 152 Antibiotic assays

Antibiotic	Ideal serum levels	Notes
*Gentamicin, tobramycin	Trough <2 mg/l Peak 4.5–10 mg/l	Repeat assays at least 2 × per week. For **synergy with penicillin in endocarditis** (≻39), aim for trough level below detectable range and low peak level (e.g. 3–4 mg/l for gentamicin). For *Pseudomonas* **spp. infection and pneumonia**, aim for peak at top of range
Netilmicin	Trough <2 mg/l Peak <12 mg/l	

continued on p. 317

Table 152 contd

Antibiotic	Ideal serum levels	Notes
Amikacin	Trough <10 mg/l Peak <30 mg/l	
Streptomycin	Peak 20–40 mg/l	
Vancomycin	Trough <10 mg/l Peak 15–30 mg/l	Assays at least 2× per week. Max safe serum level 60–80 mg/l
Trimethoprim	Trough <5 mg/l Peak 5–10 mg/l	Assays 2× per week for high dose co-trimoxazole regimens in PCP (➤119)
Sulphamethoxazole	Peak <120 mg/l	
Chloramphenicol	Trough <15 mg/l Peak 15–25 mg/l	For neonates; also preferred in those under age 4
Flucytosine	Peak 25–50 mg/l	Maximum safe serum level 80 mg/l
Itraconazole	Peak 1–2.5 mg/l (for pro- phylaxis, peak >0.5 mg/l)	Assay after 7 days' therapy, or 7 days after dose change; take peak sample 2 h after dose

*Single daily doses of aminoglycosides (e.g. single dose of 240 mg gentamicin in place of 80 mg tds) may be as, or more, effective, but cause fewer problems of toxicity; more experience with such regimens is accumulating. Probably only trough levels are required – follow advice of local microbiologists ☜

- Take the first assay sample of a course around the third or fourth dose.

Antibiotics in pregnancy

Choice of antibiotics influenced by:

- risks to fetus (teratogenesis greater in first trimester);
- effects of the pregnancy on maternal infections (asymptomatic bacteriuria ➤59, vaginal colonisation and premature labour ➤70);

Table 153 Antibiotics in pregnancy

Infection	**Safe first choices** for which there is extensive experience for common infections (possible alternatives in parentheses: ☜)
UTI	**Cystitis**: cephalexin (nitrofurantoin (may cause neonatal haemolysis if used at term), co-amoxiclav); **upper tract infection**: cefuroxime, cefotaxime (benzylpenicillin + gentamicin*)
Respiratory tract infection (RTI)	**Upper RTI with systemic symptoms**: penicillin V, erythromycin (cephalexin); **acute bronchitis**: amoxycillin (co-amoxiclav); **pneumonia**: amoxycillin + erythromycin (cefotaxime + erythromycin)
Septicaemia	Cefotaxime + metronidazole (benzylpenicillin + gentamicin* + metronidazole)
Vaginal candidiasis	Topical clotrimazole, econazole, miconazole, nystatin, or ketoconazole
Pelvic inflammatory disease	Erythromycin (add metronidazole after first trimester)

continued on p. 318

Table 153 contd

Infection	Safe first choices for which there is extensive experience for common infections (possible alternatives in parentheses: ☞)
Sexually-transmitted diseases	Syphilis or gonorrhoea: benzylpenicillin or depot preparation; syphilis + penicillin allergy: erythromycin, tetracycline + consult expert opinion; gonorrhoea + penicillin allergy: cefuroxime, cefotaxime; chlamydia: erythromycin
Prophylaxis	Surgical: cefuroxime, cefotaxime (+ metronidazole if indicated ➤312); infective endocarditis: (➤40)
Parasites	Malaria prophylaxis: consult expert opinion (➤140); falciparum malaria treatment: quinine + Fansidar + consult expert opinion; non-falciparum malaria treatment: chloroquine (give primaquine after delivery); amoebiasis: metronidazole, followed by diloxanide furoate; giardiasis: metronidazole; helminths: leave until after delivery if infection light or moderate (heavy trichuriasis: piperazine)
Tuberculosis	As for non-pregnant adults, but avoid streptomycin

*Consider avoiding aminoglycosides in second and third trimesters – possible risk of VIIIth nerve damage.

• **pharmacokinetics** (serum concentrations lower for most antibiotics in pregnancy).

In general, **full doses should be used, but course lengths kept to a minimum**. Important to **send cultures** on pregnant women to guide optimal therapy (Table 153).

Antibiotic therapy during lactation

Very few antibiotics will be taken in sufficient dosage by a suckling infant to cause harm, but information is lacking on many, and mothers may prefer to interrupt breast-feeding to avoid

Table 154 Common antibiotics to **avoid** in pregnancy

albendazole	foscarnet	primaquine
amantadine	ganciclovir	pyrimethamine
aminoglycosides (see above)	griseofulvin	quinolones*
aztreonam*	halofantrine*	rifampicin*
capreomycin	itraconazole*	sulphonamides
chloramphenicol	ketoconazole*	temocillin*
colistin	Maloprim	tetracyclines
co-trimoxazole	mebendazole*	ticarcillin*
dapsone†	mefloquine‡	tinidazole*·ǀ
Fansidar	metronidazole (avoid high dose regimens)*	trimethoprim¶
fluconazole*	nalidixic acid*	zidovudine
flucytosine	nitrofurantoin§	
Avoid live vaccines (in first trimester), povidone-iodine antiseptics and Lindane		

* Manufacturer advises avoidance, often based only on animal studies at high dose.
† May be used in third trimester – give folate supplements to mother.
‡ Avoid for prophylaxis.
§ Neonatal haemolysis may occur if used at term.
ǀ In first trimester.
¶ Theoretical risk of teratogenesis in first trimester.

any possibility of risk. Alteration of the infant's gut flora and sensitisation may occur. No antibiotic is known to inhibit lactation or the suckling reflex.

Agents **safe** because of the extremely small dosage ingested by the neonate include clavulanate, cycloserine, ethambutol, penicillins (but risk of sensitisation), pyrazinamide and rifampicin. Cephalosporins also probably fall into this group. Others that will be ingested but are not known to cause harm include erythromycin, pyrimethamine, quinidine and trimethoprim. Vancomycin, teicoplanin and aminoglycosides will not be absorbed from the infant gut. Insufficient chloroquine or proguanil is ingested to be protective. Isoniazid carries theoretical risk of convulsions and neurotoxicity, give pyridoxine to mother and infant. Nitrofurantoin is safe unless G6PD-deficient.

Avoid aztreonam, capreomycin, chloramphenicol, ciprofloxacin, clindamycin, colistin, co-trimoxazole, dapsone, Fansidar, fluconazole, foscarnet, ganciclovir, halofantrine, Maloprim, mefloquine, high-dose metronidazole (normal dose regimens safe), nalidixic acid, pentamidine, quinolones, sulphonamides, tetracyclines (although usually chelated in milk) and zidovudine. Also avoid povidone-iodine antiseptics, lindane.

33: Antibiotic Doses

Notes on tables

The recommendations in the tables are abbreviated and standardised to give individual doses and frequency; therefore they may vary slightly from those quoted in other ways in different publications, including manufacturers' recommendations. More details of dosing, adverse drug reactions and interactions can be found in the latest edition of the *British National Formulary* (which gives independent opinion) and the **ABPI** *Data Sheet Compendium*. If a reduced dose is not shown for a given degree of renal failure, the dose in the column to the left may be given. Many elderly people should be considered to have mild renal failure. In renal impairment choose antibiotics with minimal nephrotoxic potential, and avoid potentially nephrotoxic combinations (e.g. aminoglycoside + vancomycin or amphotericin or loop diuretics). For use of antibiotics in dialysis patients (➤331).

Cost: To give an indication of the relative costs of antibiotics (drug costs only), we have divided agents into three groups on the basis of the cost of 1 day's treatment at moderate–high dose: £: oral ≤£1, parenteral ≤£6; ££: oral £1.01–£2.50, parenteral £6.01–£20; £££: oral £2.51–£15, parenteral £20.01–£90. Two very expensive agents are coded $ (>£400). Many purchasers will be able to obtain antibiotics at lower prices and administration and assay costs should be remembered.

Cautions/contraindications: P: pregnancy; L: lactation; H: hepatic failure; E: epilepsy; O: porphyrias (see BNF for details); ⚠: assay needed; C: interferes with creatinine determination; ⊗: contraindicated or use not established in children below age stated in parentheses; G = caution in patients with G6PD deficiency.

Interactions: These are listed for 10 common groups of drugs. Check details in the BNF. **Any broad-spectrum agent can interfere with oestrogen absorption of the contraceptive pill and prolong prothrombin time with anticoagulants**. 1: Absorption/metabolism altered by ulcer-healing drugs, antacids, calcium/magnesium/zinc/iron salts; 2: anticoagulants; 3: antidiabetics; 4: antiepileptics; 5: carbamazepine; 6: cyclosporin; 7: digoxin; 8: rifampicin; 9: theophylline; 0: astemizole, terfenadine.

Table 155 Intravenous/intramuscular therapy. Doses and frequencies in parentheses for severe infection and to penetrate difficult sites (e.g. CSF)

Antibiotic	£	Normal doses	Modifications in renal impairment (creatinine clearance (ml/min):serum creatinine (μmol/l))			Notes
			Mild (20–50:150–300)	Moderate (10–20:300–700)	Severe (<10:>700; dialysis)	
Acyclovir	£££	iv 5(–10) mg/kg 8-hly	iv 5(–10) mg/kg 12-hly	iv 5(–10) mg/kg 24-hly	iv 2.5(–5) mg/kg 24-hly and after haemodialysis	PL
Amikacin	£££	iv/im 7.5 mg/kg 12-hly (8-hly)	iv/im 7.5 mg/kg 18-hly (12-hly)	iv/im 7.5 mg/kg 36-hly (24-hly)	iv/im 7.5 mg/kg 48-hly (36-hly)	△ P (>316) 6
Amoxycillin	£	iv/im 500 mg (1 g) 8-hly			iv/im 500 mg (1 g) 12-hly	
Amphotericin	£	iv 0.6 mg/kg (1–1.5 mg/kg; max 50 mg/day) 24-hly; 0.3 mg/kg 24-hly 'low dose' for candidiasis. 48-hly option if serum creatinine rises ≥ 200 mmol/l (>306)	Gradual work-up to full dosage in less severely ill, non-compromised patient: 1 mg in 50 ml infused over 2 h; if tolerated, give 9 mg over next 6 h; if tolerated, increase by 10 mg/day given over 6 h. Accelerated regimen for severely ill, compromised patient: first 1 mg of half full dose over 1–2 h; if tolerated, give remainder of infusion over 12 h, then give full dose from second day over 6 h		Doses as column to left, but given 36-hly	PL6
Amphotericin (liposomal)	$	iv 1 mg/kg increasing to 3 mg/kg 8-hly	iv 3 mg/kg increasing to 3 mg/kg (5 mg/kg) 24-hly			PL6
Ampicillin	£	iv/im 500 mg (1–2 g) 6-hly		iv/im 500 mg (1–2 g) 8-hly	iv/im 500 mg (1–2 g) 12-hly	
Augmentin		See co-amoxiclav				
Azlocillin	£££	iv 2 g (5g) 8-hly		iv 1 g (3 g) 8-hly	iv 0.5 g (1 g) 12-hly	Vecuronium
Aztreonam	£££	iv/im 1 g (2 g) 8-hly (6-hly)		iv/im 0.5 g (1 g) 8-hly (6-hly)	iv/im 0.25 g (0.5 g) 8-hly (6-hly)	PL2 ⊗ (1 wk)
Benzylpenicillin	£	0.6 g (2.4 g) 6-hly (3-hly). Max 14.4 g/day for short periods			0.6 g (1.2 g) 6-hly (3-hly) Max 6 g/day for short periods	
Capreomycin		im 1 g 24-hly	See dosing schedule in data sheet. Monitor renal, VIIth nerve and hepatic function			PL
Carbenicillin	£££	im/iv 5 g 6-hly (4-hly)		im/iv 5 g 24-hly (12-hly)	im/iv 5 g 48-hly (24-hly)	
Cefodizime	£££	im/iv 1 g 12-hly or 2 g 24-hly	im/iv 0.5 g 12-hly or 1 g 24-hly			O⊗ (14 yrs)

continued on p. 320

Table 155 contd

Antibiotic	£	Normal doses	Modifications in renal impairment (creatinine clearance (ml/min) : serum creatinine (µmol/l))			Notes
			Mild (20–50:150–300)	Moderate (10–20:300–700)	Severe (<10: >700; dialysis)	
Cefotaxime	£££	im/iv 1 g (2 g) 8-hly. Up to 200 mg/kg/day in meningitis	im/iv 1 g (2 g) 12-hly		im/iv 1 g (2 g) 12-hly (0.5 g (1 g) if GFR < 5 ml/min)	O
Cefoxitin	£££	iv/im 1 g (3 g) 8-hly (6-hly)	iv/im 1 g (2 g) 8-hly	iv/im 1 g (2 g) 12-hly (8-hly)	iv/im 1 g (2 g) 24-hly	OC
Cefsulodin	£££	iv/im 1 g 8-hly (6-hly) (max 6 g/day or more for short periods)		iv/im 1 g 12-hly (8-hly)	iv/im 1 g 12-hly	O
Ceftazidime	£££	iv/im 1 g (2 g) 12-hly (8-hly). Up to 150 mg/kg/day in meningitis or cystic fibrosis	iv/im 1 g (1.5 g) 12-hly	iv/im 1 g (1.5 g) 24-hly	iv/im 1 g (1.5 g) 48-hly	O
Ceftizoxime	£££	iv/im 1 g (2 g) 8-hly. Max 150 mg/kg/day		iv/im 0.5 g (1 g) 12-hly (8-hly)	iv/im 0.5 g (1 g) 24-hly	O, ⊗ (3 m)
Ceftriaxone	£££	iv/im 1 g (4 g) 24-hly	iv/im 1 g (4 g) 24-hly (reduce dose if patient has both renal and hepatic failure)			O, ⊗ (< 6 wks)
Cefuroxime	££	iv/im 750 mg (1.5 g) 8-hly (6-hly). Max 3 g 8-hly in meningitis	iv/im 750 mg (1.5 g) 12-hly	iv/im 750 mg (1.5 g) 12-hly	iv/im 750 mg (1.5 g) 24-hly	O
Cephamandole	££	iv/im 0.5 g (2 g) 8-hly (4-hly)	iv/im 0.5 g (2 g) 8-hly	iv/im 0.5 g (1 g) 8-hly	iv/im 0.5 g (1 g) 12-hly	O2
Cephazolin	££	iv/im 0.5 g (1.0 g) 12-hly (6-hly)	iv/im 0.5 g (1.0 g) 12-hly (8-hly)	iv/im 0.25 g (0.5 g) 12-hly	iv/im 0.25 g (0.5 g) 24-hly (18-hly)	⊗ (1 m)
Cephradine	£	iv/im 0.5 g (1 g) 6-hly. Max 8 g/day in severe infection		iv/im 0.5 g (1 g) 8-hly	iv/im 0.5 g 12-hly	O, ⊗ (1 m)
Chloramphenicol	££	iv/im 500 mg 6-hly (50 mg/kg/day)			iv/im 0.5 g 12-hly	PLHO △ ⊗ (neonate) 2348
Chloroquine (treatment)		iv 10 mg/kg base over 8 h, then three further infusions of 5 mg/kg base each over 8 h (>270)				HEG147

Drug	Cost				PLEG
Ciprofloxacin	£££	iv 200 mg 12-hly		iv 100 mg 12-hly	PLEG 12369 ⊗ (see data sheet)
Clarithromycin	£££	iv 500 mg 12-hly	iv 250 mg 12-hly		H ⊗ (12 yrs –iv prep.) 24567890
Clindamycin	£££	iv/im 300 mg 6-hly			PL ⊗ (1 m)
Cloxacillin	££	iv/im 500 mg (1 g) 6-hly (4-hly)			
Co-amoxiclav	££	iv 1.2 g 8-hly (6-hly)	iv 600 mg 8-hly	iv 600 mg 24-hly	H
Colistin		iv/im 2 MU 8-hly	iv/im 1 MU 18-hly (12-hly)	iv/im 1 MU 24-hly (18-hly)	PLO
Co-trimoxazole	£	iv/im 960 mg 12-hly (high dose for *Pneumocystis carinii* = 120 mg/kg/day >119)	iv/im 960 mg 18-hly	iv/im 480 mg 24-hly	PLO△ (high dose or GFR <10) 2346 ⊗ (6 wks)
Erythromycin	£££	iv 500 mg (1 g) 6-hly (IE 50 mg/kg 6-hly)			OH 24567890
Flucloxacillin	££	im/iv 500 mg (1.5 g) 6-hly (4-hly)			O
Fluconazole	£££	iv 400 mg initial dose, then 200 mg (400 mg) 24-hly	iv 400 mg initial dose then 200 mg (400 mg) 48-hly	iv 400 mg initial dose, then 200 mg (400 mg) 72-hly. On haemodialysis give one dose after each dialysis session	PL 2346890 ⊗ (1 yr)
Flucytosine	££	iv 37.5 mg/kg (50 mg/kg) 6-hly	iv 37.5 mg/kg (50 mg/kg) 12-hly	iv 37.5 mg/kg (50 mg/kg) 24-hly	iv 50 mg/kg initial dose, then assay — HPL
Foscarnet	£££	iv 20 mg/kg initial dose; 🔲 for subsequent daily doses according to serum creatinine			PL
Fusidic acid	££	Use oral route (iv 500 mg 8-hly (under 50 kg 6–7 mg/kg 8-hly))			H

continued on p. 322

Table 155 contd

Antibiotic	£	Normal doses	Modifications in renal impairment (creatinine clearance (ml/min): serum creatinine (µmol/l))			Notes
			Mild (20–50:150–300)	Moderate (10–20:300–700)	Severe (<10: >700; dialysis)	
Ganciclovir	£££	iv 5 mg/kg 12-hly	See data sheet for dosage in renal insufficiency			PL
Gentamicin	£	iv/im 1.5 mg/kg 8-hly	iv/im 1.5 mg/kg 12-hly (8-hly)	iv/im 1.5 mg/kg 24-hly (12-hly)	iv/im 1.5 mg/kg 48-hly (24-hly) and after dialysis. Assay around second dose	△ P (>316) 6
		Simple, safe aide-memoire for gentamicin dosing: give 1.5 mg/kg 8-hly for those under 55 yrs. If 55 yrs or older, or patients with mild/moderately impaired renal function, give the same dose 12-hly. Assay around third or fourth dose, and subsequently two or three times weekly. Use lower doses in endocarditis therapy (>39)				
Imipenem	£££	iv/im 500 mg (1 g) 6-hly		iv/im 250 mg (500 mg) 8-hly (6-hly)	iv/im 250 mg (500 mg) 12-hly	PLE ⊗ (3 m)
Isoniazid		iv/im 300 mg 24-hly (>33)				PLHO 1459
Metronidazole	££	iv 500 mg 8-hly			iv 500 mg 12-hly	PL 124
Miconazole	£	iv 600 mg 8-hly				PO 2340
Netilmicin	££	iv/im 1.5–2 mg/kg (2.5 mg/kg) 8-hly	iv/im 1.5–2 mg/kg (2.5 mg/kg) 12-hly (8-hly)	iv/im 1.5–2 mg/kg (2.5 mg/kg) 24-hly (12-hly)	iv/im 1.5–2 mg/kg (2.5 mg/kg) 48-hly (24-hly)	△ P (>316) 6
Ofloxacin	£££	iv 200 mg (400 mg) 24-hly (12-hly)	iv 100 mg (200 mg) 24-hly (12-hly)		iv 100 mg 24-hly	PLEG 1236 ⊗ (16 yrs)
Pentamidine	£££	For PCP: iv 4 mg/kg 24-hly for at least 14 days (>119)			iv 4 mg/kg 24-hly for 10 days then alt. die. for 4 days	PL
Piperacillin	£££	iv/im 25 mg/kg (75 mg/kg) 6-hly. For *Pseudomonas* spp. and other severe infections use 16 g/day or more	iv/im 25 mg/kg (75 mg/kg) 12-hly			🏛 ⊗ (12 yrs)

Drug	Cost					Code
Piperacillin-tazobactam	£££	iv 4.5 g 8-hly			iv 4.5 g 12-hly. Give one extra dose after dialysis	⊗ (12 yrs)
Procaine penicillin	£	im 0.4 MU 24-hly (12-hly). Gonorrhoea: up to 4.8 MU single dose. Syphilis: up to 1.6 MU 24-hly for 10 (early) or 14 (secondary or latent) days				
Quinine		iv infusion (>271)			iv infusion (>271)	HPLOG 17
Rifampicin	££	iv 0.3–0.6 g 12-hly (>33)			iv 0.3–0.6 g 12-hly (>33)	HPLO 123469
Spectinomycin	££	im 2 g (4 g) single dose			im 2 g (4 g) single dose	PL
Streptomycin		im 1 g 24-hly (500–750 mg if >40 years old or <50 kg in weight)		im 1 g 24–72-hly (500–750 mg if >40 years old or <50 kg in weight)	im 1 g 72–95-hly (500–750 mg if >40 years old or <50 kg in weight)	P△
Sulphadiazine	£	iv 1 g (1.5 g) 6-hly			iv 1 g (1.5 g) 6-hly	PLGHO △ (high dose) 2346 ⊗ (2 m)
Teicoplanin	£££	iv/im 400 mg initial dose, then 200 mg 24-hly. For severe infection: 400 mg 12-hly for three doses, then 400 mg 24-hly. For patients over 85 kg moderate infection 6 mg/kg 24-hly; severe infection 6 mg/kg 24-hly. For staphylococcal endocarditis: up to 12 mg/kg 24-hly. In renal failure give first 3 days' therapy as above, and see data sheet for subsequent dosing regimens				△ (prolonged therapy in renal failure)
Temocillin	£££	im/iv 1 g (2 g) 12-hly		im/iv 1 g (2 g) 24-hly	im/iv 1 g (2 g) 48-hly. Give one extra dose after dialysis	P
Tetracycline	££	im 100 mg 12-hly (6-hly): iv 500 mg 12-hly		Avoid if possible, otherwise restrict to im 100 mg 12-hly or iv 250 mg 12-hly	Avoid	HPL 124 ⊗ (12 yrs)
Ticarcillin	£££	iv/im 5 g 6-hly		iv/im 5 g 24-hly (12-hly)	iv/im 5 g 48-hly (24-hly)	P
Timentin (ticarcillin + clavulanate)	£££	iv 3.2 g 6-hly (4-hly)		iv 3.2 g 8-hly	iv 1.6 g 12-hly	P
Tobramycin	££	iv/im 1.5 mg/kg 8-hly	iv/im 1.5 mg/kg 12-hly (8-hly)	iv/im 1.5 mg/kg 24-hly (12-hly)	iv/im 1.5 mg/kg 48-hly (24-hly) and after dialysis. Assay around second dose	△ P (>316) 6

continued on p. 324

Table 155 contd

Antibiotic		Normal doses	Modifications in renal impairment (creatinine clearance (ml/min): serum creatinine (µmol/l))			Notes
			Mild (20–50:150–300)	Moderate (10–20:300–700)	Severe (<10: >700; dialysis)	
Trimethoprim	£	iv 150 mg (250 mg) 12-hly		iv 150 mg (250 mg) 18-hly	iv 75 mg (125 mg) 24-hly	PLGO △ (high dose, or GFR <10) 234 ⊗ (neonates)
Vancomycin	£££	iv 500 mg 8-hly (6-hly) or 1 g 24-hly (12-hly)	Begin therapy at iv 500 mg 12-hly or 1 g 24-hly, and assay on second day	Give iv 1 g single dose, and perform single assay after 48 h. Give subsequent doses when level <10 mg/l	Give iv 1 g single dose, and perform single assay after 72 h. Give subsequent doses when level <10 mg/l	△
			Nomogram in data sheet can be helpful, but each adult dose best kept at 500 mg or more. In haemodialysis patients, give iv 1 g single dose, and perform single assay after 5–7 days; give subsequent doses when level <10 mg/l			
Zidovudine		iv 1.9 mg/kg 4-hly				HPL

For abbreviations, see Notes on tables (>318).

Table 156 Oral and per rectum systemic therapy. Doses and frequencies in parentheses for more serious infection and to penetrate difficult sites, e.g. abscesses.

Antibiotic	£	Normal doses	Mild (20–50 : 150–300)	Moderate (10–20 : 300–700)	Severe (< 10 : > 700; dialysis)	Notes
			Modifications in renal impairment (creatinine clearance (ml/min) : serum creatinine (μmol/l))			
Acrosoxacin	£££	300 mg single dose				PLE 3 Ⓧ (18 yrs)
Acyclovir	£££	For HSV treatment: 200 mg (400 mg) five times daily. Prophylaxis: 200 mg (400 mg) 6-hly. Varicella and zoster: 800 mg five times daily		For HSV see left. For varicella and zoster: 800 mg 8-hly (6-hly)	For HSV treatment: 200 mg 12-hly. Varicella and zoster: 800 mg 12-hly	PL
Albendazole		400 mg 12-hly				HP
Amantadine		100 mg 24-hly (12-hly for treatment)			Avoid	P
Amoxycillin	£	250 mg (500 mg) 8-hly		250 mg (500 mg) 12-hly	250 mg (500 mg) 12-16-hly	
Ampicillin	£	500 mg (1 g) 6-hly		500 mg (1 g) 8-hly	500 mg (1 g) 12-hly	
Augmentin		See co-amoxiclav				
Azithromycin	£££	500 mg 24-hly				HPL 126780 Ⓧ (6 m)
Bacampicillin	£	400 mg (800 mg) 12-hly (8-hly)		No recommendations		
Cefaclor	£££	250 mg (500 mg) 8-hly. Also available 375 mg (750 mg) 12-hly			250 mg 8-hly or 375 mg 12-hly	O Ⓧ (1 m)
Cefadroxil	££	500 mg (1 g) 12-hly		500 mg (1 g) 24-hly	500 mg (1 g) 36-hly	O
Cefixime	£££	200 mg (400 mg) 24-hly		200 mg 24-hly		O Ⓧ (6 m)
Cefpodoxime	£££	100 mg (200 mg) 12-hly		100 mg 24-hly		O 1

continued on p. 326

Table 156 contd

Antibiotic	£	Normal doses	Modifications in renal impairment (creatinine clearance (ml/min):serum creatinine (µmol/l))			Notes
			Mild (20–50:150–300)	Moderate (10–20:300–700)	Severe (<10:>700; dialysis)	
Ceftibuten	£	400 mg 24-hly		No recommendations		O
Cefuroxime axetil	£££	250 mg (500 mg) 12-hly				O
Cephalexin	£	250 mg (1 g) 6-hly		250 mg (500 mg) 6-hly	250 mg 8-hly	O
Cephradine	££	250 mg (500 mg) 6-hly or 500 mg (1 g) 12-hly		250 mg (500 mg) 8-hly	250 mg (500 mg) 12-hly	O
Chloramphenicol	£	12.5 mg/kg (25 mg/kg) 6-hly				PLHO△ Ⓡ (neonate) 2348
Chloroquine		Treatment: 600 mg of base, then 300 mg after 6–8 h, then 300 mg 24-hly for 2 days (>270). Prophylaxis: 300 mg of base weekly				HEG 147
Cinoxacin	££	500 mg 12-hly			Avoid	PLEG 36 Ⓡ (16 yrs)
Ciprofloxacin	£££	250 mg (750 mg) 12-hly			250 mg 12-hly (consider serum assay: ↑)	PLEG 12369 Ⓡ (16 yrs)
Clarithromycin	£££	250 mg (500 mg) 12-hly				H 2456789
Clindamycin	£££	150 mg (300 mg) 6-hly				PL Ⓡ (1 m)
Clofazimine		300 mg monthly, or 300 mg 24-hly depending on combination regimen				HPL
Cloxacillin	££	500 mg 6-hly				
Co-amoxiclav	££	375 mg (750 mg) 8-hly		375 mg (750 mg) 12-hly	375 mg (750 mg) 24-hly	H

Drug	£					Notes
Co-trimoxazole	£	960 mg (1.44 g) 12-hly (high dose for *Pneumocystis carinii* = 120 mg/kg/day >119)		960 mg (1.44 g) 18-hly	480 mg (960 mg) 24-hly	PLO △ (high dose or GFR <10) 2346 ⊗ (6 wks)
Cycloserine		250 mg (500 mg) 12-hly			Avoid	PL △ 4
Dapsone		100 mg 24-hly				PLOG 8
Didanosine (DDI)		Under 60 kg, 125 mg 12-hly; over 60 kg, 200 mg 12-hly.			Under 60 kg, 75 mg 12-hly; over 60 kg, 100 mg 12-hly	HPL
Diloxanide furoate		500 mg 8-hly				
Doxycycline	£	100 mg (200 mg) 24-hly			100 mg 24-hly	PLO ⊗ (12 yrs) 12456
Erythromycin	£	250 mg (1 g) 6-hly or 500 mg (1 g) 12-hly				OH 24567890
Ethambutol	£££	15 mg/kg/day (initially 25 mg/kg/day) (>33)		15 mg/kg/36 h	15 mg/kg/48 h	P ⊗ (6 yrs)
Famciclovir	£££	250 mg 8-hly		250 mg 12-hly	See data sheet	PL
Flucloxacillin	£	250 mg (1 g) 6-hly				O
Fluconazole	£££	For superficial candidiasis and prophylaxis: 50 mg (100 mg) 24-hly. For systemic candidiasis: 400 mg first dose, then 200 mg (400 mg) 24-hly	Doses as on left, but prolong dosage interval to 48-hly		Doses as on left, but prolong dosage interval to 72-hly. On haemodialysis give one dose after each dialysis session	PL 2346890 ⊗ (1 yr)
Flucytosine	££	50 mg/kg 6-hly	50 mg/kg 12-hly	50 mg/kg 24-hly	50 mg/kg initial dose, then serum assay	HPL △
Fosfomycin	£££	3 g single dose at bedtime			Avoid	PL

continued on p. 328

Table 156 contd

Antibiotic	£	Normal doses	Modifications in renal impairment (cleatinine clearance (ml/min):serum creatinine (µmol/l))			Notes
			Mild (20–50:150–300)	Moderate (10–20:300–700)	Severe (<10:>700; dialysis)	
Fusidic acid	£££	500 mg 8-hly				H
Griseofulvin		500 mg (1 g) 24-hly				PLHO 246
Halofantrine		Three doses of 500 mg at 6-hly intervals, repeated 7 days later				PL
Hexamine (methenamine)		1 g 12-hly (8-hly)			Avoid	P
Isoniazid		300 mg 24-hly (>33)				PLHO 1459
Itraconazole	£££	100 mg (200 mg) 24-hly. Assay especially important in AIDS, neutropenia and renal failure because of unreliable absorption				PLH △ ⊗ (12 yrs) 1246780
Ketoconazole	£	200 mg (400 mg) 24-hly				PLHO 124680
Mebendazole		100 mg single dose or 12-hly according to indication				PL 1
Mefloquine (treatment)		20 mg/kg base in two divided doses, 6–8 h apart				PL 47
Mepacrine		100 mg 8-hly				H
Metronidazole	£	po 400 mg (800 mg) 8-hly, pr 1 g 12-hly (8-hly)				PL 124
Miconazole	£££	250 mg 6-hly				PO 2340
Minocycline	££	100 mg 12-hly (50 mg 12-hly for acne)			Avoid	PL 124 ⊗ (12 yrs)
Nalidixic acid	££	1 g 6-hly			Avoid	PHEG 236
Niclosamide		2 g 24-hly according to indication				

Drug	Cost	Dose			HG P (at term) ® (3 m)
Nitrofurantoin	£	50 mg (100 mg) 6-hly	Avoid		PLE 12369 ® (16 yrs)
Norfloxacin	£	400 mg 12-hly		400 mg 24-hly	PLEG 1236 ® (16 yrs)
Ofloxacin	££	200 mg (400 mg) 24-hly (12-hly)	100 mg (200 mg) 24-hly (12-hly)	100 mg 24-hly (give 200 mg loading dose)	
Penicillin V	£	250 (500 mg) 6-hly	250 mg (500 mg) 8-hly	250 mg (500mg) 12-hly	HPE
Piperazine		2250 mg–5500 mg 24-hly according to indication		Avoid	O1
Pivampicillin	£	500 mg (1 g) 12-hly	500 mg 24-hly		
Praziquantel		40 mg/kg in two divided doses 4–6 h apart (60 mg/kg in three divided doses in 1 day for *Schistosoma japonicum*). Not on UK market			
Primaquine		15 mg 24-hly		No recommendation	PLG
Probenecid		1 g single dose with β-lactam for gonorrhoea; 1 g 12-hly	Gonorrhoea as at left; avoid otherwise		PG
Proguanil (prophylaxis)		200 mg 24-hly			2
Pyrantel		5 mg/kg (10 mg/kg) 24-hly according to indication			HP
Pyrazinamide		Standard regimens: 2 g three times per week (under 50 kg in weight, 1.5 g three times per week >33)	1.5 g three times per week >33		HO
Pyrimethamine		25 mg weekly as malaria prophylaxis. For toxoplasmosis treatment >265.			PLH 3
Quinine		600 mg of hydrochloride, dihydrochloride or sulphate or sulphate salt 8-hly >271)			HPLOG 17
Rifabutin		Treatment 150–600 mg 24-hly; prophylaxis 300 mg 24-hly	75–300 mg 24-hly; prophylaxis 150 mg 24-hly		HPLO 2346
Rifampicin	££	0.3–0.6 g 12-hly (>33)			HPLO 123469

continued on p. 330

Table 155 contd

			Modifications in renal impairment (creatinine clearance (ml/min):serum creatinine (µmol/l))			
Antibiotic	£	Normal doses	Mild (20–50:150–300)	Moderate (10–20:300–700)	Severe (<10:>700; dialysis)	Notes
Sulphadiazine	££	500 mg (1 g) 6-hly				HPLOG △ (high dose) 2346 ✗ (2 m)
Sulphadimidine	££	2 g initially, then 500 mg (1 g) 8-hly (6-hly)				HPLOG △ (high dose) 2346 ✗ (2 m)
Sulphametopyrazine	££	2 g once weekly				HPLOG 2346 ✗ (2 m)
Terbinafine		250 mg 24-hly		125 mg 24-hly		HPL 1 ✗ (16 yrs)
Tetracycline (incl. oxytetracycline)	£	250 mg (500 mg) 8-hly (6-hly)	Avoid if possible; 250 mg 8-hly	Avoid (consider serum assay if essential)		HPL 124 ✗ (12 yrs)
Thiabendazole		25 mg/kg (max 1.5 g) 12-hly				HPL 9
Tinidazole	££	2 g single dose; 1 g 24-hly or 500 mg 12-hly			Avoid long-term regimens	PL ✗ (12yrs)
Trimethoprim	£	200 mg 12-hly		200 mg 18-hly	100 mg 24-hly	PLOG △ (high dose or GFR <10) 234 ✗ (neonates)
Zidovudine (AZT)	£££	250 mg 12-hly				HPL

For abbreviations, see Notes on tables (>318).

Antibiotics and haemodialysis

The extent to which antibiotics are removed by dialysis depends on many factors, particularly the degree of protein binding. Information is not readily available for many drugs; the data given below have been collated from a number of sources (see footnote to table). Where no data are available, drugs have been omitted. Prescribers should **always** consult the current manufacturer's product data sheet for any antibiotic prescribed for dialysis patients. Specific instances where additional information is known to be available in the data sheet are indicated on the chart (📄). If antibiotics are removed by dialysis a supplementary dose may be required post-dialysis, or it may be possible to schedule

drugs so that a dose falls due at the completion of dialysis. CAVH-continuous arteriovenous or venovenous haemofiltration.

Aminoglycosides (except streptomycin): Give a single dose at the end of each dialysis. For dosage see iv therapy chart (➤319), dose listed under 'Severe renal impairment'. Perform assay regularly. CAVH dose as for GFR 20–50.

Vancomycin: Not dialysed by conventional dialysis, but 20–50% removed by high-flux polysulfone dialysis. Clearance varies with age of filter. Give a single dose (1 g), then assay at the end of each dialysis and give a further dose when this trough level is < 10 mg/l (Table 157). CAVH dose as for GFR 20–50.

Table 154 Antibiotics and dialysis

Antibiotic	% removed by HD	PD	Comments
Acyclovir	> 50	5–20	2.5 mg/kg daily and after HD. CAVH 3.5 mg/kg daily
Amikacin	> 50	20–50	📄 ⚠ See comments above
Amoxycillin	20–50	5–20	Schedule dose after HD
Amphotericin	< 5		Usual regimen
Amphotericin (liposomal)			Administration should commence only after each session of HD has finished
Ampicillin	20–50	< 5	Schedule dose after HD. CAVH dose as for GFR 20–50
Azlocillin	20–50	5–20	📄 Give additional dose before each HD. CAVH dose as for GFR 20–50
Aztreonam	20–50	5–20	📄 Additional one-eighth of initial dose post-HD. CAVH dose as for GFR 20–50
Benzylpenicillin	20–50		Supplementary dose required post-HD
Cefaclor	20–50		📄 Additional dose prior to HD
Cefadroxil	20–50		Additional dose after HD
Cefamandole	20–50	5–20	📄
Cefixime			📄 No supplement required for HD
Cefotaxime	20–50	5–20	Schedule dose after HD. CAVH dose 1 g 12-hly
Cefoxitin	20–50	5–20	📄 Loading dose after each HD. CAVH dose as for GFR 20–50

continued on p. 332

Table 157 contd

Antibiotic	% removed by HD	PD	Comments
Cefsulodin	20–50		📄 Normal dose pre- and post-HD
Ceftazidime	>50	5–20	📄 Supplementary dose post-HD. CAVH dose as for GFR 20–50
Ceftizoxime			Schedule dose after HD. CAVH dose as for GFR 20–50
Ceftriaxone	<5		📄 No supplement required for HD. CAVH dose as for GFR 20–50
Cefuroxime			📄 750 mg supplementary dose post-HD. CAVH dose 1 g 12-hly
Cephalexin	20–50	5–20	📄 500 mg supplementary dose post-HD
Cephradine	20–50	5–20	
Chloramphenicol	5–20	<5	No supplement required
Chloroquine	<5	<5	
Ciprofloxacin	5–20	5–20	Schedule dose after HD
Clarithromycin	<5		
Clindamycin	<5	<5	
Cloxacillin	<5		
Co-amoxiclav	20–50	5–20	Schedule dose after HD
Co-trimoxazole			📄
Doxycycline	<5	5–20	
Erythromycin	5–20		
Ethambutol	5–20		No supplement required post-HD. CAVH dose as for GFR 20–50
Flucloxacillin	<5		📄 No supplement required for HD
Fluconazole			One dose after each HD; no doses between HD. CAVH dose as for GFR 20–50
Flucytosine	>50	20–50	📄 ⚠ Supplementary 20 mg/kg post-HD. CAVH dose as for GFR 20–50
Foscarnet	>50		📄
Fusidic acid	<5		
Ganciclovir	>50		📄 Give daily dose after HD on dialysis days
Gentamicin	>50	20–50	📄 ⚠ See comments above
Imipenem	>50	5–20	📄 Dose post-HD and at 12-h intervals. CAVH dose as for GFR 20–50

continued on p. 333

Table 157 contd

Antibiotic	% removed by		Comments
	HD	PD	
Isoniazid	>50	20–50	Usual dose post-HD
Kanamycin	>50	20–50	📄 ⚠ See comments above
Ketoconazole	<5	<5	
Metronidazole	>50	5–20	Schedule dose after HD. CAVH dose as for GFR 20–50
Miconazole	<5		
Minocycline	<5	<5	
Nalidixic acid	>50		
Netilmicin	>50		📄 ⚠ See comments above
Norfloxacin	<5		
Piperacillin	20–50		📄 Supplementary dose post-HD. CAVH dose as for GFR 20–50
Piperacillin-tazobactam	20–50		📄 Supplementary dose post-HD. CAVH dose as for GFR 20–50
Rifampicin	<5		
Streptomycin	>50		📄 CAVH dose as for GFR 20–50
Teicoplanin	<5		📄 ⚠ Give one third usual dose; CAVH dose as for GFR 20–50
Temocillin	20–50		📄 Supplementary dose post-HD
Tetracycline	5–20	5–20	
Timentin (ticarcillin + clavulanate)	20–50	5–20	
Tobramycin	>50	20–50	📄 ⚠ See comments above
Trimethoprim	20–50	<5	Schedule dose after HD. CAVH dose as for GFR 10–20
Vancomycin	<5	20–50	📄 ⚠ See comments above. CAVH dose as for GFR 20–50
Zidovudine	<5		

Sources: *Introduction to Dialysis*, eds. Cogan MG, Schoenfeld P. 2nd edn. Churchill Livingstone, London, 1991. *Textbook of Nephrology*, Massry SG, Glassock RJ. 2nd edn. Williams and Wilkins, London, 1989. *Drug Prescribing in Renal Failure*, eds. Bennett WM, Aronoff GR, Golper TA, Morrison G, Brater C, Singer I. 3rd edn. American College of Physicians, Philadelphia, 1994. ABPI *Data Sheet Compendium*.

📄: See data sheet; ⚠ : monitor serum levels; HD: haemodialysis; PD: peritoneal dialysis.

Section 4:
Appendices

Appendix A: Immunisation Schedules

Department of Health guidelines for the immunisation of children (Table 158)

Table 158 Department of Health guidelines for the immunisation of children

Vaccine	Age
Diphtheria, tetanus, pertussis, polio, *Haemophilus influenzae* type B (Hib)	Three doses at monthly intervals, starting at 2 months
Measles/mumps/rubella (MMR)	12–18 months
Diphtheria, tetanus, polio booster. MMR if not previously given	4–5 years
Rubella	10–14 years, girls only*
BCG	10–14 years or infancy*†
Tetanus and polio boosters	15–18 years

*An interval of 3 weeks should separate rubella and BCG immunisation.
†Indications for BCG in infancy are contact with case of tuberculosis, or membership of a high-risk ethnic group (➤34).

The policy of administering MMR to toddlers left a vulnerable cohort of young teenagers who were too old to have received the vaccine and remained susceptible to measles. A school-based immunisation programme to vaccinate all these children was performed in Nov. 1994.

Table 159 Vaccines for groups at special risk

Vaccine	Indications	Interval
Influenza (➤247)	Patients with cardiac, renal and pulmonary disease (including asthma), diabetes mellitus and other endocrine disorders, the immunocompromised, and residents of old people's homes and nursing homes. Influenza vaccination is also advocated for patients on long-term aspirin treatment in an attempt to reduce the risk of Reye syndrome	Annually in late October/early November. Adults: single dose. Children aged 4–12 years: dose is repeated after 4–6 weeks if receiving vaccine for the first time
Streptococcus pneumoniae (polyvalent)	Sickle-cell disease, splenectomy, chronic renal disease, immunodeficiency (incl. HIV), chronic heart, lung or liver disease, diabetes mellitus	Single dose, repeated 5–10 years later in asplenic patients and those with nephrotic syndrome
Neisseria meningitidis (groups A and C)	Control of outbreaks and contacts of cases (groups A and C only). For travellers to endemic areas (➤142)	Single dose repeated after 2 years for those still at risk

Appendix B: Glossary

aerobe—a bacterium that can grow in oxygen. Many are **facultative anaerobes**, indicating that they can grow in anaerobic conditions as well. A few are **strict aerobes**, indicating that they require the presence of oxygen for growth

anaerobe, obligate—a bacterium that can only grow in the absence, or virtual absence, of oxygen

antagonism—the reduction of activity of one antibiotic by another

antigen—a substance against which an antibody may be raised. Often used here in the context of 'antigen detection' to indicate laboratory detection of bacterial or viral proteins by immunological tests

antiseptic—a disinfectant which is safe to use on skin, mucous membranes and some tissues

aseptic—complete absence of infectious organisms. **Aseptic technique:** avoiding contamination by all infectious organisms

bactericidal (➤309)

bacteriostatic (➤309)

carrier—indicates that a particular organism is persistently present in a patient, often with the potential for transmission to others

cohorting—nursing patients with the same infection together (with the same staff looking after them and not other patients), rather than isolating them individually

coliform (➤184)

colonisation—see **carrier**

commensal—an organism which forms part of the normal flora

coryneform (➤176)

diphtheroid (➤176)

disinfection—killing or removing enough organisms from an article to render it sufficiently safe for its intended purpose. In practice this usually means removing or killing vegetative bacterial forms, but not affecting spores

endogenous—used here to indicate infection by organisms from the patient's own flora, often from the gut

nosocomial—hospital-acquired (infection)

opportunist—an organism that only causes disease when host defences are impaired

phage (bacteriophage)—a virus that infects bacteria. Often used in typing schemes

prophylaxis—treatment given to prevent infection. May be **primary**, if given before infection has occurred, or **secondary**, if given to prevent recurrence

pseudomonad (➤199)

saprophyte—a soil-dwelling organism; usually extended to include any environmental organism

sterilisation—total removal or killing of all infectious organisms

superinfection—infection of a patient by one organism during infection by or treatment for another organism

synergy—combination of two (or more) antibiotics giving enhanced activity over that of either used individually

vegetative form (of bacteria)—the multiplying form usually associated with disease production; distinguished from the resting resistant spore form of some bacteria

virulence—strictly, those factors that distinguish a pathogen from non-pathogenic members of the same genus or species. Used loosely to indicate all bacterial pathogenic mechanisms

zoonosis—an infection acquired from vertebrate animals, or with a life cycle in which vertebrate animals play an important part

Index